The Origins of AIDS

It is now thirty years since the discovery of AIDS but its origins continue to puzzle doctors and scientists. Inspired by his own experiences working as an infectious diseases physician in Africa, Jacques Pepin looks back to the early twentieth-century events in Africa that triggered the emergence of HIV/AIDS (human immunodeficiency virus/acquired immune deficiency syndrome) and traces its subsequent development into the most dramatic and destructive epidemic of modern times. He shows how the disease was first transmitted from chimpanzees to man and then how urbanisation, prostitution and large-scale colonial medical campaigns intended to eradicate tropical diseases combined to disastrous effect to fuel the spread of the virus from its origins in Léopoldville to the rest of Africa, the Caribbean and ultimately worldwide. This is an essential new perspective on HIV/AIDS and on the lessons that must be learned if we are to avoid provoking another pandemic in the future.

JACQUES PEPIN is a Professor in the Department of Microbiology and Infectious Diseases at the Université de Sherbrooke, Canada, where he is also Director of the Center for International Health. He has conducted research on infectious diseases in sixteen African countries and, during the 1980s, worked for four years as a medical officer in a Zaire bush hospital.

The Origins of AIDS

JACQUES PEPIN

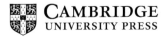
CAMBRIDGE
UNIVERSITY PRESS

CAMBRIDGE UNIVERSITY PRESS
Cambridge, New York, Melbourne, Madrid, Cape Town,
Singapore, São Paulo, Delhi, Mexico City

Cambridge University Press
The Edinburgh Building, Cambridge CB2 8RU, UK

Published in the United States of America by Cambridge University Press,
New York

www.cambridge.org
Information on this title: www.cambridge.org/9780521186377

© Jacques Pepin 2011

First published 2011
5th printing 2012

Printed in the United States of America by Edwards Brothers

A catalogue record for this publication is available from the British Library

Library of Congress Cataloguing in Publication data
Pepin, Jacques, 1958–
The origins of AIDS / Jacques Pepin.
   p. ; cm.
Includes bibliographical references and index.
ISBN 978-1-107-00663-8 (hardback) – ISBN 978-0-521-18637-7 (pbk.)
1. HIV infections – Africa.   2. HIV infections – Etiology.   3. AIDS (Disease) –
Africa.   4. Emerging infectious diseases – Africa.   I. Title.
[DNLM: 1. HIV Infections – etiology – Africa.   2. HIV Infections – history –
Africa.   3. Acquired Immunodeficiency Syndrome – history – Africa.
4. Communicable Diseases, Emerging – history – Africa.   5. Disease Vectors –
Africa.   6. HIV-1 – pathogenicity – Africa.   7. History, 20th Century – Africa.
WC 503.3]
RA643.86.A35P465   2011
362.196′97920096–dc22
                                                                    2011007350

ISBN 978-1-107-00663-8 Hardback
ISBN 978-0-521-18637-7 Paperback

Contents

List of figures, maps and table   *page* vii

Acknowledgements   ix

List of abbreviations   xi

Note on terminology   xiii

Map of Africa   xv

    Introduction   1

1 Out of Africa   6

2 The source   18

3 The timing   32

4 The cut hunter   43

5 Societies in transition   59

6 The oldest trade   84

7 Injections and the transmission of viruses   103

8 The legacies of colonial medicine I: French Equatorial
    Africa and Cameroun   118

9 The legacies of colonial medicine II: the Belgian Congo   143

10 The other human immunodeficiency viruses   168

11 From the Congo to the Caribbean   180

12 The blood trade   197

13 The globalisation   209

14   Assembling the puzzle   221

15   Epilogue: lessons learned   235

References   238
Appendix   282
Index   284

Figures, maps and table

Figures

1 Phylogenetic analysis showing the relationship between
  $SIV_{cpz\text{-}US}$ and $SIV_{cpz\text{-}gab1}$ and isolates from humans infected
  with HIV-1   *page* 25
2 Phylogenetic analysis showing the relatively distant
  relationship between SIV_{cpz} isolates obtained in Tanzania
  from *P.t. schweinfurthii* chimpanzees and isolates from
  humans infected with HIV-1   27
3 Phylogenetic analysis showing the relationship between
  SIV_{cpz} from *P.t. troglodytes* chimpanzees in Cameroon or
  Gabon and isolates from humans infected with HIV-1   28
4 Population of colonies of central Africa, 1922–60   69
5 Léopoldville's population, 1923–59: (a) adult men, adult
  women and children; (b) ratio of adult men to adult women   72
6 Age pyramids of Léopoldville in 1955   77
7 Migrations and births in Léopoldville–Kinshasa   80
8 Satellite photograph of Kinshasa and Brazzaville, early
  twenty-first century   81
9 Prevalence of HCV infection at various sites in Cameroon
  by year of birth   112
10 Incidence of African trypanosomiasis (sleeping sickness) in
   Cameroun Français and AEF-3, and use of trypanocidal
   drugs   126
11 Incidence rates (per 1,000 inhabitants per year) of African
   trypanosomiasis, yaws and syphilis in Cameroun Français,
   AEF-3 and Tchad   129
12 New cases of yaws and syphilis and consumption of
   antitreponemal drugs in Cameroun Français and AEF-3   132
13 Cases of leprosy under treatment, and new cases of
   tuberculosis diagnosed in Cameroun Français and AEF-3   135

14 Number of individuals vaccinated against smallpox and
    yellow fever in Cameroun Français and AEF-3   139
15 Number of new cases of endemic diseases in the Belgian
    Congo   147
16 Annual incidence of endemic diseases in the Belgian Congo   149
17 Annual incidence of yaws in various regions of the Belgian
    Congo   149
18 Number of new cases of gonorrhoea and syphilis,
    injections of various drugs and number of visits for free
    women at the Dispensaires Antivénériens of Léopoldville   161

Maps

1 Map of Africa   xv
2 Genetic diversity of HIV-1 in sub-Saharan Africa   15
3 Distribution of the four subspecies of *Pan troglodytes* and
   the *Pan paniscus* bonobo   19
4 Itinerary of the Brazzaville–Pointe-Noire and Léopoldville–
   Matadi railways   35
5 Map of Cameroun Français and the four colonies that
   comprised the Afrique Équatoriale Française federation   113
6 Map of the Belgian Congo (current names in brackets)   144
7 Historical range of the sooty mangabey (*Cercocebus atys
   atys*) in West Africa   171

Table

1 HIV-2 prevalence in Guinea-Bissau by age, 1987–2007   174

Acknowledgements

I am grateful to several persons who helped me through the various steps of writing up this book. I will list them in chronological order.

At a very proximal stage, my career in the tropics (and thus my interest and competence in writing this book) would not have been possible without the support and patience of the late Christian Fisch and Jean-Louis Lamboray. I am also indebted to my former mentors and colleagues at the Université de Sherbrooke (especially Raymond Duperval), the University of Manitoba, where I learned respectively to practise medicine and infectious diseases, the Medical Research Council Laboratories in The Gambia, where I understood how to do research, and the London School of Hygiene and Tropical Medicine, where I studied epidemiology. For more than fifteen years, the Canadian International Development Agency (CIDA) sponsored public health interventions in Africa during which I discovered a lot about sex workers. CIDA had also funded the primary healthcare project in Zaire where I became fascinated by African trypanosomiasis and other tropical diseases.

Over the seven years that I ultimately spent collecting the historical documents listed in the references section, I was assisted in an ever friendly way by the librarians of the following institutions (also in chronological order): Widener Library of Harvard University; Canada Institute for Scientific and Technical Information in Ottawa; British Library and School of Oriental and African Studies in London; Institute of Tropical Medicine in Lisboa (when I was mostly interested in HIV-2); Institut de Médecine Tropicale du Service de Santé des Armées in Marseilles (where I discovered that what was true for HIV-2 also applied to HIV-1 and suddenly realised that there was enough material for a book, rather than a few standard 3,000-word scientific papers, which had been my initial goal); Archives Nationales d'Outre-Mer in Aix-en-Provence; Belgian Ministry of Foreign Affairs, the Royal Library and Université Libre de Bruxelles, in Brussels; Louvain University and Université Catholique de Louvain; Institute of Tropical

Medicine in Antwerp; United Nations Library and the World Health Organization in Geneva; Bibliothèque Nationale de France in Paris; University of Ottawa, Université Laval in Quebec City, Université de Montréal and Université du Québec à Montréal and my own institution, the Université de Sherbrooke.

During the lengthy process of writing up the manuscript, I became especially indebted to Bernadette Wilson, who expertly edited the many chapters that I had written in English, and translated a few more written in French, and to Christian Audet, who professionally designed the illustrations.

When I finally reached the stage of seeking a publisher, Michael Watson of Cambridge University Press was kind enough to look at my manuscript and to find it worthy of publication. He then guided me through the difficult but necessary process of further editing the work. Like most academic authors, I initially saw this last step as a multi-organ amputation, but it turned out to be just a long-overdue haircut. Chloe Howell assisted with the finishing touches.

This having been said, the most important person who helped me through this whole adventure will be acknowledged in the Introduction.

Abbreviations

AEF	Afrique Équatoriale Française
AIDS	Acquired immune deficiency syndrome
CDC	Centers for Disease Control and Prevention
CFA	Colonies Françaises d'Afrique/Communauté Financère Africaine
CFCO	Chemin de Fer Congo–Océan
CIA	Central Intelligence Agency
CRF	circulating recombinant forms
DNA	desoxyribonucleic acid
DRC	Democratic Republic of the Congo
EIC	État Indépendant du Congo (Congo Free State)
GPA	Global Programme on AIDS
HBV	hepatitis B virus
HCV	hepatitis C virus
HIV	human immunodeficiency virus
HTLV	human T-cell lymphotropic virus
ID	intradermal(ly)
IDU	injection drug user or intravenous drug user
IM	intramuscular(ly)
IV	intravenous(ly)
KS	Kaposi's sarcoma
MMWR	*Morbidity and Mortality Weekly Report*
NIBSC	National Institute for Biological Standards and Control
ONUC	Organisation des Nations-Unies au Congo
OPV	oral polio vaccine
SC	subcutaneous(ly)
SFV	simian foamy virus
SIV	simian immunodeficiency virus
STD	sexually transmitted disease

UNESCO	United Nations Education, Science and Culture Organization
WHO	World Health Organization
WWI	World War I
WWII	World War II

Note on terminology

Before we move on, I want to point out that for readers unfamiliar with virology, the Appendix provides a brief overview of the viruses that we will be discussing. In a few chapters where this is necessary, elements of molecular biology will be discussed. I aimed to explain them succinctly to readers who have no training in this field.

With regard to toponymy, in English-language publications West Africa generally encompasses all countries on the Atlantic coast of Africa, plus some in the corresponding hinterland. I will rather use French terminology whereby West Africa starts in Mauritania, ends with Nigeria and also includes the corresponding hinterland. Central Africa (in colonial times, Equatorial Africa) starts with Cameroon and Chad, goes all the way to Rwanda and Burundi and also encompasses the two Congos, Gabon, the Central African Republic and Equatorial Guinea. Most of the story told in this book occurred in central Africa.

In former French colonies, city names did not change much after independence. Gabon's major port is still called Port-Gentil, despite the latter character's dubious human rights record. However, in the former Belgian Congo, these traces of the colonisers were enthusiastically erased so that Léopoldville became Kinshasa, Stanleyville became Kisangani, Elisabethville was renamed Lubumbashi, and so on. The country itself was successively known as the Congo Free State, the Belgian Congo, the Democratic Republic of Congo (DRC) after 1960 (or Congo-Léopoldville, and then Congo-Kinshasa), Zaire under Mobutu's dictatorship and then DRC again after Mobutu was overthrown.

The federation of Afrique Équatoriale Française (AEF) included four distinct colonies: Moyen-Congo (present day Republic of Congo, or Congo-Brazzaville), Oubangui-Chari (Central African Republic), Gabon and Tchad. AEF disappeared as a geographic entity shortly before 1960 when independence was granted to the four countries. To avoid confusion between the two Congos, I will use the term Congo-Brazzaville (it also changed names a few times) to designate the independent country that succeeded Moyen-Congo. Cameroun Français, or just Cameroun with the French spelling, refers to the part of current day Cameroon that was administered by France under a mandate from the League of Nations after World War I (WWI) and the United Nations after World War II (WWII), until the country became independent in 1960. The maps in this book use the names of countries and cities as they were known at the time of the events in question, and in principle the location of each city, district, region, river or park mentioned anywhere in the book should be shown on at least one of the maps.

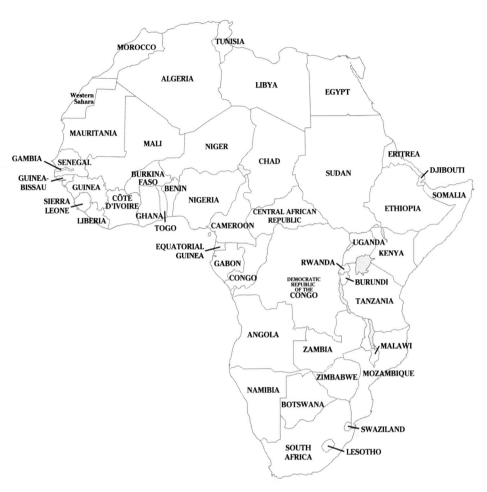

Map 1 Map of Africa.

Introduction

June 1981 is the official birth date of the AIDS epidemic. In a short article published in the Centers for Disease Control's *Morbidity and Mortality Weekly Report* (*MMWR*), American clinicians described a cluster of five cases of *Pneumocystis carinii* pneumonia, an infection of the lungs hitherto seen only in patients with severe impairment of their immune system. These five initial cases had been diagnosed in 1980–1 among gay men, all living in Los Angeles, who had been previously healthy and were not receiving drugs that suppressed the body's immune response. At the time, the standard treatment for *Pneumocystis* pneumonia was an old drug called pentamidine, developed during WWII for the treatment of sleeping sickness, which happened to be highly active against *Pneumocystis*. Pentamidine was not commercially available and had to be distributed centrally from the CDC in Atlanta. An astute CDC technician found it strange to have received several requests for pentamidine within a short period of time from hospitals in California and, a bit later, from New York as well. This became the first step in the identification of the new syndrome by this federal agency.[1-2]

Nobody could have imagined that, within three decades, more than twenty-nine million individuals would have died of AIDS, leaving in the process sixteen million orphans. By 2009, another thirty-three million were living with its HIV aetiological agent, making it by far the most dramatic epidemic since the Black Plague devastated Europe 500 years ago. Since that fateful day in 1981, more than 300,000 scientific articles and thousands of books have been published on HIV/AIDS. Most are biomedical but others analyse the psychosocial, historical, economic, geographic and even photographic features of AIDS. Thus the history of HIV/AIDS from 1981 to 2011 has been described in great detail. Randy Shilts' *And the band played on* and Laurie Garrett's *The coming plague* contain captivating descriptions of the early years of the pandemic in the US and Europe. Some books have chronicled the AIDS epidemic in

Africa after the initial description of the disease, its devastating impact
on the lives of so many, a few success stories and unfortunately many
more failures in the response to HIV/AIDS, most tragically in South
Africa. For a summary of the dissemination of the virus between 1981
and 2006, I recommend John Illiffe's *The African AIDS epidemic. A
history.*[2–10]

However, what happened before 1981 – how did the human race
reach that point? – has, to my knowledge, only been addressed in
Edward Hooper's *The river. A journey back to the source of HIV and
AIDS.* This book was written in support of the hypothesis that the
emergence of HIV/AIDS was triggered by the contamination of an
oral polio vaccine with a simian immunodeficiency virus through the
use of chimpanzee cells during vaccine production. There is now overwhelming evidence that this did not happen, as we will see later.[11]

This book will summarise and assemble various pieces of the puzzle
that have gradually been delineated over the last decade by a small
group of investigators, to which I have added historical research of
my own. Some elements are irrefutable, such as the notion that the
Pan troglodytes troglodytes chimpanzee is the source of HIV-1. Other
elements are less clear, for example the exact moment of the cross-
species transmission (sometime in the first three decades of the twentieth
century). My own contribution focused around the idea that medical
interventions requiring the massive use of reusable syringes and needles
jumpstarted the epidemic by rapidly expanding the number of infected
individuals from a handful to a few hundred or a few thousand. This set
the stage for the sexual transmission of the virus, starting in core groups
of sex workers and their male clients and later spreading to the rest of
the adult population. Some parts of the story rely on circumstantial
evidence, such as the links between the Congo and Haiti and the
potential contribution of the blood trade in triggering the epidemic in
Port-au-Prince, from where it moved into the US. Potentially sceptical
readers should look at the whole story before making a judgement. I
believe it is coherent, and that the weaker parts are supported by a
strong body of evidence immediately before or after these uncertain
areas.

My own background is that of an infectious diseases physician and
epidemiologist. I started my career in the early 1980s as a medical
officer in a bush hospital in Zaire, where I spent the four most challeng-
ing years of my life. The type of medicine that I practised there was not

much different from that of my colonial-era predecessors: approximate diagnoses, empirical treatments, lack of human and material resources, systematic re-use of syringes, needles and other medical supplies. I developed a fascination with sleeping sickness, a disease which happened to be epidemic in my district and around which I conducted research for the next twenty years. After completing my training in infectious diseases in Canada, I went back to Africa, this time as a clinical researcher at the Medical Research Council Laboratories in The Gambia, working on the epidemiology of HIV-2 infection and its interaction with sexually transmitted diseases (STDs). I returned to Canada in 1990 as an academic infectious diseases physician, but I also coordinated AIDS control projects in central and West Africa, which provided preventive and curative care to a large number of sex workers. During a sabbatical, I studied for a master's degree in epidemiology. Epidemiology is a science which connects exposures (for instance, to some infectious agent) and outcomes (developing AIDS or cancer, death, etc.). I will not use much epidemiology in this book though I confess to an inborn love of numbers which, Mark Twain notwithstanding, can often prove or disprove an argument.

Eventually, these various professional interests coalesced, when I belatedly understood that there was probably a link between HIV-2 infection in Guinea-Bissau, its epicentre, and programmes to control sleeping sickness during the colonial era, when that country was known as Portuguese Guinea. An epidemiological study among elderly individuals in Bissau confirmed that subjects who had been treated for sleeping sickness or tuberculosis decades before were more likely than others to be HIV-2-infected (in contrast with HIV-1, HIV-2 infection is compatible with prolonged survival, which enabled us to document such associations).[12]

I realised that during my time in Zaire patients under my care were probably infected with HIV-1 during health care. In the rather primitive 110-bed Nioki hospital, in the Mai-Ndombe region about 500 kilometres north-east of Kinshasa, we used glass syringes and reusable needles. Normally, these would go through the hospital's autoclave after each use, which should have killed all pathogens, including viruses. However, I did not pay too much attention to how long they were boiled for by the nurses in between patients when the hospital ran out of electricity so that the autoclave could not be used. Power outages could last up to two months at a time, when the whole country was short of the diesel fuel needed for generators.

For sleeping sickness patients (up to 400 per year), we mostly relied on 6–12 intravenous (IV) injections of an old arsenical drug called melarsoprol. Melarsoprol was in short supply, so that even 0.1 ml remaining in the vial after administering the dose for a first patient would be used for the next. I also remember the unfortunate tuberculosis patients, who were given intramuscular (IM) injections of streptomycin every day for sixty days (or even longer for those who did not tolerate one of the oral antituberculous drugs), with fairly dramatic adverse effects (the drug was toxic to the inner ear, and many patients had a hard time walking, some of them permanently). At the time, 'international health' resources were an order of magnitude lower than they are today, and the much more effective and less toxic treatment for tuberculosis, comprising only oral meds, was deemed far too expensive at $50 per patient, compared to $10 for the streptomycin-based regimen. Potentially even worse, in the twenty or so rural health centres which I supervised, several of which could only be reached by dugout canoe, formol tablets were put into a metal box along with the syringes and needles as a sterilisation measure. Abscesses following injections were rare, so this process killed the bacteria, but what about the viruses?

I do not believe that transmission via medical interventions plays an important role in HIV dynamics today and I agree with the experts who maintain that it contributes to less than 5% of recent HIV infections, although even a single case is unacceptable. However, I became convinced that transmission during health care contributed to the simultaneous emergence of HIV-1 and HIV-2 in different parts of the African continent fifty to seventy-five years ago.[13]

These were sobering thoughts, and I started trying to connect the dots in the history of HIV. This book is the result of these efforts over the last five years. It would not have been possible without the support of my wife Lucie, a Congolese nurse, who kept my interest for Africa very much alive. Several friends and relatives died of an AIDS-like illness before and after the disease was identified in Africa.

Some may say that understanding the past is irrelevant, what really matters is the future. I disagree. There are at least two good reasons for attempting to elucidate the factors behind the emergence of the HIV pandemic. First, we have a moral obligation to the millions of human beings who have died, or will die, from this infection. Second, this tragedy was facilitated (or even caused) by human interventions:

colonisation, urbanisation and probably well-intentioned public health campaigns. Hopefully, we can gain collective wisdom and humility that might help avoid provoking another such disaster in the coming decades.

1 | *Out of Africa*

Ex Africa semper aliquid novi

Out of Africa, there is always something new, wrote historian Pliny the Elder more than 2,000 years ago. He was quite right. As early as 1984, just three years after the first description of the new disease, it was suspected that HIV, its recently discovered aetiological agent (then known as human T-cell lymphotropic virus (HTLV)-III in the US, LAV (lymphadenopathy-associated virus) in Europe), originated in central Africa. This was mainly because the first studies in Africa, conducted in Zaire and Rwanda, showed that AIDS was common in Kinshasa and Kigali, where nearly 90% of sex workers were infected. These field studies were prompted by the observation that of the first few hundred cases of AIDS diagnosed in Europe, about half occurred among patients coming from central Africa, mostly from Zaire. Over the following years, the epidemiology of HIV-1 infection in Kinshasa would be described in great detail by a group of American, Belgian and Congolese researchers known as Projet Sida, based at Hôpital Mama Yemo (Mama Yemo was dictator Mobutu's mother, a former sex worker, and she suffered the same fate as the Belgian colonists after her son was overthrown: this institution is now called Hôpital Général de Kinshasa). Projet Sida came to an abrupt end in 1991, when the whole of Kinshasa was looted by the city's poor people. During the same period and until the 1994 genocide, similar epidemiological work was conducted in Kigali, 1,500 kilometres east of Kinshasa.[1–3]

In retrospect, this early vision of central Africa as the source of HIV-1 was rather naive. Researchers assumed that since this was at the time the region with the highest prevalence (i.e. the proportion of the population that is infected) among groups representative of the general adult population, the virus must have originated there. There were at least two problems with this assumption.

First, there was an obvious bias, as little information on HIV prevalence was available from other parts of the continent, especially East and southern Africa. Belgian researchers, the most prominent being Peter Piot, from the Institute of Tropical Medicine in Antwerp (who would later become the founding executive director of UNAIDS, the UN programme specifically dedicated to the control of HIV/AIDS), had naturally initiated HIV research in the former Belgian colonies where their institutions had maintained networks and contacts over the preceding decades. Much to their credit, Zaire and Rwanda were open to AIDS research from the start, but this was not the case in other countries such as Burundi and some English-speaking countries of East Africa, where there was a strong temptation to keep AIDS under wraps: if we ignore it, perhaps it will go away.

Second, the relationship between HIV prevalence and duration of the epidemic is not straightforward: it all depends on the annual incidence (the proportion of previously uninfected individuals who acquire HIV each year). We now know that in Kinshasa the HIV incidence among the general adult population was probably never higher than 1% per year. However, in some countries of southern Africa, annual incidence reached the extraordinary level of 5% in the 1990s (one seronegative adult out of twenty got newly infected with HIV each year). A prevalence of 10% could reflect an annual incidence of 1% continuing for more than ten years, or an incidence of 5% over just a couple of years. However, even if these assumptions about a central African origin of HIV/AIDS were naive, eventually they proved to be correct, showing that in the scientific domain intuition can sometimes be trusted!

Archival samples

Additional support for a central African origin of HIV-1 came from the testing of archival samples of blood. In the mid- and late 1980s, to understand the dynamics of HIV in the recent past, researchers tried to locate collections of sera obtained earlier for other purposes and kept frozen. Scientists tend to clean out their freezers once in a while to make room for new samples, or their samples are destroyed when they retire or move on to other positions. However, sometimes samples are forgotten for a long time or deliberately conserved. In Kinshasa, among mothers attending a well-baby clinic in the Lemba district, HIV-1 prevalence was 0.25% in 1970 (n=805) and 3.0% in 1980 (n=498). In the remote Catholic mission of Yambuku and surrounding communities of the Equateur province of Zaire, 0.8% of 659 samples collected in 1976 during an investigation of an epidemic of Ebola fever were found to be HIV-1 seropositive when tested ten years later. This proved that the virus had existed in this part of the world for some time, but not necessarily that it originated there; testing of archived samples of serum from American gay men who participated in epidemiological studies of hepatitis B also retrospectively documented cases of HIV-1 in the late 1970s, and even earlier for drug addicts.[4–8]

The Yambuku epidemic of Ebola fever which had prompted the collection of these samples had largely been 'iatrogenic' (healthcare related). In this small rural hospital, syringes and needles were scarce and constantly re-used, fuelling transmission of the blood-borne Ebola virus between patients attending the hospital for other reasons (malaria, gonorrhoea, etc.). The nuns issued only five syringes to the nurses each morning, which were then used and re-used on the 300 patients attending each day. Three-fourths of the first 100 cases of Ebola in Yambuku were infected through injections received at the hospital. The epidemic came to an end after the hospital was closed following the death of several nurses and nuns, infected by their patients. Clearly, noble intentions for providing health care to the underprivileged could have disastrous consequences when the risk of transmission of blood-borne viruses was not appreciated. This unfortunate situation was not new or specific to the Yambuku hospital, and had already had infinitely more dramatic consequences, although this was not known at the time, than these few hundred deaths from Ebola fever. It was decided to call this new disease after a nearby river rather than after the Yambuku mission, to avoid further stigmatisation after all it had gone through. The contrast between the two diseases is an excellent illustration of the genius of HIV. People infected with the Ebola virus quickly fall ill and die. This causes a spectacular epidemic, which triggers a massive (and always successful) reaction to control it. People infected with HIV, on the other hand, can live and quietly pass on the virus for ten years or more, and it will take even longer before physicians can recognise the emergence of this new disease, because symptomatic cases are not clustered within a short period of time.[9,10]

Elsewhere in Africa, no trace of HIV was found before the 1980s, which increasingly pointed to a central African origin of this 'new' virus. In West Africa, out of more than 6,000 samples obtained in Nigeria, Liberia, Ivory Coast, Togo, Senegal, Sierra Leone, Mali, Niger and Ghana in the 1960s and 1970s, not a single case of HIV-1 infection was found. A few cases of HIV-2 infection were documented, however. Among 789 samples obtained in Senegal in 1981, one was positive but it is unclear whether this corresponded to HIV-2 or HIV-1.[11-16]

Meanwhile in East and southern Africa, in samples obtained from low-risk groups between 1959 and 1981, HIV was not found in Mozambique, Zimbabwe, Zambia, Uganda, Tanzania and northern Kenya, nor in mine workers in South Africa (who originated from Mozambique, Malawi, Lesotho, Botswana, Angola, Swaziland and South Africa itself). The earliest evidence of HIV in East Africa comes from Nairobi in 1980–1 where 1% of patients with STDs and 5% of sex workers were HIV-1-infected. Just three years later, 82% of Nairobi sex workers were HIV-1-infected. This exponential transmission among prostitutes is central to the story and will be examined later.[14,17-19]

Documentation of early cases of full-blown AIDS was also achieved retrospectively. First, let me say that no conclusions can be drawn from isolated cases of apparently immunocompetent patients found to have had, many years ago, a diagnosis of a condition now frequently associated with AIDS such as *Pneumocystis* pneumonia, if this is not substantiated by a specimen positive for HIV in the patient or his/her spouse. This is because there are rare non-infectious diseases of the immune system which lead to very low counts of CD4 lymphocytes (the cells which are the main target for destruction by HIV), and subsequently to any of a long list of opportunistic infections. Short of an archived specimen positive for HIV, the clustering of cases, geographically or temporally, or within a couple, is more suggestive of AIDS but never conclusive.[20-21]

Valuable journalistic information about some documented early cases can be found in *The river* as well as in *And the band played on*. The most interesting is that of a Norwegian family (father, mother and nine-year-old daughter), who all tragically died in 1976 from AIDS caused by HIV-1 group O, and whose sera were found to be HIV-positive when tested twelve years later. The child was born in 1967, which implies that the mother was already HIV-infected by then. The father had been a sailor, visiting a number of ports in Africa in the early 1960s, where he developed STDs, presumably after contacts with prostitutes. He probably acquired HIV-1 group O in Nigeria or Cameroon, where his boat stopped for a few days in 1961–2. A Danish surgeon died of AIDS in 1977, after working at the Abumonbazi rural hospital in Zaire in 1972–5 and in Kinshasa in 1975–7, following an earlier stint in the same country around 1964. An eight-year-old Zairean child, infected perinatally in 1974–5, died in Sweden in 1982, and AIDS was serologically proven later on. A very unfortunate Canadian pilot involved in a plane crash in 1976 in northern Zaire, where he had surgery and received a blood transfusion, died of AIDS in 1980; his serum was later found to be HIV-1-positive (transfusion-acquired HIV infection progresses rapidly to AIDS, because of the huge quantity of viruses present in the blood bag). Former physicians at the university hospital in Kinshasa reported seven cases of AIDS diagnosed retrospectively, five of them confirmed serologically, which had been acquired sexually in the DRC (or Burundi in one case) in the late 1960s or the 1970s, mostly among Belgian nationals. Then in 1979, cases of AIDS started trickling down among the small proportion of Zaireans rich enough to seek health care in Belgium.[22–30]

We do not know whether other researchers tested ancient samples from other parts of Africa without reporting their findings. Studies with negative results tend not to be published in scientific journals, a phenomenon known as 'publication bias'. Thus although sketchy, testing of archival samples suggested that HIV-1 was present in the 1960s and 1970s, albeit at a low prevalence, in several locations in central Africa but not in West or East Africa.

The next step came from the documentation of the earliest case of HIV-1 infection in a sample obtained in the Belgian Congo around 1959, during the course of a study on genetic diseases of red blood cells. Of 672 samples, collected in Léopoldville and other locations, and miraculously kept (probably forgotten) in a freezer, one was found twenty-six years later to contain antibodies against HIV-1. Apparently, the HIV-1-positive specimen came from a male adult recruited in Léopoldville. HIV genetic material was amplified from this sample, and analyses confirmed that this was indeed the oldest HIV-1 isolate ever documented. It was named ZR59.[31–33]

It took more than twenty years for another ancient specimen containing HIV-1 to be located. Finding old tissue blocks collected between 1958 and 1960 and kept at the pathology department of the University of Kinshasa, scientists discovered HIV-1 sequences in a lymph node biopsy obtained in 1960 from an adult woman. It was given the name DRC60. Twenty-six other specimens (lymph nodes, livers and placentas) did not contain HIV. DRC60 and ZR59 differed by about 12%. It was calculated that DRC60 and ZR59 shared a common ancestor around 1921, as we will discuss later. Although the exact time of its introduction into human populations remains debated, there is no doubt that HIV-1 was present in Léopoldville by 1959–60.[34]

Viral diversity

Now we will examine how the genetic diversity of HIV-1 in different parts of the world helped scientists trace back the origins of the virus. But first, we need to review quickly what 'sequencing' is all about. Sequencing is the identification in their proper order of the series of 'nucleotides' that constitute a gene. There are four types of nucleotides: adenine (A), thymine (T), guanine (G) and cytosine (C). The genome of any living organism is a long list of these four letters. When scientists compare viruses, the similarity between sequences is called 'homology', and non-similarity 'divergence'. If 90% of the nucleotide sequences between two isolates are the same, they have 90% homology or 10% divergence. This degree of divergence is used to decide whether two isolates constitute subtypes of one viral species, or two distinct species. For instance, sequences of HIV-1 and HIV-2 differ by more than 50%.

Based on such analyses, HIV-1 is now divided into four 'groups': group M (main), which is responsible for the current pandemic and causes more than 99% of all HIV-1 infections in the world, group O (outlier), group N (non-M non-O) and group P, which did not spread outside central Africa, for reasons still unclear.

HIV-1 group M is further subdivided into nine 'subtypes': A, B, C, D, F, G, H, J and K (the alphabet is not respected because subtypes E and I were found not to be real subtypes and have been renamed). HIV-1 often makes mistakes when replicating, a phenomenon compounded by the high level of viral production throughout the long natural history of the infection. Up to ten billion copies of the virus are produced every day, and the potential for errors in replication is commensurate. Over time, the accumulation of these errors leads to viral diversity. When around 20% of the nucleotide sequences of the initial virus have undergone replication errors, the result will be a new subtype, as defined arbitrarily by scientific consensus.[35–36]

High-risk individuals (especially in Africa) can get infected with a first subtype, and later with a second subtype, which can recombine into 'circulating recombinant forms' (CRF): part of their genome is derived from the first subtype, part from the second. Recombinants can be transmitted forward. Forty-eight recombinants have now been recognised. Their names correspond to the two subtypes involved in the recombination, for example CRF02_AG is a recombination of subtypes A and G. Some recombinants have generated their own epidemic in specific countries or regions.[37]

There is no clear-cut difference between subtypes with regard to their propensity to cause AIDS, with one exception: individuals infected with subtype D die faster than others. Do subtypes differ in their transmissibility? Shedding of HIV-1 in the genital tract of women infected with subtype C is higher than for other subtypes, which would imply more effective female-to-male sexual transmission. With subtype C, the high degree of 'viraemia' (the quantity of virus in the blood) that characterises acute infections may be worse than with other subtypes, increasing its infectiousness. Subtype C spread like wildfire in southern Africa, even if other subtypes had been introduced at the same time. These findings do suggest that subtype C is transmitted more efficiently than the others, which might explain its current worldwide preponderance.[38–42]

Some subtypes are associated in specific locations with particular modes of transmission. This represents a founder effect within specific risk groups: a subtype originally introduced in a group of intravenous drug users will continue to be transmitted preferentially to other addicts, another subtype originally introduced in sexual networks of homosexuals will be transmitted preferentially to other gay men, and so on. A good example of this is South Africa, where subtype B is found in 96% of white homosexuals (probably after it was imported from the US in the 1970s–80s), while subtype C accounts for 81% of infections of black heterosexuals. There is limited mixing between these two groups: few homosexual Afrikaners have sex with heterosexual Zulus! To date, there is no evidence that some subtypes are intrinsically better transmitted by one route than another. As the relative contribution of some modes of transmission varies over time, depending on the effectiveness of control efforts targeting a specific risk group, the distribution of subtypes within a given country can also change.[43]

HIV-1 evolves at a rate about one million times faster than that of animal desoxyribonucleic acid (DNA). This means that, in just over a decade, HIV-1 will change as much as all the genetic changes and the ensuing diversity that accrued among the common predecessors of *Homo sapiens*, chimpanzees and gorillas over ten million years. The longer HIV-1 has been present somewhere, the more opportunities it will have had to undergo a series of mutations which will eventually allow it to evolve into different subtypes, and the more likely it is that recombinants will be created. Conversely, if we were to examine all of the HIV-1 isolates in a city or country in which the very first case was introduced only a year earlier, for example in a population of drug addicts, we would find little genetic variation and the viruses of all the individuals infected after this first case would still belong to the same original subtype, the founder. There would not have been enough replication errors to result in new subtypes.

Because HIV evolves in only one direction, from a single model of virus to an increasingly complex differentiation into numerous subtypes and recombinants, we can reconstruct the sequence of its progress in a particular region or country by examining the local distribution of subtypes. Starting in the early 1990s, as new tools made it easier to examine nucleotide sequences from a large number of HIV-1 isolates obtained in various locations, an additional and most convincing argument emerged which supported a central African origin: the extreme genetic diversity of HIV-1 isolates from this part of the world.

Worldwide, subtype C accounts for about 50% of all HIV-1 infections, followed by subtypes B and A (10–12% each), G (6%), CRF02_AG (5%), CRF01_AE (5%) and D (2.5%), while subtypes F, H, J and K have undergone limited transmission (each fewer than 1% of cases). However, the contribution of each subtype varies dramatically from region to region.[44–45]

In North America and Western Europe, respectively 98% and 88% of HIV-1 infections correspond to subtype B, which is clearly the subtype that was originally introduced into these two continents, the founder strain. Subtypes other than B are usually found in migrants, who acquired HIV-1 in their countries of origin. In contrast, in Eastern Europe and central Asia, subtype A accounts for 79% of HIV-1 infections: clearly, this epidemic had a different origin than that of Western Europe, and it spread initially through needles rather than gay sex.[36,44–46]

In Latin America and the Caribbean, subtype B accounts for respectively 75–80% and 95% of strains. Cuba stands out as the country with not only the lowest HIV prevalence in the Americas but also the highest diversity: about half of Cuban isolates are either non-B subtypes or recombinants. This reflects the acquisition of multiple subtypes of HIV-1 (or recombinants) by some of the *internationalistas*, the soldiers that Castro sent to fight alongside the leftist Movimento Popular de Libertação de Angola during the civil war in Angola, and very limited opportunities for transmission upon their return to the island. The whole Cuban population was screened for HIV in 1986–9; seropositives were quarantined for years in AIDS sanatoria and brainwashed with preventive messages (Cuba was indeed the only country that tried to control HIV like an infectious disease, rather than making it a human rights issue). At the peak of their intervention in 1986, 35,000 Cuban troops were stationed in Angola, which became one of the most corrupt and capitalist regimes in Africa, while smaller numbers of Cuban soldiers were stationed in sixteen other African countries. Recent studies documented a high diversity in HIV-1 isolates in Angola, where all non-B subtypes found in Cuba are present. This illustrates how political and military events, even ideologies, had a measurable impact on the transmission of HIV.[47–52]

In southern Africa, subtype C corresponds to 92–8% of HIV-1 infections. This implies that the virus was introduced relatively recently into this region now so afflicted by AIDS, a finding corroborated by epidemiological investigations. Subtype C accounts for 99% of infections in Ethiopia and also predominates in Zambia, while subtype A accounts for 70% of infections in Kenya. In Tanzania, subtypes A, C and D are the major players. In Uganda, which borders not only Tanzania and Kenya but also the DRC, there is more diversity, with a high prevalence of A, D and recombinants, and lower frequencies of C, B and G. In West Africa, all the way from Nigeria to Senegal, CRF02_AG predominates, implying that this part of the continent was infected only after subtypes A and G had had the opportunity to recombine.[36,45,46]

Countries of central Africa (the two Congos, Cameroon, Gabon, the Central African Republic and Equatorial Guinea) display by far the widest diversity in HIV-1 subtypes. All subtypes of HIV-1 group M and many recombinants have been found in this region, where there is also more genetic diversity within each subtype. Map 2, reproduced from a 2003 review paper, illustrates the extreme genetic variation of HIV-1 in central Africa compared to other parts of the continent. Additional studies published since might indicate small changes in the distribution of this or that subtype, without modifying the general pattern. The conclusion is crystal clear: HIV-1 must have originated in central Africa, where it has had more time to diversify genetically.[45]

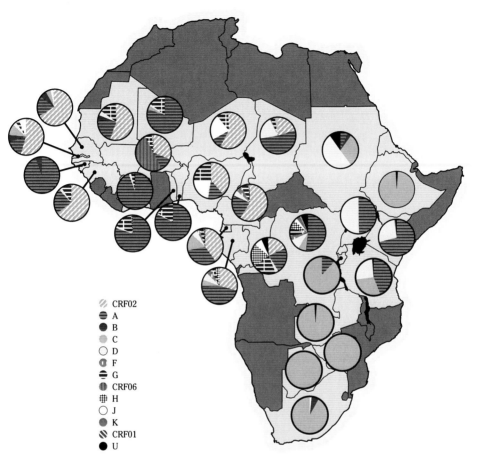

Map 2 Genetic diversity of HIV-1 in sub-Saharan Africa. The circles show the distribution of HIV-1 subtypes in various countries (U stands for unknown).
Adapted from Peeters.[45]

Within central Africa, however, there are differences between countries, which help us to track past events. In Cameroon, the CRF02_AG recombinant is by far the predominant subtype, as in Nigeria to the north and Gabon and Equatorial Guinea to the south. This means that most of the HIV-1 transmission occurred relatively recently in these countries, without excluding the possibility that the initial case occurred there.[53–56]

In the Central African Republic, there is a strong preponderance of subtype A. In Chad, a country not inhabited by the *Pan troglodytes troglodytes* chimpanzee, there is diversity but the distribution differs:

subtype A represents only 20% of isolates, while 40% are recombinants. This suggests that the virus disseminated there later than in the DRC.[57,58]

HIV-1 isolates obtained in 1997 from Kinshasa, Bwamanda and Mbuji-Mayi (all in DRC) were characterised. In Kinshasa, by descending order these were subtypes A (44%), D (13%), G (11%), H (10%), F (6%), K (3%), J (4%) and C (2%), while 8% could not be properly subtyped. Of note, only one subtype B strain was found, from a patient in Bwamanda in the Equateur region. This broad distribution of subtypes proved similar to what was measured retrospectively in samples collected in Kinshasa in the mid-1980s by Projet Sida: HIV-1 diversity in Kinshasa twenty-five years ago was far more complex than among strains currently found in any other parts of the world![59,60]

Only recently has HIV-1 diversity in Congo-Brazzaville been evaluated on a large number of isolates, obtained mainly in Brazzaville. A pattern similar to that of Kinshasa was found: a predominance of A and G but few CRF02_AG recombinants and no subtype B. So in the final analysis, the two Congos are the countries with by far the greatest diversity of HIV-1 subtypes. This implies that the oldest epidemic did in fact start in the DRC and Congo-Brazzaville.[61]

The genetic diversity of HIV-1 in a given location is influenced not only by how long it has been there, but also by how efficiently it propagated. An HIV-1 strain producing only one case of secondary infection every five years would present fewer variations after fifty years compared to the same strain which, introduced into another environment, would have generated a secondary case every three months, with each secondary case in turn producing a tertiary case every three months, and so on. The more people are infected, the more copies of the virus are produced each day, which increases the number of mutations and differentiation into subtypes. In practice, what the great genetic diversity of HIV-1 in Kinshasa and Brazzaville means is that for the first time the virus found in this large urban area conditions conducive to its dissemination on a scale that enabled it to flourish and differentiate, after an initial phase of stagnation or very slow multiplication, which could have occurred elsewhere in any of the countries inhabited by its simian source.

It is still a mystery why subtype B remained rare in central Africa, where it represents only 0.2% of all HIV-1 infections, but spread so successfully into the Americas and Western Europe. Presumably, chance (the founder effect) played a major role, depending on whether a given subtype was introduced into some mechanism of amplification, sexual or otherwise, which gave it the initial boost after which it could disseminate slowly but effectively.

2 | *The source*

So, HIV-1 originated from central Africa. But then, one may ask, why central Africa? The answer, as we will see, is because this region corresponds to the habitat of the simian source of the virus.

Our closest relatives

Chimpanzees are the closest relatives of humans, sharing between 98 and 99% of their genome with us, and are considered the most intelligent non-human animal. Chimpanzees and humans shared a common ancestor and are thought to have diverged between four and six million years ago. In fact, chimpanzees are so close to humans that it was recently proposed to move them into the genus *Homo*. Long-term studies in the Gombe reserve of Tanzania revealed that, like humans, chimpanzees have their own personalities. Some are gentle, others are more aggressive. Some have a good relationship with their parents or other members of the troop while others are loners. Some have a strong maternal instinct, others do not. This marked individualisation and their ability to laugh are what make chimpanzees most like humans. Rather than reacting predictably and instinctively to a given situation, chimpanzees show intelligence and spirit and experience all kinds of emotions.[1–3]

According to current taxonomy, there are two species: *Pan troglodytes*, the common chimpanzee, and *Pan paniscus*, the bonobo. Based on analyses of mitochondrial DNA (DNA that comes solely from the mother), there are now four subspecies of *Pan troglodytes*: *Pan troglodytes verus* (western chimpanzee), *Pan troglodytes ellioti* (Nigerian chimpanzee, until recently *P.t. vellerosus*), *Pan troglodytes schweinfurthii* (eastern chimpanzee) and *Pan troglodytes troglodytes* (central chimpanzee) (Map 3).[4]

Chimpanzees are poor swimmers, so that large rivers like the Cross, Sanaga, Ubangui and Congo became natural boundaries between the

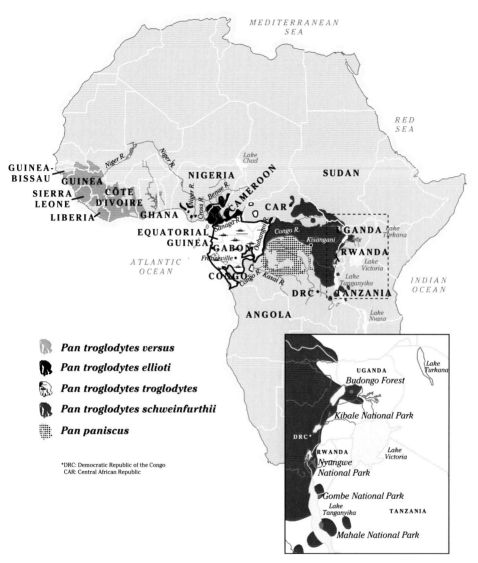

Map 3 Distribution of the four subspecies of *Pan troglodytes* and the *Pan paniscus* bonobo.

habitat of various species and subspecies. *Pan troglodytes verus* (total population in 2004: between 21,300 and 55,600, according to the International Union for Conservation of Nature) inhabits West Africa, from southern Senegal to the west bank of the Cross River in Nigeria;

most of its population is now found in Guinea and Ivory Coast. *Pan troglodytes ellioti* (total population: 5,000–8,000) is found from east of the Cross to the Sanaga River in Cameroon, its southern boundary. *Pan troglodytes schweinfurthii* (total population: 76,400–119,600) inhabits mostly the DRC, east of the Ubangui and north of the Congo rivers, but its range extends into the Central African Republic, southern Sudan and eastwards to Uganda, Rwanda and Tanzania.[5]

Pan troglodytes troglodytes (total population: 70,000–116,500) inhabits an area south of the Sanaga River in Cameroon and extending eastward to the Ubangui and Congo rivers, spread over seven countries: southern Cameroon, Gabon, the continental part of Equatorial Guinea, Congo-Brazzaville, a small area in the south-west of the Central African Republic, the Cabinda enclave of Angola and the adjacent Mayombe area of the DRC. The largest populations are found in Gabon (27,000–64,000), where unfortunately they are rapidly declining, Cameroon (31,000–39,000) and Congo-Brazzaville (about 10,000). Other countries have fewer than 2,000 each, with probably less than 200 in the DRC. It is estimated that *P.t. troglodytes* and *P.t. schweinfurthii* diverged approximately 440,000 years ago.[5,6]

Chimpanzee populations in the first half of the twentieth century were certainly higher than now, because there had been relatively little opportunity for human activities to disrupt the natural equilibrium of the species. Human populations were much smaller than today, with fewer hunters and fewer clients willing to purchase bush meat. As an educated guess, some experts suggested that, combining all subspecies, there was around one million chimps in 1960. The subsequent decline was particularly severe for *P.t. verus*, and is generally attributed to the destruction of its habitat by increasing human populations who farmed or logged and hunted for bush meat, to diseases like Ebola fever, and captures for medical experiments.[6–10]

The rest of this section will focus on the central *P.t. troglodytes* chimpanzee, but the morphologic, demographic and behavioural differences between the four subspecies of *Pan troglodytes* are minor, at least for the non-expert. *P.t. troglodytes* chimps have a life expectancy of 40–60 years. An adult male weighs 40–70 kg, a female 30–50 kg. They live in rather loose communities ('troops') of 15 to 160 individuals, with a dominant male leader. When they reach sexual maturity, males generally remain in the community into which they were born, while females often join other troops. This intuitive exogamy maintains the genetic diversity of the sub-species and avoids the potentially devastating effects of inbreeding.

Chimpanzees are largely diurnal. To sleep at night, each individual builds a nest in a tree, complete with a pillow, 9–12 metres above the ground, which is normally used only once. For this reason, scientists have used nests to estimate chimpanzee populations, based on counts by surveyors who walk on line transects through forested areas as a sampling method. Population density of *P.t. troglodytes* is generally between 0.1 and 0.3 km^2. Most communities live in forested areas, and a minority in savannahs.

Chimpanzees are intensely territorial and most troops spend their entire lives within a 20–50 km^2 area. Adult males are aggressive, and spend much of their time patrolling their small territory. Males of one troop can form raiding parties to attack lone males (or couples) from other troops. *P.t. troglodytes* chimpanzees usually have a hostile and violent attitude towards members of other communities. Among their *P.t. schweinfurthii* counterparts in Tanzania, primatologists documented a war between two neighbouring communities which, after three years of attacks and killings, ended with the complete annihilation of the weaker troop.[1,11–13]

P.t. troglodytes chimpanzees are able to develop and use tools, mostly sticks to procure food (for instance, to dig out ants or termites or extract honey from hives). Unlike gorillas, chimpanzees are omnivorous, with a highly diversified diet consisting mostly of fruits, leaves, seeds, plants, insects and eggs, but they occasionally eat vertebrates, including monkeys, antelopes and warthogs.

An infant chimp spends the first five years of its life completely dependent on its mother. Like humans, they become progressively autonomous during adolescence, reaching sexual maturity at age 12–13. Chimpanzees are promiscuous, and most of their sexual activity takes place when the adult female is in heat and her vulva swells, which attracts the males, who copulate with her quickly, one after the other. As many as six different males may copulate with the same female in just ten minutes. Some males establish an exclusive relationship with a female of their choice, presumably for reproductive purposes, and take her on a 'honeymoon' far from the other chimpanzees. This usually only lasts for a week or two during which they copulate as often as five times a day. So while their behaviour limits the transmission of pathogens between troops, sexually transmitted infectious agents will easily disseminate within a given troop once they have been successfully introduced.

P.t. troglodytes chimps have low fertility: on average, 800 matings occur for each conception. During their reproductive years (from age 14 to 40), females give birth to a mean of 4.4 babies, half of which die before reaching maturity. Each female has a lifetime reproductive success of only 2.3. A small increase in mortality, due to hunting or diseases, is sufficient to reduce this number to less than two and for the population to contract.[14,15]

Like humans, chimpanzee communities are occasionally stricken by epidemics. In Gombe, during an outbreak in the region's human population, poliomyelitis caused four deaths and left some chimpanzees permanently paralysed. Respiratory infections followed, also with fatal consequences. This reflects not just the communal nature of life among the chimpanzees, which have frequent and close contacts with other members of their troop, but also their biological similarity to humans, whose microbes can be transmitted to chimpanzees and vice versa.[1]

All kinds of trees

We will now examine how it gradually became clear that one subspecies of chimpanzees was the source of HIV-1. But first, let us review quickly a science called phylogenetics. Phylogenetics uses nucleotide sequences to reconstruct the evolutionary history of various forms of life, including microbial pathogens. A 'phylogenetic tree' superficially resembles a genealogical tree. However, phylogenetic trees describe the relatedness between living organisms (and their classification) rather than ancestry. They measure the genetic distance between organisms, and identify the nearest relatives. Because ancestors are not available to be tested, ancestry is assumed rather than proven. Each division in the tree is called a 'node', the common ancestor of the organisms or the isolates identified to its right. After such branching, the organisms and their sequences evolve independently. The 'root' (at the extreme left) is the assumed common ancestor of all organisms in the tree. To construct a phylogenetic tree, molecular biologists compare the differences in nucleotide sequences of many isolates of putatively related organisms. This exercise is repeated for various genes; if the findings are the same for two or three genes, scientists are confident that they have produced the right phylogenetic tree.

An 'isolate' corresponds to a given pathogen obtained from one specific patient or animal at a specific point in time. If substantial laboratory work is done on any isolate, it will be given a name corresponding either to the initials of the patient, the name of the city or country where it was obtained or whatever the researcher decides to call it. Like children's names, these names serve only one purpose, to distinguish isolates from each other.

For two isolates belonging to the same species, a greater degree of divergence, corresponding to a larger cumulative number of errors in replication, indicates that their common ancestor was further back in time compared to isolates with a lesser degree of divergence. This is like brothers and sisters, born of the same mother and father, being more similar to each other than distant cousins who only share, say, great-grandparents. In practice, phylogenetic trees tell us that certain viruses are closely related and have a relatively recent common ancestor (these are said to 'cluster'), like brothers or first cousins, while for other viruses the relationship is similar to that of tenth cousins, whose common ancestors lived many generations ago.

The first report of the isolation of a simian immunodeficiency virus (SIV) from a chimpanzee born in the wild came in 1989. This isolate, given the name $SIV_{cpz-gab1}$, was obtained from a chimpanzee kept at the primate centre of Franceville, Gabon, where fifty chimps had been tested with assays used for the detection of anti-HIV antibodies in humans. Only two carried such antibodies; from one of them, the virus could be grown in cell culture, and its proteins were analysed. This chimpanzee, captured at six months of age, was four years old when the blood sample was obtained and seemed healthy despite presenting enlarged lymph nodes. Based on the crude methods available at the time, this SIV isolate was described as related although not identical to HIV-1. Phylogenetic analyses suggested that $SIV_{cpz-gab1}$ was closer to HIV-1 than to HIV-2 and to SIVs from African green monkeys, mandrills and other monkeys.[16–17]

It was not possible to isolate the virus from the second seropositive chimp, a two-year-old animal shot by hunters and that died of its wounds shortly after being brought to Franceville for care. A few years later, thanks to technological advances, nucleic acid amplification was used on this chimp's lymphocytes (which had been kept frozen), in order to sequence parts of the viral genome. This isolate became known as $SIV_{cpz-gab2}$. It was phylogenetically close to $SIV_{cpz-gab1}$. In 1992, a third isolate ($SIV_{cpz-ant}$) was obtained from Noah, a five-year-old chimpanzee captured in the wild and impounded by customs officers in Brussels upon illegal arrival from Zaire. His isolate was somewhat divergent from HIV-1 and from the two previous SIV_{cpz} isolates.[18–20]

In 1999, a fourth isolate, SIV_{cpz-US}, was obtained from Marilyn, caught in the wild in an unknown African country and imported into the US as an infant in 1963. Marilyn was used as a breeding female in a primate facility until she died in 1985 at the age of twenty-six, after delivering still-born twins. During a survey of captive chimpanzees, Marilyn was the only one that was seropositive for HIV-1 antibodies. She had not been used in AIDS research, but had received human blood products between 1966 and 1969. During this early period, it is very unlikely that the blood products contained HIV-1, so there was a good chance that Marilyn had acquired her SIV_{cpz} infection in Africa. SIV sequences were amplified from the spleen and lymph node tissues procured at autopsy. Using mitochondrial DNA analyses, researchers identified the subspecies of chimpanzees from which this recent and the previous three isolates had been obtained.[21–22]

As could have been expected from the geographic distribution of *Pan troglodytes* subspecies, Noah (from Zaire) was a *P.t. schweinfurthii* while the other three, including Marilyn, were *P.t. troglodytes*. As illustrated in Figure 1, phylogenetic analyses revealed that the three SIV isolates obtained from *P.t. troglodytes* were similar to each other, and similar to HIV-1 strains from humans, while Noah's $SIV_{cpz-ant}$ diverged from these and lay outside this cluster, as did HIV-2 and SIVs obtained from other non-human primates.

Thus, naturally occurring SIV_{cpz} strains fell into two related but highly divergent, chimpanzee subspecies-specific, lineages: one for *P.t. troglodytes* and another for *P.t. schweinfurthii*. It was bravely concluded that *P.t. troglodytes* was the primary source of HIV-1 group M and its natural reservoir, and that there had been host-dependent evolution of SIV_{cpz} in chimpanzees resulting in *P.t. troglodytes* and *P.t. schweinfurthii* being infected with different lineages of SIV. Scientists could not rule out the possibility that other chimpanzee subspecies, especially *P.t. schweinfurthii*, could have transmitted their viruses to humans. This prudence was justified because a single isolate of SIV_{cpz} from *P.t. schweinfurthii* was

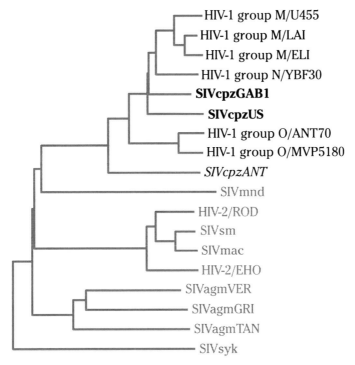

Figure 1 Phylogenetic analysis showing the relationship between SIV$_{cpz-US}$ and SIV$_{cpz-gab1}$ obtained from *P.t. troglodytes* chimpanzees (bold) and isolates from humans infected with HIV-1 (group M, group N, group O). The SIV$_{cpz}$ isolates obtained from *P.t. troglodytes* cluster within the HIV-1 isolates, while SIV$_{cpz-ant}$ obtained from a *P.t. schweinfurthii* chimpanzee (italics) lies outside. Other SIV isolates obtained from monkeys and human isolates of HIV-2 lie further away.

Adapted from Gao.[21]

available. It was possible that in the future other isolates of SIV$_{cpz}$, more similar to the human isolates of HIV-1, might be found in *P.t. schwein-furthii*. Additional isolates of SIV$_{cpz}$ were later obtained from captive *P.t. troglodytes* in Cameroon, some of which were similar to those human HIV-1 isolates from the same country, reinforcing the view that HIV-1 originated in chimpanzees.[21,23]

Since this initial work was conducted mostly with chimpanzees which had been in captivity for some time, it was questionable whether the apes had acquired their SIV$_{cpz}$ naturally in the wild or artificially in their cages where they had been in contact with other primates. In the first case, the puzzle was close to being solved while, in the second, researchers had ventured down the wrong track. Non-invasive technologies were then developed to measure the presence of SIV antibodies and nucleic acids among chimpanzees living in the wild using urine and faecal samples, since obtaining blood samples was neither feasible nor ethically acceptable (some animals may have been hurt or killed in the process). We can but admire the motivation and expertise of these researchers and especially their trackers, roaming through the forest looking for chimpanzee urine or stools, which they had to distinguish from those of other animals. Urine samples proved inferior to faeces and were abandoned.

Among 100 wild *P.t. schweinfurthii* from Uganda and Tanzania, only one was infected with $SIV_{cpz-tan1}$. This isolate was similar to the previous $SIV_{cpz-ant}$ isolate from Noah, the Zairean *P.t. schweinfurthii*. More isolates were later found among *P.t. schweinfurthii* chimps in Gombe, where SIV_{cpz} prevalence was estimated to be around 20%. Phylogenetic analyses showed that these isolates clustered with $SIV_{cpz-ant}$ and diverged from the *P.t. troglodytes* isolates and from HIV-1 (Figure 2), confirming that *P.t. schweinfurthii* was not the source of HIV-1. Testing of additional *P.t. schweinfurthii* chimps from the Budongo forest of Uganda, the Mahale park in Tanzania and the Nyungwe reserve in Rwanda (Map 3) failed to identify a single animal infected with SIV_{cpz}. This heterogeneous distribution of SIV_{cpz}, which has recently been mirrored in a study of *P.t. schweinfurthii* in the DRC, probably reflects the community structures of chimpanzee populations and their behaviour: they have few contacts with chimpanzees belonging to other communities, except during territorial fights or when adolescent females migrate to other troops. But once SIV_{cpz} is successfully introduced into a community, there seems to be substantial transmission between its members, sexually or otherwise.[24–28]

SIV is non-existent among captive *P.t. verus* (the western chimpanzee), about 1,500 of which were tested and found to be uninfected. Surveys of wild *P.t. verus* and *P.t. ellioti* also failed to find a single case of SIV_{cpz} infection. Why is SIV_{cpz} absent within these two subspecies? Presumably, because SIVs were introduced into *P.t. troglodytes* and *P.t. schweinfurthii* only after these subspecies had diverged from *P.t. verus* and *P.t. ellioti* half a million years ago. Such a scenario would imply that there has been little contact between the subspecies ever since, which is possible since the large rivers of Africa constitute watertight barriers.[29]

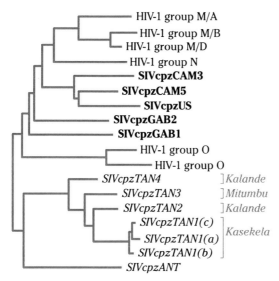

Figure 2 Phylogenetic analysis showing the relatively distant relationship between SIV$_{cpz}$ isolates obtained in Tanzania from *P.t. schweinfurthii* chimpanzees (italics) and SIV$_{cpz\text{-}ant}$ obtained from a *P.t. schweinfurthii* chimp from the DRC (italics), clearly separated from the HIV-1 group M isolates. The latter are close to SIV$_{cpz}$ isolates obtained from *P.t. troglodytes* (bold). HIV-1 group O lies outside the other HIV-1 isolates (in contrast to HIV-1 group N, which lies inside).

Adapted from Santiago.[26]

Prevalence of SIV$_{cpz}$ among wild populations of *P.t. troglodytes* was then measured in an extraordinary study performed in ten forest sites throughout southern Cameroon. To make sure that the faeces originated from *P.t. troglodytes* and to avoid counting stools from any individual chimp more than once, the researchers amplified a number of host DNA sequences for species, gender and individual identification. In other words, they used the chimpanzee cells present in stools to fingerprint molecularly each and every individual ape who had defecated. After excluding degraded specimens, those that contained gorilla (the trackers' noses may not always be perfect!) or *P.t. ellioti* DNA, specimens were available from 106 individual *P.t. troglodytes* chimpanzees. Sixteen were infected with SIV$_{cpz}$. Again, there was a lot of variation in SIV$_{cpz}$ prevalence between the study sites: in four of them not a single infection was found; in three sites prevalence was over 20% and the highest was 35%.[25]

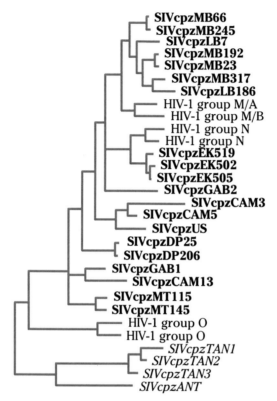

Figure 3 Phylogenetic analysis showing the relationship between SIV$_{cpz}$ from *P.t. troglodytes* chimpanzees in Cameroon or Gabon (bold) and isolates from humans infected with HIV-1 group M, HIV-1 group N and HIV-1 group O. SIV$_{cpz}$ isolates obtained from *P.t. troglodytes* cluster with the HIV-1 group M and N isolates, while HIV-1 group O remains an outlier. SIV$_{cpz}$ obtained from *P.t. schweinfurthii* chimpanzees in Tanzania or DRC (italics) lie further away.

Adapted from Keele.[25]

Phylogenetic analyses (Figure 3) showed that all sixteen new SIV$_{cpz}$ isolates were closely related to SIV$_{cpz}$ isolates from captive *P.t. troglodytes* chimps and to HIV-1 groups M and N, but not to HIV-1 group O (always the outlier) or SIV$_{cpz}$ obtained from *P.t. schweinfurthii*. This phylogenetic proximity confirmed – now irrefutably – that the SIV$_{cpz}$ of *P.t. troglodytes* of central Africa was indeed the source of HIV-1 group M. Game over for this part of the story.

Chimpanzee populations separated by long distances or natural barriers like rivers harboured distinct lineages while adjacent troops harboured viruses closely related to each other. More detailed analyses of the genome showed strong clustering of human HIV-1 groups M and N viruses with the SIV_{cpz} lineages obtained from some specific *P.t. troglodytes* troops in southern Cameroon. In other words, in these rural communities, the local strains of HIV-1 infecting humans genetically resembled the local strains of SIV_{cpz} from the chimpanzees living close by. The SIV_{cpz} isolates from south-east Cameroon, towards the border with Congo-Brazzaville and the Central African Republic, were most closely related to HIV-1 group M, while those from south-central Cameroon were closer to HIV-1 group N.[30]

Additional faecal samples from *P.t. troglodytes* were collected over the following years, mostly in Cameroon, where the prevalence of SIV_{cpz} infection is now estimated to be 5.9%, a figure that I will use for calculations in forthcoming chapters. In the Central African Republic, no SIV_{cpz} infection was found but fewer than fifty specimens have been tested.[31]

SIV infection was found among faeces from western gorillas (*Gorilla gorilla gorilla*); a virus which was called SIV_{gor}. SIV_{gor} is very similar to HIV-1 group O, rather than to group M. Thus gorillas are not the source of the HIV-1 group M pandemic. Without getting into the details, chimpanzees may be the source of HIV-1 group O as well, which they transmitted to humans and to gorillas independently, or to gorillas first, which then infected some humans.[31–33]

Until proven otherwise, it is most likely that the modes of transmission of SIV_{cpz} between chimpanzees are the same as in humans: sexual intercourse, from mother to child and possibly through blood–blood contacts. There is much sexual promiscuity in chimpanzees. For instance, one adult male in Gombe is known to have mated since puberty at least 333 times with 25 different females, and of course only a very small proportion of all matings can be observed. A female called Flo was once observed to copulate fifty times within a twenty-four-hour period. The substantial genital swelling of females during oestrus may facilitate transmission of viruses by making the mucosa more fragile. Most of this sexual activity takes place within the closely knit community. A study of paternity among chimpanzee communities showed that only 7% of offspring had a father from outside the troop. Transmission between troops could occur via out-migration of adolescent females, or during fights between males when blood-borne viruses could be exchanged.[3,11,12]

The fourth ape

A weakness in the investigations of SIV among chimpanzees is the dearth of virological information about the fourth ape, the *Pan paniscus* bonobo. Previously called the pygmy chimpanzee, this was a misnomer since the difference in size compared to *Pan troglodytes* is minor. It inhabits parts of the DRC south of the Congo but north of the Kasaï–Sankuru river system, in the Congo central basin which has low human populations but is linked by rivers to Léopoldville–Kinshasa, the main market for its farming and fishing products.

Bonobos are less aggressive and more mutually tolerant than *P.t. troglodytes*, and males and females have similar social ranks (some primatologists even describe an unusual situation of female dominance). Bonobos are not territorial so that males do not stalk or attack males from other troops and interactions with other communities are generally peaceful. They have a particularly intense, peculiar – and dare I say – quasi-human sexual activity: they do it for fun rather than just for reproductive purposes, and they have sex mostly in what biologists call a 'ventral–ventral mount' (the 'missionary position'). Among other practices that have been described by highly dedicated primatologists, they practise mutual genital–genital rubbing, genital massages, mouth kisses and even oral sex. Another unique feature of bonobos is their bisexuality, seen in both males and females.[34–36]

About half of intercourses are preceded by some form of courtship, but once they copulate fifteen seconds suffice. Intercourse is used to solve conflicts and maintain social interactions, and female bonobos are known to accept sex in exchange for food, a process quite similar to some human behaviour that we shall describe later. The period of sexual receptivity of female bonobos is twice as long as for *Pan troglodytes* and bonobos are more likely to have promiscuous matings outside their own group. In principle, these factors could facilitate the sexual transmission of viruses.

Until recently only thirty-two bonobos, all but four living in zoos or primate centres in Europe and the US, had been tested for SIV_{cpz} infection and none was infected. The main problem in studying bonobos in the wild is that they are close to extinction, with between 10,000 and 20,000 individuals scattered around a large area of the DRC. Their distribution is discontinuous and bonobos are well aware that their main predator is humans. Just last year, samples from around sixty wild-living bonobos, obtained from two sites in the DRC, have finally been tested and were all negative for SIV. Given the heterogeneity in the distribution of SIV among *Pan troglodytes*, one would like a larger number of *Pan paniscus* troops to be tested, but in the meantime it is fair to say that there is no evidence that this primate played a role in the emergence of HIV-1.[28,37–38]

Origins of SIV in chimpanzees

What was the source of SIV_{cpz} infection in chimpanzees lies outside the scope of this book, which is to understand the early twentieth-century events that led to the current HIV-1 pandemic. To finish the story quickly, I will just add that, as reviewed elsewhere, SIV_{cpz} probably originated from the recombination of distinct SIVs infecting smaller monkeys, principally the SIV_{rcm} of red-capped mangabeys and a SIV which seems to infect greater spot-nosed monkeys, moustached guenons and mona monkeys. The most likely opportunity for such a recombination occurred when chimpanzees hunted and ate smaller monkeys. Perhaps the two SIVs that gave rise to SIV_{cpz} were transmitted independently to different chimpanzees and spread for some time before an ape became infected with both, allowing recombination to occur. Alternatively, one of the SIVs could have established itself within the chimpanzee population, the recombination occurring when one of the chimps infected with the original SIV acquired a second SIV from a small monkey, again via predation.[25–27,39]

3 | *The timing*

Having identified the source of HIV-1, the next question is: *when* did the virus manage to cross species from chimps to humans? It has often been said that AIDS was a new disease on the African continent. Apart from the published cases mentioned in Chapter 1, clinicians working in central Africa, for instance Dr Bila Kapita, chief of internal medicine at Hôpital Mama Yemo in Kinshasa, reported that, at least since the mid-1970s, they started seeing cases that in retrospect were very likely to have been AIDS. This would be consistent with some degree of dissemination of the virus during the mid-1960s, given the average ten-year interval between infection and symptomatic disease. But could the disease have been present even earlier?[1,2]

Bush medicine

In most district or regional hospitals of countries inhabited by *P.t. troglodytes*, the diagnostic facilities during the colonial era (and even now) were so minimal that it would have been difficult, even for astute and experienced clinicians, to recognise the emergence of a new disease characterised by intermittent fevers and profound wasting. Most such institutions did not have any kind of half-decent microbiology laboratory. No cultures were done, either for common bacterial pathogens or the agent of tuberculosis, and diagnoses were based on stains made directly on the specimens, or solely on the combination of symptoms and signs found during the clinical examination. Fifty years later, I found the same situation at the Nioki hospital in Zaire: nothing had changed. This approach was relatively effective for diagnosing parasitic diseases (malaria, sleeping sickness, filariasis, intestinal parasites) but very insensitive for most bacterial diseases. Little radiological investigation was available either; only in the best hospitals was it possible to get something as elementary as a chest x-ray. The first x-ray machine in Brazzaville was installed in 1931, two years before one became available in Léopoldville.

Thus a patient with fever, chronic diarrhoea and wasting might initially have been administered an antibiotic active against, say, typhoid fever. An old antibiotic, chloramphenicol, used to be popular for this indication. If this did not work, then extra-pulmonary tuberculosis would be suspected and the patient started on antituberculosis drugs (only after 1950 because, prior to that, there was no drug treatment for tuberculosis). Several weeks would be required to determine whether the patient improved on this second empirical medication. Some responded, and probably indeed suffered from occult tuberculosis. Others did not and would slowly die, often at home after it had become clear that the hospital could not provide a solution, and the families did not want to waste all their meagre resources on unsuccessful therapeutic trials. The doctors would presume that these patients died from some form of cancer, the diagnosis of which was well beyond the scope of bush hospitals. A final diagnosis would never be made, as doctors had too many other things to worry about to try to determine the actual cause of a particular death by performing an autopsy. The capacity to recognise an emerging disease was minimal, for the simple reason that there was a long list of serious diseases, already recognised in every medical textbook of the time, that these hospitals could not diagnose.

In the capitals, diagnostic facilities were better but still far from the European standards of the time, even in the clinics whose main (or only) role was to provide care for Europeans. These hospitals had a few specialists, mostly surgeons who could carry out biopsies if some form of cancer was suspected. The histopathological slides would be sent to a collaborating hospital in Europe, and the results would come back months later. One such surgeon who worked in Brazzaville thought he had perhaps recognised a new disease, as we will see now.

A colonial tragedy

Léon Pales was not an ordinary colonial doctor. He graduated from Bordeaux in 1929, aged twenty-four. During his medical studies, to earn some money Pales worked as an anatomical assistant at the medical school, helping with autopsies and the dissection of cadavers for medical students learning anatomy, an experience that would later prove very useful. While the usual MD thesis at the time consisted of a 60–80 pages literature review of some narrow medical topic, his was

429 pages long and addressed a very unusual field, palaeopathology: the study of diseases of prehistoric humans through examination of their bones. It would remain the standard French-language textbook for three decades. One of its main themes was that the study of ancient diseases could provide knowledge useful in understanding modern health problems. After the tropical medicine course in Marseilles, Pales was posted to Moyen-Congo (1931–3) and Tchad (1934–7). Back in France, he worked in Marseilles, taught anatomy and ethno-anthropology at the École du Pharo, and directed a field surgical unit during the invasion of France in 1940. Made a prisoner, he was repatriated to France the following year. He became assistant director of the Musée de l'Homme in Paris but does not seem to have been involved in the resistance movement organised around this institution. After WWII, the rest of his career (in France, and a few years in West Africa) would be devoted to palaeopathology, his first love, to anthropology and nutrition.[3,4]

During his two-year term in Brazzaville, Pales' career intersected with a colonial tragedy for the sake of 'economic development': the building of a railway between Brazzaville and Pointe-Noire, the Chemin de Fer Congo–Océan (CFCO), whose main purpose was to avoid depending on the Belgian railway. In a region with little infrastructure, a second railway was built only 100 kilometres from the Matadi–Léopoldville line, at the same time as the latter was expanded (Map 4). Started in 1921, the 511-kilometre railway would not be completed until 1934. Ninety-two bridges or viaducts had to be erected, as well as twelve tunnels, with the longest stretching over 1.5 km. During construction, the regions immediately west of Brazzaville and east of Pointe-Noire presented no major logistical problem; food could easily be delivered and the sick evacuated. In the middle, however, the 100-kilometre stretch in the Mayombe, a dense and hilly equatorial rain forest, became a nightmare. The Mayombe was thinly populated and the workforce had to be imported, creating a huge melting pot of all AEF ethnic groups, forced to live in squalid conditions highly propitious for the spread of microbial agents, perhaps including HIV-1.[5]

Initially in Moyen-Congo, and later in Oubangui-Chari and Tchad, 127,250 adult men were conscripted to work on the CFCO. Paid 1.5 francs per day, less than 1% of what their French foreman received, they worked ten hours a day, six days a week. Daily rations of food were inadequate, and the workers often received less than they were

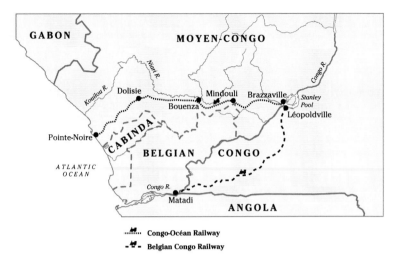

Map 4 Itinerary of the Brazzaville–Pointe-Noire and Léopoldville–Matadi railways.

supposed to. They were housed in mud-brick buildings, where 50–60 men slept in the same room. As rumours spread concerning the fate of CFCO workers, it became increasingly difficult for the local chiefs to recruit their target numbers, for many fled to safer areas. The colonial authorities lowered the age limit, increased the duration of forced labour and coerced some unfortunate men in returning up to five times. Some workers absconded, usually in groups, but escape was harder to envision for men from Oubangui-Chari and Tchad. How could they possibly get back to their villages, a thousand kilometres away, without a penny in their pockets or any understanding of the local languages?[6,7]

Slave owners had an obvious interest in keeping their slaves alive: it was expensive to replace those who died. The situation was different with the CFCO. By contract, the AEF government had to supply the Société de Construction des Batignolles with 8,000 workers year round. Their recruitment, transportation, lodging and feeding was the responsibility of the state. As soon as a worker died, the state had to provide another and pay a penalty to the company if the minimum number of workers was not available. This was an early example of a public–private partnership in which the private company got excellent terms.

Grossly underpaid, underfed, overworked and housed in appalling conditions, between 15,000 and 23,000 workers died in the process, ten times the death toll of the Léopoldville–Matadi railway thirty years earlier. The most murderous section, and the most difficult from the engineers' point of view, was the Mayombe. On top of the work accidents, epidemics broke out in the workers' camps. Mortality among the Mayombe workers was a staggering 496 per 1,000 men-years in 1926 (in other words, half would be dead within a year), 454 in 1927 and 384 in 1928. It declined to 173 per 1,000 men-years in 1929, when sanitary conditions improved after this scandal was revealed in France by writer André Gide and journalist Albert Londres. In absolute terms, the peak mortality occurred in 1927, when 2,892 workers died: eight per day. Mortality was highest among those recruited in Tchad.[6–9]

Inspection missions were sent by the French government to investigate whether the newspaper reports were true, and to come up with solutions. Two military doctors, General Lasnet and Lieutenant-Colonel Ferris, led these inspections. Ferris described the pathetic conditions of the primitive hospitals set up near the building sites, where huts erected for twelve patients could house thirty, causing transmission of pathogens between patients. Someone admitted for pneumonia ended up with dysentery a few days later, or vice versa. The main causes of mortality were: dysentery (bloody diarrhoea), caused by *Shigella dysenteriae*, endemic in the Mayombe; pneumonia, caused by a bacterium known as the pneumococcus; beriberi, a vitamin B1 deficiency which causes heart failure; other ill-defined febrile illnesses; and what the doctors called 'physiological misery', with some features (apathy, nostalgia) suggestive of major depression.[6,10]

The scandal in France and the inspection visits forced the AEF government to improve the workers' sanitary conditions. Governor Raphael Antonetti knew that he was in trouble and spent months writing detailed replies to the inspectors' reports. Instructions about how to take proper care of the workers were issued. Wages were increased, and some women were allowed into the workers' camps. Naturally, prostitution quickly developed, and STDs, hitherto inexistent, appeared among the workers. Prostitutes were noted to collect 'their fees on paydays amidst long palavers'.[9]

Instructive autopsies

When Léon Pales arrived in Brazzaville in 1931 as the colony's surgeon and obstetrician, the CFCO workers' health situation had already improved. Surgical facilities in Brazzaville were limited, so Pales had a lot of free time to do what he had learned in Bordeaux and which nobody in AEF had done before: autopsies. He had access to the Institut Pasteur laboratory, where bacteriological cultures were available (for instance, to look for pathogens causing diarrhoea, such as *Shigella* and *Salmonella*) and where guinea pigs could be inoculated to look for the aetiological agent of tuberculosis. The Pasteur laboratory was even able to characterise pneumococci (the main agent of pneumonia) into serotypes.

Pales eventually published a few scientific papers on this necropsic work. First, he reported the findings from eighty-five patients who had died from pneumococcal infections, sixty-four of whom were CFCO workers. The pneumococcus was grown from the blood cultures, the cerebrospinal fluid, pleural fluid, pericardial fluid or other specimens obtained either pre-mortem or during autopsy. Pales described the autopsy findings, from the adrenals to the brain, which often revealed disseminated pneumococcal infections. This did not imply that the patients were immunologically impaired, but reflected the absence of an effective treatment which allowed this virulent pathogen to spread throughout the body. It certainly demonstrated Pales' unique competence and motivation in performing detailed autopsies and his access to the only laboratory in AEF where bacteriological cultures could be performed.[11-12]

He subsequently published a paper on tuberculosis in AEF, and more detailed information is available from a thesis written by medical student Jean Auclert in Marseilles using material provided by Pales. Pales described a new condition that he called Cachexie du Mayombe. Cachexia means profound weight loss. Adult male patients with Cachexie du Mayombe weighed as little as 30–5 kg, and were described as 'an assembly of bones held together by skin ... whose only sign of life lay in their gaze'. They had a normal appetite and experienced no vomiting but suffered from chronic non-bloody diarrhoea. However, repeated examination of their stools failed to reveal a parasitic agent, and stool cultures performed at the Institut Pasteur were negative for the enteric pathogens known at the time, especially the *Shigella dysenteriae* which had killed many of the CFCO workers.[13-14]

Pales autopsied fifty such patients who, by his definition of the syndrome, had worked on the Mayombe part of the railway and sought care in Brazzaville after being declared unfit for service due to poor health. In thirteen autopsies, he found confirmation of a tuberculosis that had been diagnosed pre-mortem, in seven others he found occult tuberculosis undiagnosed pre-mortem (tuberculosis of the intestine or the intra-abdominal lymph nodes), in four he found other diseases which killed the patient, but in twenty-six autopsies he did not find any macroscopically obvious medical condition explaining the profound wasting. He did note, however, that many of these patients had cerebral atrophy, very unusual for young adults, and that they also had generalised lymphadenopathy, including large mesenteric (around the small bowel) lymph nodes, which failed to reveal the tuberculosis bacillus via staining and/or guinea pig inoculation. We do not know the actual incidence of the Cachexie du Mayombe, but Pales presumably autopsied only a small fraction of cases, as many must have died elsewhere than at the Brazzaville hospital.

This new syndrome was certainly suggestive of AIDS. We can be pretty sure that these twenty-six patients did not have disseminated tuberculosis or cancer, which should have been easy to recognise during the autopsy. Severe malnutrition was also unlikely, because the patients' condition should have improved when properly fed in Brazzaville. The concentration of cases among patients who had worked in a well-defined area suggests a transmissible agent. Brain atrophy is common in patients with AIDS, and leads to a complication called AIDS dementia. Generalised lymphadenopathy is a hallmark of HIV infection, caused either by the virus itself or a variety of opportunistic infections which supervene. Such findings, as well as their chronic diarrhoea, would not have been noted had the patients died of major depression or some other severe psychological disturbance related to the hardship they had to endure.

One could speculate that the extremely high male/female ratio in the Mayombe work camps (ten men for each woman) and the intense prostitution that ensued would have facilitated the transmission of HIV-1, possibly from a single worker who had been infected with SIV_{cpz}. The time between the workers being sent to the CFCO camps and the development of their disease was not indicated in Auclert's thesis, but was probably less than the ten years we usually see today between getting HIV-1 and the first symptoms of AIDS. This does not exclude anything: for complex virological reasons, it is possible that this incubation period was actually shorter soon after the virus was introduced into human populations. And even nowadays, some unfortunate patients develop AIDS within two years after their infection.[9]

Unless the original tissue blocks or some of the slides prepared from the biopsies performed during these autopsies could be miraculously located, this will remain a hypothesis. I contacted the Pales family, the Institut Pasteur, the Musée de l'Homme and Le Pharo, and no such material seems to have survived over the past seven decades. Unfortunately, there is no longer an Institut Pasteur in Brazzaville, and whatever archives may have existed seem to have been destroyed during the long periods of civil strife this country went through. So we will never know for sure. But the point that can be made from this story is that the supposed absence of a clinical condition recognised by early twentieth-century doctors cannot be used as a strong argument for dating the emergence of HIV.

Molecular clocks

We have just seen the limitations of what can be extrapolated from reports or publications by colonial-era clinicians. Fortunately, molecular biology offers some help with dating. For readers who are unfamiliar with molecular biology, this is the last section where we will need to talk about these particular concepts.

First we will review what scientists call 'molecular clocks'. Their principle is simple, and is based on an assumption that the rate of genetic change is fairly constant over time. From a known mean rate of substitutions (which correspond to replication errors: mutations, deletions, etc.) within each gene, it is possible to estimate the chronology of the evolution of the organism. In its simplest form, if we assume a rate of evolution of, say, 0.002 substitutions per nucleotide per year at some given part of a gene and find, say, a 10% (0.1) difference in sequences between two isolates, we can back-calculate that they shared a common ancestor fifty years earlier, after which they diverged, each undergoing its own series of genetic changes. Of course, if the isolates were not obtained at roughly the same time, this will be taken into account.[15]

Viral recombination between two different subtypes of HIV-1 is the most difficult obstacle for molecular clocks. For instance, CRF02_AG isolates have part of their genome that originated from a subtype A, and part from a subtype G. It is not always clear which is which in the specific parts of the genome whose substitutions will be used to calculate molecular clocks. It is then impossible to evaluate how long the process of evolution has been going on, because the starting point is unclear. The counter-strategy is simple: all inter-subtype recombinant viruses must be excluded. This works well as long as the recombinants are identified, which is not always easy. Other challenges associated with molecular clocks are reviewed elsewhere.[15]

In a landmark paper that tried to address these limitations through complex analytical strategies, scientists at the Los Alamos National Laboratory estimated that the most likely date for the common ancestor of all HIV group M isolates (that is, all subtypes and recombinants within group M) was 1931. This common ancestor corresponds to the root in phylogenetic trees, the point after which all divergence occurred. As in opinion polls, they calculated a 'confidence interval', which in this case was pretty wide, from 1915 to 1941. In other words, there were nineteen chances out of twenty that the true date of the common ancestor was somewhere within this range.[16]

To verify the validity of this dating, they back-calculated the date of the oldest HIV-1 sequences (ZR59) obtained in Léopoldville in 1959, as well as the date of isolates from Thailand, a country where HIV-1 was introduced in 1986–7 according to extensive epidemiological studies. They dated the Léopoldville sequence between 1957 and 1960, while for Thailand the common ancestor was calculated as having existed in 1986. So in both cases their dating was similar to what could be inferred from historical information, which suggested that their 1931 dating for the common ancestor of HIV-1 group M was relatively accurate.

However, the researchers could not directly address the question of when the cross-species transmission, from chimpanzee to man, had occurred. If the 1931 common ancestor was a human virus, the cross-species event would have occurred in the preceding decade (otherwise the patient would not have survived until 1931). But could the 1931 common ancestor still have been a simian virus at the time? This latter scenario was thought to be highly unlikely since it would have required multiple and close to simultaneous cross-species transmissions, all after 1931, that were all epidemiologically successful. On the contrary, analyses suggested that each group of HIV-1 (M, N, O and now P) represented a distinct cross-species transmission event, and that for pandemic HIV-1 group M the most likely number of such events was one. In other words, the 1931 ancestor indeed lay within a human host – and from this single individual, the true 'patient zero', more than sixty million people across the world were subsequently infected![17–20]

Then, from a database of HIV-1 isolates from the DRC, and using a sophisticated mathematical approach, the population dynamics of HIV-1 in that country were reconstructed by estimating, year after year, the number of infected individuals. This showed a very slow growth between 1930 and 1940, with an exponential growth later on. Prior to 1930, the number of HIV-1-infected individuals in the Belgian Congo was estimated at somewhere between 0 and 100.[17]

For a long time, ZR59 was the only ancient specimen of HIV-1. The recent discovery of DRC60, obtained from a lymph node biopsy performed in Léopoldville in 1960, provided additional information. ZR59 and DRC60 diverged by 12%, and were clearly phylogenetically distinct: ZR59 is an ancestor of subtype D while DRC60 is related to subtype A. This implies that HIV-1 group M began to diversify into human populations and entered Léopoldville a few decades before 1960. The inclusion of DRC60 changed the measure of the most recent common ancestor of HIV-1 group M, which was now dated at 1921 (confidence interval: between 1908 and 1933). Other models yielded slightly different dates. Reconstruction of the HIV-1 dynamics in the Belgian Congo was again compatible with a total of fewer than 100 HIV-1-infected individuals for a long time, then a very slow increase in the number of infected individuals until the mid-1950s, when exponential growth supervened.[21]

This gives us an appreciation of the lack of certainty in such measures. The addition of a single isolate, DRC60, changed the estimates by ten years, and the confidence interval remained wide. In practice, the common ancestor of all the subtypes of HIV-1 group M probably existed sometime in the first three decades of the twentieth century. To keep things simple, I will use '1921' from now on, but this should be viewed as indicating a period rather than a specific year.

For how long has SIV$_{cpz}$ been present in chimpanzee populations? The same methods were used, based on sequences in the Los Alamos database. The results varied according to which gene was used for the molecular clocks and lacked precision. By and large, they suggested that the emergence of SIV$_{cpz}$ in chimpanzees preceded its cross-species transmission to humans by something in the order of a few hundred years, not thousands or tens of thousands. This is probably why SIV$_{cpz}$ is not found in *P.t. verus* and *P.t. ellioti* populations: the virus appeared long after these subspecies diverged from *P.t. troglodytes*.[22]

To summarise, there is compelling evidence that the common ancestor of HIV-1 existed in a human being sometime in the first three decades of the twentieth century, and that the whole group M pandemic was started by a single cross-species transmission. Now we will try to understand how the virus crossed species, what happened after 1921, and how HIV-1 eventually expanded into a global pandemic.

4 | *The cut hunter*

The next question to be addressed is: how did the virus cross species to infect humans? How did the simian immunodeficiency virus of *P.t. troglodytes* chimps become the human immunodeficiency virus type 1? Again, science started out with an intuition: this must have occurred through the handling of chimpanzee meat by hunters, or their wives who would cut up the animals before cooking them. We will now examine whether this theory remains plausible after reviewing the various pieces of evidence accumulated over the past decade.

Hunters and their prey

Hunters and/or cooks can acquire infectious agents from their prey, including primates. For instance, Herpes B virus is a rare but highly lethal infection of individuals who handle monkeys, and especially laboratory technicians working with rhesus and cynomolgus macaques. Monkeypox is a smallpox-like but benign viral infection associated with exposure to monkeys. Highly lethal Ebola and Marburg haemorrhagic fevers have been reported in veterinarians and villagers who handled the carcasses of apes that had died in the wild from these infections. Recently, a retrovirus called simian foamy virus (SFV) has been associated with human exposure to monkeys and apes, and its sequencing allows the identification of the exact simian source. American veterinarians and animal caretakers working in primate centres or zoos were found to be infected with SFV acquired from chimpanzees. Fortunately, this virus does not seem to be pathogenic for humans, and no person-to-person transmission has ever been documented.[1–3]

Because of their intelligence, agility and aggressiveness, chimpanzees have no predators in the forest apart from leopards and, of course, humans. However, they are by no means easy prey for hunters, and rarely a specific target unless the apes had the bad idea of destroying the crops in plantations near the villages. Although they might occasionally fall into wire snares, lianas knots, nets or pits of all kinds set up for other game animals, chimpanzees can escape from many such traps. Pygmies hunted year round with bows, crossbows and assegais. Targeting chimps would have been a dangerous undertaking, but the fact that pygmies could hunt elephants without firearms (albeit at considerable risk) was testament to their skills. For reasons still unclear, HIV-1 has remained remarkably rare among pygmies, and when present seems to have been acquired through their contacts with Bantus rather than from apes. Bantus hunted mostly during the dry season when the forest was easier to penetrate and when they had less farm work to do and needed additional sources of food until the next crop. If the hunt was successful, carcasses of great apes were generally first cut up in the forest to make them easier to carry, and then cut into smaller pieces in the village before being sold and eaten.[4–8]

It is difficult to hunt chimpanzees without firearms, and the firearms with small pellets generally available in the bush are not powerful enough to kill an ape. French colonisers had to deal with a number of armed rebellions from populations who opposed their rule, especially in the south-west of Oubangui-Chari and adjacent areas of the Moyen-Congo. Therefore, regulations made it difficult for the natives legally to procure powerful weapons. In France's annual reports to the League of Nations concerning Cameroun Français, the exact number of firearms and bullets imported into the country was spelled out (for instance, in 1922, 789 shotguns, 41 revolvers and 6,740 kg of ammunition). Africans could, however, own locally made piston firearms for small game hunting.[6,9,10]

In the Belgian Congo, regulations were looser. In 1927 an astounding 122,804 firearms permits were issued. This number gradually increased to 245,644 (a quarter of a million!) by 1945. The situation was made worse by a regulation forcing employers to provide their workers with meat at least once a week: hunting was much cheaper than farming. By 1925, Professor Leplae of Université Catholique de Louvain, an expert who also worked for the Ministry of Colonies, was complaining that many species of game animals were being butchered at such a rate that extinction would soon ensue. He estimated that 25,000 elephants were killed each year in the Belgian Congo, often with automatic rifles. Thirty years later, game animals of all kinds were indeed nearly extinct, and this was attributed to a combination of factors: the regulations concerning meat for workers, the development of large cities which created lucrative markets for hunting products, the widespread availability of firearms and all kinds of materials that could be used for trapping, the bad example set by some European hunters and the disappearance of customary hunting regulations through which an equilibrium was maintained between human populations and game animals in the pre-colonial era.[11–13]

In edicts in April 1901 and December 1912, the Belgian Congo's governor prohibited the hunting of a number of animals, including chimpanzees, by both natives and Europeans. The ban was upheld in subsequent amendments of the law in 1934 and 1937, which divided game animals into four categories: gorillas belonged to category I and could not legally be hunted apart from what was required by scientific institutions, while chimpanzees, listed in category II, could be hunted by those who could afford to buy the appropriate, more expensive, permit. A tax also had to be paid for each animal killed: 1,500 francs ($30) for a *P.t. schweinfurthii*, and 3,000 francs for a *Pan paniscus*. That was far more expensive than the 50 francs charged for a monkey but a lot less than the 25,000 francs to be paid for a white rhinoceros. In practice, only expatriates could afford to pay such a high tax for killing a chimp. However, the extent to which the regulation could be enforced in such a huge territory was an entirely different matter.[14]

In French colonies of Africa, decrees issued in April 1930 and November 1947 prohibited the hunting of some species including chimpanzees. Sanctions for offenders included fines from 50 to 2,000 francs, confiscation of firearms or jail terms from six days to six months. The French colonial administrations did not have either the human resources or the will to enforce such regulations in remote, self-subsistent, communities but these decrees made it more difficult for hunters to sell chimpanzee meat openly in the markets of small provincial towns or in the workers' camps of private companies established in rural areas for logging or agriculture.[15]

Furthermore, in several ethnic groups of central Africa there were traditional cultural taboos against the consumption of chimpanzee meat because of their similarity to humans. For instance, among the Bayombe of the DRC and the Bakota of Gabon, eating apes is culturally prohibited for fear that women will give birth to apes, or to children with a simian face. In the Equateur region of the Belgian Congo, the bonobo was considered a human which had been transformed in the distant past.[6,16–18]

Thus, apart from pygmies, who lived in the forests, hunted daily and were not too concerned about government regulations (but were limited by their lack of firearms), the above factors tended to limit the number of natives who might potentially handle chimpanzee carcasses and acquire SIV_{cpz} from scratches or cuts on their hands. This may have changed in recent decades, as human populations increased and moved deeper into forested areas, using the dirt roads built by logging companies.

Quantifying the exposure

Now we will try to estimate the number of individuals who could have been occupationally infected with SIV_{cpz} in the 1920s. We will need to review findings from several studies which we will then assemble.

A few years ago, researchers visited remote villages in the Cameroonian rain forest and identified people who reported having had contacts (bites, scratches, wounds or other injuries) with animals at any time in their lives. This mostly involved a contact with small monkeys or non-primate animals, from rats to leopards and elephants. Twenty-nine individuals reported contact with gorillas or chimpanzees, up to fifty-three years earlier, and some had the scars to prove it. Antibodies against SFV, an innocuous retrovirus highly prevalent among apes and monkeys, were more common among villagers exposed to apes than those exposed to monkeys, presumably because the wounds, bites or scratches inflicted by the former were more severe.[1]

The exposure to apes was better quantified in seventeen other Cameroonian villages, where almost 4,000 adults were interviewed. A large majority of the exposures to primates involved monkeys rather than apes. Hunting was limited to men, 10% and 12% of which reported having hunted gorillas and chimpanzees respectively. Similar proportions of men and women reported having butchered these apes at least once in their lives. However, when asked about direct contact with primate blood or saliva (scratches, bites or other injuries) during hunting and butchering, only four men reported such exposures to chimpanzees, and seven to gorillas. No woman did so. In other words, only 0.1% of adults reported having had at least one direct contact with chimpanzee blood or body fluids, and 0.2% with gorillas.[19]

This enables us to estimate roughly the number of individuals living in the relevant parts of central Africa around 1921 who might have had at least one contact with SIV_{cpz}-containing chimpanzee blood at some point in their lives. Let us assume that no exposure occurred among children under sixteen, that only exposure to chimpanzees was relevant (the prevalence of SIV_{gor} infection in gorillas is lower and its relevance to human transmission unclear) and that the frequency of lifetime exposure to chimpanzee blood among inhabitants of areas populated by *P.t. troglodytes* was the same in 1921 as in the recent past.

Around 1930, when reliable censuses became available, about 2.3 million persons lived in the areas inhabited by *P.t. troglodytes*: 900,000 in Cameroon south of the Sanaga River, 387,000 in Gabon, 664,000 throughout Moyen-Congo, 120,000 in continental Equatorial Guinea, 130,000 in the south-west of the Central African Republic, and at most 100,000 in the Cabinda enclave and the adjacent Mayombe area of the Belgian Congo. At the time, the natural growth of central African populations each year (the difference between the birth and death rates) was 0.6%, so we can estimate that the relevant populations in 1921 were around 2,177,000. Of all inhabitants, 62% were aged sixteen years or over (the population was older than today because of the high child mortality). If we multiply 2,177,000 by 62% by 0.1%, it can be estimated that 1,350 adults living in 1921 had been exposed to chimpanzee blood at least once in their lives.

Of course there are many sources of error: inaccuracies in the censuses, lower exposure to chimps in the 5% of the population that was truly urban, no exposure in parts of Moyen-Congo where there were no *P.t. troglodytes*, exposures among adolescents, recall biases in the estimate of the proportion exposed to chimpanzee blood, etc. However, this provides us with an order of magnitude of the number of individuals potentially exposed to SIV_{cpz}. This number must now be multiplied by the percentage of chimpanzees infected with SIV_{cpz} and by the probability of transmission during each exposure, if the source chimpanzee was indeed infected with SIV_{cpz}.

We will assume that the SIV_{cpz} prevalence in 1921 among *P.t. troglodytes* communities of central Africa was similar to what it is today. In Cameroon, 5.9% of wild *P.t. troglodytes* are infected with SIV_{cpz}. Thus, of the 1,350 adults exposed to chimpanzee blood, about 80 were exposed to a SIV_{cpz}-infected ape. Then how many of these 80 individuals did acquire SIV_{cpz}? This depends on the probability of transmission during each exposure.[20]

This probability must have varied according to the degree of viraemia, i.e. the quantity of SIV_{cpz} present in the ape's blood. The higher the viraemia, the more infectious a given amount of blood was. In humans, the degree of HIV-1 viraemia increases markedly as the disease progresses towards AIDS. Although it was initially assumed that SIV_{cpz} is not pathogenic to chimpanzees, there is now much evidence supporting the opposite view. Experimental HIV-1 infection of chimpanzees can lead to rapid loss of their CD4 lymphocytes and full-blown AIDS with opportunistic infections. More recently, it was proven that SIV_{cpz} was pathogenic in wild *P.t. schweinfurthii*. In the Gombe reserve, ninety-four chimpanzees habituated to human contact were followed for nine years. Analyses of their stools showed which chimpanzees were infected with SIV_{cpz}. Over this period, the mortality rate in the seventeen chimpanzees infected with SIV_{cpz} was ten times higher than that among the non-infected animals. Although based on a limited number of observations, this relative mortality was similar to what happens in humans infected with HIV-1. An autopsy, done on three of the infected chimpanzees, revealed a reduction in the number of their CD4 lymphocytes. In one case, less than three years had elapsed between the infection with SIV_{cpz} and death. This suggested that SIV_{cpz} infection in chimpanzees could lead to immunodeficiency and high viraemia, which would make these animals more infectious, not just to other chimps, but to humans as well. It remains unknown whether SIV_{cpz} is as pathogenic in *P.t. troglodytes* as in their cousin *P.t. schweinfurthii*.[21–28]

So how much virus is there in their blood? In an early study using insensitive methods, our friend Noah, naturally infected with $SIV_{cpz-ant}$, was found to be viremic at a low level. Using the blood of Noah injected IV, a second chimp, Ch-Ni, was experimentally infected with $SIV_{cpz-ant}$. Very much like humans who develop acute HIV infection, Ch-Ni developed very high viraemia (5×10^6 viral copies/ml), which declined markedly in the ensuing months, eventually reaching levels similar to those of Noah. A few years later, using modern viral quantification methods, Noah was shown to have persistent and rather high viraemia (10^5 copies/ml). Ch-Ni maintained stable but lower viraemia (10^4 copies/ml). In humans, such levels are found at an advanced stage of HIV-1 infection, with a diagnosis of AIDS. Higher HIV-1 levels (10^5–10^7 copies/ml) are seen for a few weeks during acute infection and much later as a pre-terminal condition in untreated patients or in those whose virus has become resistant to all available therapies. To summarise, we can assume that in chimpanzees the degree of viraemia, and thus the potential for bloodborne transmission, is similar to that in humans.[23,29–31]

To estimate the frequency of SIV$_{cpz}$ transmission when someone is exposed to chimpanzee blood, we can extrapolate from studies among healthcare workers exposed to blood from an HIV-1-infected patient, which correspond fairly well to what we are interested in here: the risk of transmission after a single accidental exposure through the skin. Since the mid-1990s, healthcare workers exposed to HIV-1 have been given preventive antiretroviral drugs, which decrease the probability of transmission by 80%. Before such prophylactic methods became widely used, the overall risk of transmission was 0.3% per exposure, but was modulated by factors reflecting the quantity of viruses inoculated during the injury. Transmission was much less common (0.03%) for exposures that involved only non-penetrating contact (say, a splash) between blood and mucous membranes (the mouth or eyes) or non-intact skin. The risk when blood came into contact with intact skin was near zero. Conversely, with deeper injuries, or accidents during which a larger quantity of blood was inoculated, the risk of transmission could be as high as 25%, especially when the incident involved a patient with terminal illness.[32,33]

When a hunter or cook was exposed to chimpanzee blood containing SIV$_{cpz}$ in the bush of central Africa, some exposures would have been similar to those of healthcare workers, while others were far worse, for example a deep injury with a knife used for butchering or a traumatic wound inflicted by a struggling chimpanzee. Overall, the risk of transmission was probably higher than among healthcare workers sustaining needle pricks, because the injuries were more severe. As an educated guess, let us say that it was between 1 and 3%, that is, up to ten times more frequent than in occupationally exposed healthcare workers.

We had calculated that eighty adults living in central Africa in 1921 had been exposed to blood containing SIV$_{cpz}$ while handling chimpanzee carcasses or hunting. With 1% transmission, the result is one human infected from chimps, and two or three if the risk of transmission per exposure was closer to 3%. Obviously, there are several sources of errors so these estimates cannot be taken at face value, but the bottom line is that the number of persons infected naturally with SIV$_{cpz}$ around 1921 must have been small, and almost certainly less than ten.

We know that over several decades a cross-species transmission occurred at least four times for HIV-1, i.e. once for each of groups M, N, O and P, each of which is thought to reflect distinct cross-species transmission events rather than evolution within humans. It occurred at least eight times for each of the different groups of SIV$_{smm}$, which became HIV-2, as we will see later. Thus, the epidemic of HIV-1 group M was triggered not because a lot of humans were infected directly from chimpanzees but because a rare case of infection managed to spread and multiply, something which all the others that preceded it had not managed to do. In the following chapters, we will try to understand why this time the subsequent human-to-human transmission was so effective. But apart from the occupational infections of hunters or cooks, could other modes of transmission have been responsible for the first case(s) of SIV$_{cpz}$ transmission from chimpanzee to man? We will now review three such hypotheses.

The river

Oral poliovirus vaccines (OPV) distributed in the 1950s and early 1960s were massively contaminated with a simian virus (simian vacuolating virus 40), which originated from the macaque cells used to grow the vaccinal virus. Fortunately, this virus was not pathogenic for humans. In an article published in *Rolling Stone* in 1992, journalist Tom Curtis proposed the theory that HIV-1 came from the contamination of OPV with SIV from African green monkeys. Of course, it was later shown that African green monkeys were not the source of HIV-1, as their own SIVs were too different from HIV-1. Then in 1999, Edward Hooper published a book entitled *The river. A journey back to the source of HIV and AIDS*, which focused on the theory that chimpanzee cells had been used to produce an experimental oral polio vaccine called CHAT, developed by Hilary Koprowski at the Wistar Institute in Philadelphia. Koprowski had collaborated with Belgian scientists from the Stanleyville public health laboratory in the Belgian Congo. Clinical trials of the CHAT vaccine were conducted between 1957 and 1960 in the vicinity of Stanleyville, in the capital Léopoldville, as well as in the Ruzizi valley of Ruanda–Urundi. Eventually, the Koprowski vaccine proved inferior to the other OPV developed by his competitor Albert Sabin, and CHAT was never commercialised.[34]

The Stanleyville laboratory set up a colony of chimpanzees (presumably, all *P.t. schweinfurthii* or *Pan paniscus*) nearby, at a place called Camp Lindi, primarily to verify experimentally not just the efficacy but also the neurological virulence of the CHAT vaccine. Experimental oral polio vaccines were based on live viruses which had been empirically attenuated through repeated passages over various cell cultures, and scientists were worried that these viruses could eventually regain their original virulence, in which case the vaccine would cause the disease rather than prevent it. Camp Lindi chimps were given the CHAT vaccine, then the wild polio virus, and monitored clinically for neurological deficits. Others were sacrificed for their spinal cord to be examined after intraspinal injection of the CHAT virus. In addition, about thirty chimpanzees were used for hepatitis research, in an attempt to identify the agents of viral hepatitis through inoculation of stool suspensions from human patients.

The main theory in *The river* was that the Stanleyville laboratory had supplied the Wistar Institute with chimpanzee tissues obtained from sacrificed animals, which had then been used in Philadelphia to produce the CHAT vaccine so that SIV_{cpz} had been introduced into some vaccine lots, which were then sent back to the Congo where their oral administration in the late 1950s started the pandemic. A number of elements described in the book itself made this theory implausible, most importantly the fact that Koprowski had conducted very large trials of the same CHAT vaccine in his native Poland, where HIV-1 did not emerge. It would have been an extraordinary coincidence for SIV_{cpz}-contaminated vaccines to be re-exported from Philadelphia only to the very country where, allegedly, the SIV_{cpz}-infected chimpanzee tissues had been obtained. Then Hooper changed his hypothesis somewhat, and suggested that the Stanleyville laboratory had produced batches of the vaccine locally, using cells from locally procured chimpanzees, which led to contamination with SIV_{cpz} in Stanleyville rather than in Philadelphia.

Many circumstantial elements argued against either version of the hypothesis. There is no documentary evidence that chimpanzee cells were ever used, anywhere in the world, to produce OPV. Scientists had easy access to small monkeys of the *Macaca* genus, which were abundant in Asia, cheaper and easier to handle than chimpanzees, raised fewer ethical issues and worked well in cell culture systems. In 1955, up to 200,000 rhesus monkeys were imported into the US for medical research. Furthermore, as noted by the late Dr Paul Osterrieth, a scientist who worked at the Stanleyville laboratory for a few years, it was technically impossible for this rather basic facility to produce any kind of novel viral vaccine. The laboratory just did not have the human and material resources for such an endeavour. The annual reports of the

Stanleyville laboratory for the crucial years never mentioned any local production of OPV, something that, had they achieved it, the laboratory workers would certainly have been proud of. Neither did the reports of the colony's health system mention any local production of OPV – while the same reports provided much information about other vaccines produced by the network of public health laboratories of the Belgian Congo. Hooper seems to have confused *conditionnement*, which meant local dilution of concentrated frozen vaccine stock or its distribution from a large container to smaller containers, with local production or amplification of the vaccine strain.[35-37]

Nevertheless, to test this hypothesis once and for all, old vials containing the CHAT vaccine, which had been kept frozen for decades, were located. Some came from the Wistar Institute, where CHAT had been developed and produced, and conspiracy theorists could argue that this institution had a vested interest in supplying vials which they already knew were not contaminated with HIV-1. But other CHAT vials were fished out of freezers at the CDC in Atlanta and at Britain's National Institute for Biological Standards and Control (NIBSC). Some vials contained the very batches (10A-11 and 13) that had been used in the Belgian colonies. Samples were tested by several institutions, including the NIBSC, the Institut Pasteur, the Max Planck Institute, the Karolinska Institute, the New York University School of Medicine and Roche Molecular Systems. All reached the same conclusions: there was no HIV or SIV nucleic acids in these vials; there was no chimpanzee DNA, only DNA from rhesus (*Macaca mulatta*) or cynomolgus (*Macaca fascicularis*) monkeys and, in one batch which had been grown on human diploid cells, *Homo sapiens* DNA; and there was poliovirus, which meant that there had not been extensive degradation of viral nucleic acids over the very long storage period.[38-40]

Furthermore, 131 faecal samples were collected from chimps in the forested areas around Kisangani (ex-Stanleyville), where the laboratory and chimpanzee colony had been located: only one was SIV-positive. This virus, obtained from a *P.t. schweinfurthii*, was called SIV$_{cpz-DRC1}$. In phylogenetic trees, it was close to the *P.t. schweinfurthii* viruses obtained from Uganda and Tanzania and with Noah's SIV$_{cpz-ant}$, and clearly distinct from all *P.t. troglodytes* SIVs.[41]

Therefore, there is no evidence that chimpanzee cells were used in the Stanleyville laboratory to prepare batches of OPV vaccines, or that any OPV was produced there. And even if chimpanzee cells had been used in

Stanleyville, they could not have contained the *P.t. troglodytes* SIV_{cpz} that triggered the pandemic. There is no evidence either of any retrovirus having been present in the old batches of CHAT available for testing. Furthermore, even when taking into account the margin of error on these estimates, SIV_{cpz} emerged in human populations at least twenty-five years before the CHAT trials. This theory can be firmly rejected.

Bold experiments

Because of their similarity to humans, chimpanzees have been used for almost a century as animal models of many infectious diseases, to prove that a putative pathogen is the cause of a given disease, to evaluate new vaccines, etc. In the course of these experiments, chimpanzees have been injected with various amounts of human blood or other types of human specimens, containing a wide diversity of infectious agents: viruses (HIV-1 of course, poliomyelitis virus, hepatitis B virus (HBV), hepatitis C virus (HCV) and yellow fever virus), prions (proteins causing kuru, Creutzfeldt-Jakob disease and scrapie), bacteria (the aetiological agents of tuberculosis, leprosy, gonorrhoea and trachoma) and parasites (causing malaria and the Guinea worm). There was even a chimpanzee model of alcoholism and addiction to narcotics!

However, it is rather extraordinary that, on several occasions, the reverse was done: the IV injections of chimpanzee blood in humans. The first such experiment was performed in Sierra Leone by Donald Blacklock and Saul Adler, who injected two Europeans (presumably, themselves) subcutaneously (SC) and intravenously with small quantities of blood from a chimpanzee infected with malaria parasites. They did not develop malaria. We do not know what happened next but they certainly got worried when the donor chimpanzee died a few days later, with the autopsy showing a disseminated *Strongyloides* infection, with this intestinal worm being present in the chimp's bloodstream! Shortly thereafter, at the Institut Pasteur in Paris, a man was injected IV with 40 cc of chimpanzee blood as part of a comparative study of blood groups of chimpanzees and humans. The volunteer apparently tolerated the procedure well. With great foresight, the Pasteur scientist noted that such experiments should be avoided in the future, 'to keep off potentially transmitting to humans hitherto unknown infectious pathogens of chimpanzees'![42–45]

This advice seems to have fallen on deaf ears. Renowned parasitologist Jérôme Rodhain, director of the Tropical Medicine Institute in Brussels and then in Antwerp, studied whether malaria parasites of primates were transmissible to man. As a secondary interest, or perhaps as a moral justification, he also investigated whether fever induced by malaria could have a beneficial effect on patients with late-stage syphilis. Such work would be unthinkable today but in those days there were no ethics committees and each scientist could decide whether an experiment was morally acceptable. Similar investigations were conducted in other parts of the world, especially India, with inoculation to humans of blood obtained from Asian apes and monkeys.[46]

Rodhain carried out a series of experiments in which chimpanzee blood (5–10 cc) was injected IV in humans, most of them patients with syphilitic dementia. The chimpanzees (Thomas, Suzanne, Simone ...) originated from the Belgian Congo; although Rodhain alluded to them as *P.t. verus*, in retrospect they were probably *P.t. schweinfurthii*. Between 1938 and 1940, Rodhain injected chimpanzee blood to twenty-six patients. He did prove that some of these malaria parasites were infectious to humans, and that the parasite named by others *Plasmodium rodhaini*, in his honour, was in fact *Plasmodium malariae*. We should give him a lot of credit for being humble since he himself killed the chance of his name going down in history as the name of a species. Rodhain conducted similar experimentations with other species of malaria parasites, most notably *Plasmodium reichenowi*, a parasite of chimpanzees and gorillas. In 1954–5, he injected chimpanzee blood in four more psychiatric patients, and managed to transmit *Plasmodium schwetzi*.[47–52]

These experiments were done in hospitals in Antwerp and clearly could not have led to the emergence of HIV-1 in Africa. Furthermore, as the apes originated from the Belgian Congo, they were all presumably *Pan troglodytes schweinfurthii* (Rodhain would not have confused *P.t. verus* with *Pan paniscus*, the other ape potentially available from his Belgian collaborators). It seems unlikely that other scientists carried out similar experiments for malaria research, since Rodhain would have mentioned this in the detailed reviews of the subject that he wrote in the discussion section of his own papers. Of course, one could hypothesise that similar experiments were carried out in the nascent research institutions in Africa and the results never disseminated, but this would be pure speculation. There is no evidence of similar experiments being conducted in the Léopoldville research laboratory, where Rodhain had worked during the early part of his career and which he continued to visit intermittently from his academic posts in Belgium.

At the Institut Pasteur in Paris, Auguste Pettit worked for sixteen years on developing a therapeutic serum containing high titers of antibodies against the poliomyelitis virus, to be given to patients with this disease. As it was difficult to obtain large enough quantities of serum from human cases recuperating from polio, he produced animal sera, which were then used on humans. Antipoliomyelitis serum was prepared from horses, monkeys and chimpanzees, and then administered to at least eighty patients. Two chimpanzees were used for this purpose; the first one was bled to death and the second was bled repeatedly over a two-and-a-half-year period. They were *P.t. verus* chimps from Guinea, and the patients were in France not Africa. So once again, this could not have led to the emergence of HIV-1.[53]

Eternal youth

Among French surgeons of the early twentieth century, Serge Voronoff had a most unusual résumé. Born in Russia, he emigrated to France as a teenager, changed his name to conceal his Judaism, got a medical degree in Paris in 1894, trained as a surgeon and worked in Egypt for fourteen years for the Khedive, the local monarch. There, according to his biographer, he was struck by the short life span of eunuchs among the Khedive's servants. His return to France in 1910 coincided with the emergence of a new speciality, endocrinology: the science of hormones. Hormones are secreted by some gland, transported via the bloodstream and have their main effect on distant organs. At the time, there was no hormone replacement therapy, neither for hypothyroidism, nor for diabetes, pituitary insufficiency and so on.[54]

Voronoff was given a chair of experimental surgery at the Collège de France in Paris, something to be taken with a pinch of salt since the Collège did not have a medical school. He did not choose the easiest route for treating patients with endocrine dysfunction. While the obvious solution (soon to be available) was to find animal sources of the defective hormone, concentrate it and administer the product to patients orally or by injections, Voronoff attempted to tackle their problems by transplanting animal organs. He trained for a few months in the US under Alexis Carrel, soon to be awarded a Nobel for his pioneering work on organ transplants and vascular anastomoses.

Upon his return to Paris, Voronoff undertook experimental organ transplantations in animals, first within a given species and then between different species. In 1913, he performed his first xenotransplant (xeno- means foreign, in this case a foreign species), implanting a chimpanzee thyroid in a young man with congenital hypothyroidism. According to his surgeon, the patient improved. He performed a few more thyroid transplants, but this came to a stop when thyroid hormones were synthesised. During WWI, Voronoff grafted animal bones (in at least one case, from a chimpanzee) in soldiers with post-traumatic bone defects, but it was soon shown that in many cases bone could be obtained from the patient himself, at some other site.

Perhaps drawing on his earlier observations of eunuchs, Voronoff became convinced that the male hormones were necessary not only for sexual activity and phenotypes, but also for preserving various functions of the body, and especially the brain. Ageing was seen as a consequence of a degeneration of the testes. In his laboratory, he attempted to transplant testes from young animals to their older counterparts. Eventually, in 1920 this culminated in his first interventions on two humans, one of whom received the right and the other the left testes of the same baboon. These did not work well, and Voronoff attributed the failure to the use of organs from a species too different from humans. He decided to use chimpanzees instead.

Over the next two years, Voronoff performed twelve testicular transplants, from chimpanzee to man. It was not possible at the time to perform microvascular surgery, and Voronoff thought he could avoid the necrosis of the transplanted organ by actually grafting thin slices, with the assumption that small new blood vessels would form to revascularise the organ. That was very optimistic. Furthermore, nobody at the time had any understanding of the immunological rejection of a transplanted organ, presumably very severe when that organ was not of human origin. To maximise the use of the precious organs, each patient received half a testicle; from one chimpanzee donor four transplantations could be conducted. Finding chimpanzees was difficult. A Catholic order sent him a few dozen from Guinea. Through the Ministry of Colonies, he tried to arrange the shipment of chimps from Gabon but apparently none survived the journey. French newspapers reported that entrepreneurs in the Congo had sensed the potential for a quick profit so that the price of a chimpanzee had increased ten-fold on the local market, but it is unclear whether any of these animals made it to the old continent. To maintain his supply, Voronoff visited Guinea, Senegal and Mali in the mid-1920s.[55–57]

Like many experimental surgeons, Voronoff claimed that his procedure was successful in more than half his patients. It is hard to say whether this claim was the result of unwarranted enthusiasm, the lack of objective measures, the placebo effect of surgery, data manipulation for commercial reasons or perhaps even a genuine effect. Despite the necrosis and immunological rejection, it is possible that for a few weeks, as the transplanted organ was disposed of by the recipient body's defence mechanisms, there was some absorption of the huge quantities of hormones present in the graft, some of which were not too dissimilar from the human ones.

Even if Voronoff might have had sincere scientific aims initially, he quickly realised the immense commercial potential of the procedure. Here was a renowned surgeon, holding a chair at the Collège de France, who had invented a procedure that could act not only as a surgical Viagra but prolong life and enhance quality of life for decades. Many rich and old men were willing to pay a fortune for a shot at eternal youth. Voronoff even travelled to India in 1929 to perform a testicular transplant on a maharajah. Although some of his fortune may have been inherited from his second wife, Voronoff certainly made a lot of money out of this surgical adventure, allowing him to spend the last three decades of his life in a fancy villa on the Italian Riviera, where he had set up a chimpanzee breeding colony, probably as a public relations ploy.

Such a lucrative business interested colleagues in France and overseas, and Voronoff's biographer estimated that about 2,000 testicular transplants were performed in Paris, Bordeaux, Nice, Lille, Alger, London, Rome, Turin, Milan, Genoa, Vienna, Madrid, Lisbon, Porto, Berlin, Alexandria, Constantinople, Chicago, New York, San Francisco, Buenos Aires, Valparaiso, Rio and even in Hanoi. Voronoff himself claimed to have performed 475 transplants. Eventually, the procedure was completely discredited for a number of reasons, including the fact that Voronoff had started performing ovarian transplants (inserting a chimpanzee ovary into a woman and vice versa), which raised extremely serious ethical concerns (could one of these females become pregnant with a half-chimp, half-human baby?). Voronoff became the butt of popular humour in France and abroad. He died in 1951, aged eighty-five. We do not know whether he believed in the procedure strongly enough to have it performed on him, but he did transplant one of his older brothers, who came all the way from Russia for the surgery.[54,57]

So to get back to the question, could some of these chimpanzee organs have contained SIV_{cpz}, which may have infected the recipient, starting a chain of transmission? That seems unlikely for a number of reasons. First, all of the procedures seem to have been performed in countries unrelated to the emergence of HIV-1. Second, most of the recipients were elderly men, who were unlikely to have infected many sexual partners, even if re-invigorated by the procedure. Third, at least according to what was documented, Voronoff's chimps came from West Africa, thus were *P.t. verus*, a subspecies not infected with SIV_{cpz}. Fourth, it appears that in some of these procedures, the profit-seeking surgeons used testes from monkeys rather than apes due to a shortage of the latter. Therefore, this bizarre scenario can also be rejected.

In summary, there is now a reasonable body of evidence suggesting that the initial intuition of early researchers, the cut hunter theory, was correct and there is no alternative hypothesis that can be supported after a careful examination of the facts. Such occasional cases of cross-species transmission must have been occurring for hundreds of years, as humans and *P.t. troglodytes* chimpanzees have coexisted in the forests of central Africa for many generations. For a long time these ancient cases of SIV_{cpz} becoming HIV-1 did not manage to disseminate successfully. What happened in the early twentieth century for HIV-1 to spread successfully into human populations, while HIV-2 managed the same feat, albeit on a much more limited scale, in West Africa? We will start by briefly reviewing in the next chapter the history of European colonialism in central Africa, and how it created conditions propitious to the emergence of HIV.

5 | *Societies in transition*

This background chapter aims to describe the settings in which the rest of the story took place. Africans understandably resent and reject as arrogant, or at least Eurocentric, historical accounts of their continent which consider the European penetration as the starting point and describe this process as discovery rather than what it really was: a military conquest for the purpose of economic exploitation. However, since the events relevant to the emergence of HIV-1 occurred during the colonial occupation of central Africa, and were facilitated by the profound social and economic changes brought about by colonisation, especially around the pool on the Congo River, we will focus on this period, but after a short detour which will enable us to examine how history confirms the molecular clocks of Chapter 3.

The slave trade and the exportation of infectious diseases to the Americas

The arrival of the Bantus in central Africa is, on the scale of human history, relatively recent, having occurred about 2,000 years ago, when migrants from around Lake Tchad managed to dominate the truly indigenous pygmy populations and for the first time introduced various forms of agriculture. In some areas, organisation was limited to small tribes that occupied geographically limited territories. Elsewhere, kingdoms were established, such as the Kongo kingdom, a loose confederation of tribes which corresponded to parts of current day Congo-Brazzaville, DRC, Angola and Gabon. These societies were not technologically advanced, which made it easy for Europeans to conquer the heartland of Africa once they found solutions to the health problems (mostly malaria) that decimated their early soldiers and settlers, many of whom died within two years of their arrival. But central African people had strong values, beliefs and traditions centred on the extended family, the clan. And there was already a fair amount of trading between ethnic groups within the Congo basin.[1]

For a long time, the European presence was limited to coastal areas, where forts were established for buying slaves. First in the region were the Portuguese, soon followed by the Dutch, Spanish, English, French and even Danes. Over three and a half centuries, 10.3 million slaves survived the journey and arrived in the Americas. Information on two-thirds of the voyages is available in a database prepared by the W. E. B. Du Bois Institute of Harvard University. It contains details on only 31,000 slaves embarked in Cameroon, and it is not possible to figure out how many more were embarked via Nigeria. About 35,000 were shipped from Gabon. However, the numbers embarked further south on the Congo coast were far greater: 79,000 from Loango, 107,000 from Malembo, 274,000 from Cabinda and 120,000 from the mouth of the Congo. It can be extrapolated that around 800,000 slaves originating from regions inhabited by *Pan troglodytes troglodytes* arrived in the Americas.[2–4]

These massive movements of human populations were responsible for the introduction of parasitic diseases from Africa into discrete areas of the Americas, where they found the necessary ecological conditions and/or suitable vectors to sustain their transmission until today. River blindness was exported to Guatemala, Mexico, Venezuela and Ecuador. Schistosomiasis (which causes inflammation of the rectum and fibrosis of the liver) managed to establish its cycle of transmission in the eastern regions of Brazil, in some Caribbean islands and Venezuela. Lymphatic filariasis, a disease causing massive swelling of the legs and genitalia, became endemic in Haiti, the Dominican Republic, Guyana and Brazil.[5–8]

Viral diseases were also exported. Slaves with yellow fever would die before reaching their final destination, but its mosquito vector travelled in the same ships and managed to establish transmission of the virus into the Americas. Phylogenetic studies demonstrated that some strains of HCV found today in Martinique as well as strains of HBV currently infecting Haitians were imported during the slave trade. But the virus for which transcontinental transmission has been documented best is HTLV-1, the first retrovirus isolated from humans. Like HIV-1, HTLV-1 (which does not cause AIDS) originated in primates, including *P.t. troglodytes*. Phylogenetic studies indicated that some lineages of HTLV-1 found in the Americas were imported along with the human cargo. Using the same methods, researchers investigated whether HIV-1 or HIV-2 were imported into the Americas during the transatlantic slave trade. The conclusion is that this did not happen. This indicates that HIV-1 must have been rare or inexistent among central African populations until the middle of the nineteenth century, and that events subsequent to this period facilitated its emergence.[9–15]

A pool on the river

The desire to penetrate Africa's heartland appeared in the last quarter of the nineteenth century, as European powers hoped to find exploitable resources and set up new colonies after most of the American colonies had established themselves as independent states, or become less lucrative after the abolition of slavery. The same powers which had traded millions of slaves over 350 years then used the abolition of slavery as moral justification for this new colonial conquest: their stated goal was to bring civilisation and morality to these primitive populations that did not yet know Christianity.[16]

In central Africa, French settlements were initially concentrated around the Gabon estuary. Christian missions were established, leading to the foundation of Libreville in 1849. Among its first inhabitants were a few hundred slaves whose ship had been intercepted by the French navy. It was not possible to take the slaves back to their homeland, so they were settled in what became Libreville, literally 'free town'. The French presence in Gabon remained modest.

No Europeans had reached the inland pool on the Congo River since some brave Capucin priests in the seventeenth century. As the latter's goals were spiritual rather than temporal, their achievement was quickly forgotten. Pierre (originally Pietro) Savorgnan de Brazza, born into a Roman aristocratic family, became an officer of the French navy to fulfil his desire for discovery and adventure. He first travelled upriver on the Ogooué in Gabon in 1872, aiming to reach the pool of the Congo, which would provide access to its basin, assumed to be rich in minerals, agricultural products and ivory. To Brazza's disappointment, journalist Henry Stanley managed to cross the continent, from Zanzibar all the way to Boma near the mouth of the river, where he arrived in 1877 in pitiful condition, having descended the Congo from its source. Stanley was soon hired by Leopold II, the king of Belgium, who dreamed of establishing a large colony, for his own profit. Belgium itself had no interest whatsoever in acquiring colonial possessions. It would later change its mind.

In 1880, Brazza managed to reach the Congo by land. He arrived at the pool, thirty-five kilometres long and twenty-four kilometres wide, where 20,000 Bateke lived in trading and fishing villages on both sides of the river. The pool was the terminus for all navigation on the Congo, because a series of rapids starts a few kilometres downstream. During the slave trade, the area had been used as a depot for slaves purchased in the Congo basin, before they were sent to a coastal port. Brazza signed a treaty with a chief on the north side of the river, and planted the French flag. The chief could not read French and did not realise that he had conceded a large piece of land to France rather than merely getting some kind of protection and trading rights. Meanwhile, on the south side of the river, Stanley signed a similar treaty with another chief.[17]

Stanley worked for an individual, Leopold II, who was to become sole owner of the État Indépendant du Congo (EIC, Congo Free State), the largest private property in history, while Brazza worked for France, a parliamentary democracy. Stanley was an adventurer motivated by greed, who killed hundreds during his journeys. Brazza was an atypical nineteenth-century explorer, motivated by humanitarian concerns, per-haps naively as France had other ambitions. These nuances were not lost on the local populations, and the city of Brazzaville still bears his name and erected a monument to honour Brazza's memory, while across the border Stanleyville became Kisangani thirty-five years ago. The former Stanley Pool on the Congo is now known as the Malebo Pool.[18]

Back in France, Brazza had a hard time convincing the French gov-ernment to ratify the treaty and invest in the development of a new colony in central Africa, which was quite a gamble since nobody knew whether this huge territory contained valuable resources apart from rubber and ivory. France had its hands full digesting the parts of Indochina it had recently conquered. Reluctantly, Brazza was given limited resources and 400 West African mercenaries to set up small outposts. This mission ended when the Berlin treaty was signed in 1885. European powers had divided most of Africa, with France acquiring what was initially called the Congo Français. But the true winner was Leopold, who grabbed the centre of the continent, designed as a buffer zone between the territorial ambitions of France, Britain, Germany and Portugal.

The task of establishing a French administration was given to Brazza himself, as commissioner-general of the Congo Français. Additional colonial posts were founded, more treaties signed, decrees promulgated, maps drawn, taxes levied and a number of skirmishes were fought against rebellious tribes. French rule was progressively expanded north of Brazzaville, reaching Bangui in 1889 and Tchad in 1900, which allowed, at least on paper, equatorial Africa to be connected with French West Africa. Treaties with other powers further defined its boundaries, but failed to provide the Congo Français with access to the mouth of the river. For a few decades its exports had to travel on the Belgian railway between Léopoldville and Matadi, or on the backs of porters, 7,000 of whom worked between Loango and Brazzaville, a twenty-five-day journey.

The other important protagonist in the early history of the Congo Français was Prosper Augouard. Born in 1852, ordained in the congregation of the Holy Spirit, he arrived in Gabon in 1877. Missionaries of the time had to be highly motivated for their life expectancy in Africa was just three years. Augouard was more robust than average, used quinine readily for self-treatment of malaria and would spend the next forty-four years in central Africa. Having a strong personality, resourceful and energetic, he had much of a say in how the colony was run. Unlike the civil servants who tried to get promoted to richer and more comfortable colonies, Augouard had no desire to move. Unusually for a missionary of the time, he went back to Europe regularly. He understood early on that public relations, political lobbying and fundraising were essential components of his evangelical ministry. Numerous French ministers of colonies considered him the most senior adviser concerning all matters related to the Congo Français.[19–22]

In 1881, barely a few months after Brazza had signed the treaty, Augouard arrived at the pool after a 560-kilometre walk from the coast, to prepare the ground for a Catholic mission, buying a piece of land around the village of Mfoa. He was the true founder of Brazzaville, for the explorer had left just a hut with a Senegalese sergeant to guard the post. Augouard built the parish of Brazzaville, while Brazza spent most of his time in Libreville, then the capital. French, Dutch and Portuguese companies established trading posts. In 1890, Augouard became the first bishop of Brazzaville, with a territory extending all the way to the Oubangui-Chari, which he crisscrossed constantly in a flotilla of small steamboats. A good architect and builder, skilled manager, excellent writer and a geographer, Augouard was always ready to go hippopotamus hunting when the mission fridges were empty. In 1892, its first physician was posted in Brazzaville. Within a few years, a brick cathedral was built, with a belltower twenty metres high, topped by a crucifix and the French flag. Schools were added, housing for the teachers, technical buildings and so on. Augouard was a nationalist, who often said to his Christians that 'to learn how to love God required learning how to love France'. A journalist of the time wrote that there had been an error in casting: Augouard should have been governor while Brazza, the idealistic humanitarian, could have been an excellent bishop if only he had believed in God. In 1898, Brazza was fired, primarily because the colony's finances were in a parlous situation. He certainly had been more of a visionary than a manager.[19,23]

Emile Gentil was appointed commissioner in 1903, a year before Brazzaville became the capital of the entire Congo Français, renamed in 1910 Afrique Équatoriale Française (AEF). AEF was made up of four colonies: Gabon, Moyen-Congo, Oubangui-Chari and Tchad, following the model of the two other colonial federations, Afrique Occidentale Française and Indochine. The AEF territory was considered 'pacified'. Its militia consisted mostly of West African mercenaries and conscripts, who were more willing to obey their French officers than locally recruited soldiers. Gentil divided the Congo Français into forty blocks, each allocated to a concessionary company, which was given a monopoly of all trade on a well-defined area. The natives could only sell their crops to the local company, and they could not opt out of the cash economy because they also had to pay head taxes. The largest companies operated their own private militias, and atrocities were committed by their European agents. Some of these crimes were reported in the French press in 1905, the most famous case being that of a poor man who was blown up with dynamite inserted in his rectum. Others were executed for petty crimes without any formal judgement. In Bangui, forty-five women, who had been jailed because their husband failed to bring back enough rubber, died in detention within a five-week period. These scandals preoccupied the French government, which sent a mission of inquiry headed by Brazza himself, who had by then retired in Algiers.

He travelled through Matadi, Léopoldville, Brazzaville and all the way to the upper Chari, finding large areas of the colony depopulated, as the villagers had fled from the violence and taxes imposed by the concessionary companies. Unfortunately, Brazza became sick with dysentery, and died in Dakar on his way back to France. His report, highly critical of the abuses of the Gentil administration, was buried with him. Many of his enemies attended his national funeral in Paris, and spoke highly of him. His wife was not amused, and remained convinced until her death that Brazza had been poisoned. In AEF, the concession system did not change much for a decade. Eventually, it was criticised by the French socialists and replaced by a more normal market economy. Some companies had already gone bankrupt, as the area they had been allocated proved less wealthy than anticipated.[24-25]

French officials had no scruples about using forced labour. Military raids were conducted on villages and local chiefs were requested to provide a number of young men, who would spend the next few years transporting goods on their backs and building roads or telegraph lines for a miserable salary. The telegraph came first, with several thousand kilometres of lines installed in 1909–11, allowing communications between the major trading posts. After a few decades, the Africans at last derived some benefits from the colonial system: primary school education, control of communicable diseases, a communication network which facilitated trading with some wealth eventually trickling down to the local populations. In 1927, it was possible for the first time to drive from Bangui up to the port of Douala, and there were 6,000 kilometres of laterite roads in Oubangui-Chari. The Bangui airport was opened in 1930, and the first commercial route to Europe was inaugurated in 1939. The urbanisation and social changes that were to foster the emergence of HIV-1 had appeared, and this was not limited to the territory of the AEF.[24-26]

Kamerun, Cameroun and Cameroons

Around the time of the 1884–5 Berlin conference, Chancellor Bismarck, until then preoccupied mainly with Germany's expansion within Europe, decided that Germany should have African colonies too. His emissaries managed to grab some nice pieces of land. While his British competitor was busy making deals in the Niger delta, Gustav Nachtigal, imperial consul for the west coast of Africa, signed a treaty that paved the way for the German occupation of Cameroon, which was to last only thirty years. In fact, the chiefs of the Douala tribe had signed a protocol with a private trader from Hamburg, who transferred his rights to Germany the very next day. It had been a pretty good week for Nachtigal, for just a few days earlier he had signed another treaty establishing a German protectorate in Togo.[27]

Germany invested heavily in developing Kamerun's infrastructure (ports, roads, bridges, two railways, etc.) but committed its own colonial atrocities, especially under governor von Puttkamer, Bismarck's nephew. Germany increased the size of Kamerun by 50% in 1911 through a controversial deal with France: Germany abandoned its claims to Morocco, and in exchange the French gave the Germans substantial parts of AEF. German occupation of this new territory did not last long. At the outset of WWI, Kamerun was invaded from the Nigerian side by British troops and from the other side by French troops from AEF assisted by soldiers from the Belgian Congo. They greatly outnumbered the Germans who fled to Spanish Guinea. A deal was made between the victors, in which France did best, getting almost all of Kamerun less a small band of land alongside the Nigerian border. The British already had their hands full taking care of Tanganyika and South-West Africa, two other former German colonies. After the war, Britain and France were given a mandate by the League of Nations to administer Cameroun Français and British Cameroons. Since our story unfolded in the southern forested areas inhabited by *P.t. troglodytes*, we will examine only the fate of Cameroun Français.

French rule was somewhat more benevolent in Cameroun than in neighbouring AEF. France had to provide a report each year to the League of Nations (later, the UN), and there was some moral pressure for basic human rights to be respected. The natives could write letters of complaints to the League. Unlike their AEF counterparts, Cameroonians could not be conscripted into the French colonial army and sent to do the dirty work in other African countries, or to die for France on the battlefields of Europe or Indochina. The terms of the mandate prohibited forced labour but the Geneva-based organisation could never enforce it and many Cameroonians were requisitioned for public works. The other major difference with AEF was the prosperity of Cameroun, built around cash crops (coffee, cocoa, rubber, timber) and the easy access to the port of Douala. The development of roads, the railway, the healthcare system and the urbanisation progressed more speedily than in AEF, but by the mid-1920s only Douala was considered to have a truly urban character.

Congo Belge/Belgisch Kongo

To bring to an end the scandals associated with the EIC and save the country's honour, Belgium purchased the Congo from its ailing king, Leopold II, in 1908. He died the following year, shortly after marrying his long-time mistress Caroline, a former prostitute. This led to an appreciable improvement in the respect for basic human rights. A colonial charter was promulgated, a ministry of colonies was created and the first holder of the post, Jules Renkin, gradually abolished the trade monopoly given to concession companies. Renkin even visited the Congo, which Leopold had never done. Fifty-two years of colonial rule followed which, like all others, was based on racism as its moral justification. After WWI, Belgian possessions were extended to the small kingdoms of Ruanda and Urundi, administered like Cameroon under a League of Nations mandate. While resource-poor Ruanda and Urundi were managed through a system of indirect rule via the traditional kings, in the Congo thousands of Belgian officials were posted at every level and in every district, in the public and private sectors.[18]

The Belgian Congo proved a very lucrative enterprise for Belgium. Often described as a 'geological scandal', the territory was rich in copper, cobalt, tin, zinc, manganese, gold, industrial diamonds and uranium to name a few. It was also very fertile, and rubber tree plantations replaced the picking of wild rubber while large quantities of coffee, cocoa, cotton and palm oil were exported. Most of the Belgian Congo's wealth was controlled by a huge and tentacular financial holding, the Société Générale de Belgique. Its most lucrative branch was the Union Minière du Haut-Katanga, which operated the mines in the southern Katanga province.[28]

Through the Société Générale and other groups, there was a steady flow of resources and money in one direction: from the Congo to Belgium. The motherland kept a monopoly over the processing of the Congo's raw products, resulting in the development of a vast industrial sector in Belgium, from metallurgy to chocolate factories. A fraction of the colony's income trickled down to the Congolese population, through the taxes and duties paid by the companies, which funded more than half of the Belgian Congo's budget. However, the Congolese benefited from the development of the country's infrastructures, even if its primary goal was to facilitate the operations of private enterprises. Up to 5,000 kilometres of railways were built, roads were kept in good condition and hydro-electric dams provided electricity to many cities. Air transportation started in 1920 with domestic flights, and by 1936 there was a service between Brussels and Léopoldville. The proportion of the Congo's population that lived in an urban environment increased from 6% in 1935, 15% in 1945, to 24% by 1955.[28–29]

Throughout central Africa, the impact of all these rapid changes on the traditional African societies was profound. Progressively, for better or worse, many Africans no longer felt bound by the customs that had regulated their lives for dozens of generations. Women acquired a degree of freedom, some of whose consequences were unexpected. While their ancestors had been generally content to procure food on a day-to-day basis and spend their evenings in endless palavers, colonisation and European examples brought materialism. Different clothes, a radio, lighting devices, a bicycle and later on a house made with cement blocks and a corrugated iron roof became the long-term goals of many workers now serving the Europeans. This hope for what was perceived as a better life lured many into the nascent cities of central Africa which, in the Belgian Congo, were quite appropriately called *centres extra-coutumiers*, centres where customs no longer held sway.

Created by Europeans, populated by Africans

Central African colonial cities were described as having been created by Europeans and populated by Africans. In the first half of the twentieth century, this process engendered communities whose lifestyle dramatically differed from that of traditional African societies, in a way that facilitated the dissemination of sexually transmitted pathogens, including SIV_{cpz}/HIV-1. Before we examine some specific cities, let us glance quickly at the populations they emerged from. Figures provided by colonial censuses, especially before 1930, need to be taken with a pinch of salt: some adult males avoided being counted for fear of taxation, forced labour or conscription, while administrators exaggerated their numbers as budgets and chances of promotion were proportional to the population. Around 1930, the population of Cameroun Français was estimated to be 2.2 million, while it was 1.26 million in Oubangui-Chari, 664,000 in Moyen-Congo and only 387,000 in Gabon (Figure 4; year-to-year variations over the following decades were caused by changes in the boundaries between colonies within the AEF). The continental part of Equatorial Guinea had only 100,000

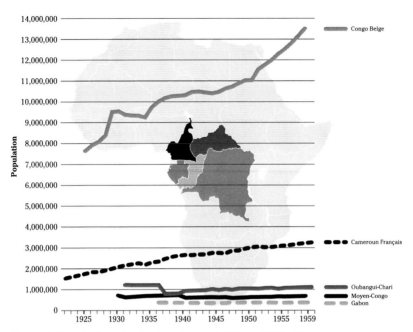

Figure 4 Population of colonies of central Africa, 1922–60.

inhabitants, and the Cabinda enclave of Angola even fewer. The population of the Belgian Congo, a 2.3 million km^2 subcontinent, was estimated to be 9.6 million in 1930, and 13.5 million in 1958. In all these colonies, population densities were low, generally between one and four inhabitants per km^2.[28–31]

We will focus on the evolution of the twin cities of Brazzaville and Léopoldville (better known as 'Brazza' and 'Léo'), founded at the same time by French and Belgian colonisers, and where ultimately the diversification of HIV-1 took place. Around 1904, when Brazzaville replaced Libreville as the AEF capital, about 250 Europeans and 5,000 Africans lived there, those necessary for the colonial administration, an embryonic private sector, and the Catholic mission which had constituted the initial nucleus. A colonial bureaucracy was slowly developed, with a residence for the governor, buildings for the telegraph, customs, barracks, a tribunal, a prison, a local Institut Pasteur, three dispensaries and so on. Meanwhile, Léopoldville had been given a major boost with the opening in 1898 of the Matadi–Léo railway, which bypassed the cataracts on the Congo. Léopoldville drained a much larger chunk of territory than its AEF counterpart. It did not make sense to manage such a huge colony out of Boma near the mouth of the river, and in 1923 Léo became the capital of the Belgian Congo. It took a few years for this administrative decision to be implemented. This attracted a further influx of migrants, initially house servants and low-level employees of the Belgian administration. Several thousand workers were coerced to come to Léo in the mid-1920s to build the new docks along the river.[32]

Brazza, the capital of an underpopulated and resource-poor colony, remained a sleepy colonial city populated by French civil servants and their house staff, missionaries, soldiers, traders and employees of a few private enterprises, while Léo thrived as the commercial hub of a wealthy colony, housing more than 600 companies by 1928. Many of these were small family-owned businesses but there were also large employers with up to 1,000 workers, such as the Lever palm oil company and the Otraco transportation utility.

In 1921, around the time that SIV_{cpz} emerged into HIV-1, only 7,000 people lived in Brazza, and 16,000 in Léo. Ten years later, Brazzaville, the largest city of AEF, had only 18,000 inhabitants while Léopoldville already had 40,000. As a proxy for colonial economic development, in 1931 there were 800 Europeans in Brazza versus 3,000 in Léo. The twin cities were followed by Douala (22,000), Bangui (17,000), Yaoundé and Libreville (6,500 each), and Pointe-Noire (5,000). Other agglomerations were in essence large villages rather than small towns. All told, less than 5% of the population of central Africa lived in an urban environment. But after this inauspicious start, the urbanisation process accelerated dramatically. Just twenty years later (1951), Douala had 81,500 inhabitants, Brazzaville 80,000, Bangui 65,000, Yaoundé 30,000, Pointe-Noire 28,500, Libreville 18,000 and Port-Gentil 11,000. Léopoldville was already in a category of its own with 222,000 inhabitants.[23,26,33–35]

Too many males

There is nothing more conducive to large-scale prostitution than bringing together, in a given location, a much larger number of young adult males than young women. Male sexual drive is highest in the twenty-five years after adolescence, and if monogamous or polygamous unions are not possible because of a lack of potential partners, sex will be purchased. This has been proven time and again, from the American military bases in Asia to colonial Nairobi and the mining areas of northern Rhodesia and South Africa. We will now examine how colonial policies created a gross gender imbalance on the banks of the Congo River, in the binational conurbation that attracted hundreds of thousands of migrants from the very areas inhabited by the *P.t. troglodytes* chimpanzee, including at least one who was infected with SIV_{cpz}/HIV-1.

During the first decades of the Belgian colony, its policy was to discourage the migration of women to the cities, and only the men needed to fill vacant positions in the private or public sectors were welcome. Any concentration of unemployed men was seen as a security risk. Workers lived in labour camps and the lack of facilities discouraged them from bringing their families along. After obtaining the administrative authorisation required for any travel more than fifty kilometres away from their village (*passeport de mutation*), adult men needed a permit to live in Léo (*permis de séjour*) and another to be employed (*carte de travail*). There were regular police checks to find illegal residents, and every adult residing in Léo was fingerprinted. Needless to say, serious crimes were uncommon. An office of manpower administered work permits and found work for the jobless. Unemployment was minimal (<1% in 1946), as those without a position had to leave, and new migrants were accepted only if workers were required by employers.[36-38]

Women's migration to the cities was restricted on 'moral' grounds. With prostitution being common in the urban areas, administrative and religious authorities tried to hamper the exodus of women from the villages for fear that they would also be tempted, apparently not understanding that these very policies were driving prostitution. It was hard to obtain a mutation passport for a woman. The evolution of Léo's population can be seen in Figure 5. In 1929, there were 26,932 adult males, 7,460 adult females, and only 2,662 children. Father Joseph Van Wing, a Jesuit who wrote copiously about Kongo culture, described Léo as 'clean but joyless and infinitely gloomy because of the dearth of children, a camp rather than a village'. Eventually, restrictions on the movement of women were relaxed, but the very nature of these booming cities perpetuated the imbalance. Young unmarried men were more likely than others to try their luck in the developing urban areas, while married men would go alone at first, get a steady job, find proper housing and accumulate savings before asking their families to follow them.[17,39,40]

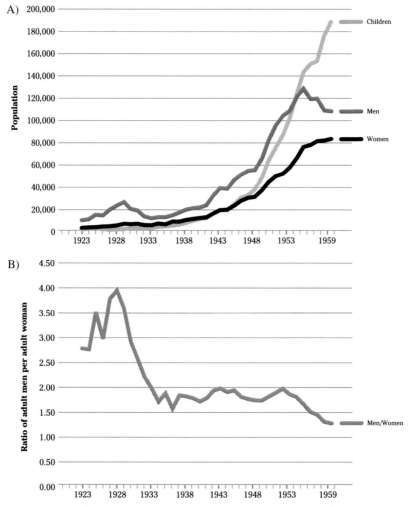

Figure 5 Léopoldville's population, 1923–59: (a) adult men, adult women and children; (b) ratio of adult men to adult women.

The economic depression of the early 1930s reverberated in central Africa, as the price of minerals and agricultural products fell dramatically. Some large companies sent back to the old continent three-quarters of their European employees and more or less the same happened to African workers. The Belgian administration preferred to return thousands of jobless men, especially the unmarried, to rural areas where they would be less likely to defy the colonial order. By 1934, the number of women had remained stable while the number of adult men had dwindled by half. Following the economic recovery and increased production during WWII, Léopoldville had 38,940 adult men, 20,234 adult women and 19,967 children in 1944. But Léo was not yet the melting pot it later became: three-quarters of its population belonged to the Bakongo cluster of ethnic groups, from the region downriver or from the northern part of Angola, while only 5% came from the eastern half of the colony.[36,41–43]

Figure 5 shows the evolution of the male/female ratio among adults in Léo. In 1928–9, there were 3.9 men for each woman, which was a substantial improvement since in 1910 there were 10 men for each woman. The gender ratio decreased to 2.0 in 1933 and fluctuated just below 2.0 until independence. In 1942, for the very first time there was at least one child per woman on average. The flow of migrations was such that in 1946 only 11% of Léo's inhabitants had been born in the city. In 1956, this proportion had augmented to 26%.[44–46]

In Brazzaville, the government also reduced its workforce during the 1930s but many were simply transferred to Pointe-Noire where opportunities were plentiful with the construction of the port. In the AEF capital, the male/female ratio was 1.9 in 1950, similar to that of Léo, but it decreased to 1.4 in 1955, as the colonial authorities were more tolerant of female migrations, even for unmarried women. Elsewhere, the male/female ratio in 1952 was 1.25 in Bangui, 1.4 in Libreville and Port-Gentil, and 1.7 in Pointe-Noire.[34,47,48]

During WWII, the Belgian Congo made an extraordinary contribution to the war effort, to a large extent through coercive measures, especially after the Japanese conquest of parts of Asia crippled the Allies' supply of rubber and tin. More wild rubber was gathered than during the EIC era, and the Congolese were forced to work for the colony 120 days per year. The production of copper, tin, zinc and manganese more than doubled, while that of uranium increased tenfold, all for export to the US and Britain. This would eventually allow Belgium to emerge from the conflict debt-free, unlike the other victors.[49,50]

Cut off from Europe, the colony needed to produce locally goods which until then had been imported. This generated an economic boom and the development of light industries. These processes accelerated the peopling of Léo, whose population doubled from 47,000 in 1940 to 96,000 in 1945, and doubled again to 191,000 in 1950. The exodus of men towards the urban areas, where they enjoyed a relative freedom, was also driven by the compulsory crops imposed on rural populations. Most of the Belgian war effort was actually borne out by poor and rural African women. Many migrants intended to stay in Léo only temporarily, but eventually settled permanently as life in the villages now seemed dull and monotonous. The intense promiscuity that resulted was seen by the missionaries as having a deleterious impact on traditional moral values. Small houses built for four persons would hold twelve people on average. The strict separation between men and women vanished.[45,51,52]

Meanwhile, the AEF under Félix Éboué, the black governor from Guyana, grandson of a slave, rallied de Gaulle's France Libre in 1940, and the population of Brazza swelled from 22,000 to 33,500. To affirm its independence symbolically from Britain and the US, de Gaulle made Brazzaville the capital of France Libre for two years. More than 85% of Free French soldiers that crossed the Sahara under general Leclerc to attack Italian positions in Libya were Africans from the AEF. The neglected Cinderella colony helped save the honour of France, creating a moral debt. At the Brazzaville 1944 conference, de Gaulle promised Africans more civil rights. The numerous post-war French governments had no choice but to respect this commitment, and forced labour was abolished in 1946. Major investments were made to develop the infrastructure of Brazzaville, including a new airport, modernisation of its river port, hydro-electricity, a water treatment plant, a stadium, large administrative buildings, etc. But as in the Belgian Congo, there was a bottleneck in the educational system. In 1952–3, there were only 1,895 secondary school students in AEF, compared to 122,951 in primary schools. The French government started giving scholarships to a small number of Africans, who were sent to France to complete secondary school and go on to university. When these countries became independent, they could at least count on a small intellectual elite.[48,53]

In retrospect, the impact of WWII was mostly psychological. The Africans had seen that their French and Belgian masters were not all-powerful, that the Europeans could behave in a way that was far from their proclaimed ideal of civilisation and that European societies were divided rather than a homogeneous block. The independence of India sent a strong signal that colonial domination was not necessarily for ever. And anger grew against the blatant racism underlying colonialism. This came as no surprise to France and Belgium, whose governments in exile had vetoed the use of African troops to liberate the motherland, knowing full well that this would alter the sense of inferiority that was essential to the survival of the colonial system.

On the other side of the Congo, the Belgians, although reluctant to grant any kind of political autonomy, made day-to-day life easier for the Congolese and started to consider that one of the colony's missions was to improve the living conditions of the natives. Governor Pierre Ryckmans, who had driven the war effort, understood that the patience of the Congolese had been stretched to the limit and a more benevolent attitude was imperative. Small-scale revolts, mutinies and labour conflicts during WWII had indicated that a wind of change was about to blow. Forced labour was abolished, African trade unions were permitted and minimum wages set. Schools, maternity hospitals and dispensaries were erected throughout the colony. Perhaps due to a gradual change in the type of manpower needed by industry (more specialised and skilled than in the early days when a pair of biceps sufficed), large employers realised that it was in their interest to stabilise their workers' situation by facilitating familial reunification.[49-50]

The amount of decent urban housing was increased through a massive construction effort, and loans were made available to help people buy houses. From 1945, electricity, hitherto reserved for the Europeans, was distributed in the African sectors of Léo. Starting in 1953, family allowances were provided to married workers so that they could afford to bring their wives and children to the cities. There, up to 80% of adult men were wage earners who benefited from these allowances if their children lived with them. Urbanisation having caused hyperinflation in the value of bridewealth, leading some men to delay the age of marriage, large companies instituted a loan programme for their employees, to help them pay the bridewealth. Despite these measures, there were so many male migrants that the gender imbalance persisted. The population of Léo added 25,000 new inhabitants each year (compared to 3,500 per year in Brazza), to reach 477,000 by 1960 versus only 120,000 in Brazza and 80,000 in Yaoundé. The European population of the Belgian Congo also expanded considerably, reaching 113,000 in 1958, with one third living in Léo, one third in the Katanga province and one third in the rest of the country.[39,48,50,54]

The post-war period saw the emergence in Léo and Brazza of a vibrant urban popular culture dominated by rumba music, a process facilitated by the extraordinary proliferation of bars of all kinds: one per 651 adults in Brazza, and one per 947 adults in Léo. This had followed the abolition in the early 1930s of restrictions on the sale of alcohol to natives. In 1946, Emmanuel Capelle, the Léopoldville district officer, estimated that up to 25% of income was spent on beer. In 1954, there were no fewer than 315 bars in Léo, up from about 100 ten years earlier. The triad of music, beer and dance were the pillars underlying the party atmosphere of Léo, in which the *ndumbas* (free women) were major actors, along with musicians and their bands like Papa Wendo, Joseph Kabasele's African Jazz and Franco's OK Jazz. Free women and musicians were positioning themselves, consciously or not, outside the colonial order whereby everyone in the cities needed to have a well-defined occupation.[36]

The most successful free women became bar owners, now selling beer rather than their bodies. Bars became focal points for opponents to colonialism, a place where they could discuss in Lingala without Europeans minding. Patrice Lumumba, the Congo's future prime minister, spent a lot of time building support in the bars of Léopoldville and Stanleyville. In the early 1950s, the income of wage earners in Léo increased quickly and became equivalent to that in AEF and British colonies. The gross national product of the Belgian Congo shot up by a staggering 57% between 1950 and 1954.[54–59]

The particular situation in Léopoldville with regard to the surplus of adult men over adult women, presumably the strongest driver of prostitution, is evident in the data gathered in 1955 through a census of a representative fraction of the population of the Belgian Congo (a sample of 10% in rural and 15% in urban areas). In Léopoldville (population: 272,954), for adults the male/female ratio was 1.72. In other large cities, this ratio was 1.24 in Elisabethville (population: 140,104), 1.25 in Stanleyville (72,237), 1.16 in Jadotville (64,937), 1.60 in Matadi (54,840), 1.32 in Luluabourg (43,341), 1.26 in Coquilhatville (30,542), 1.27 in Bukavu (30,296) and 1.24 in Boma (24,906), the only city located close to areas inhabited by the *P.t. troglodytes* source of HIV-1. Of course, in rural areas the opposite was seen: a surplus of women. Figure 6 illustrates the sex and age distribution of Léopoldville's population at the time of this census.[60,61]

The distribution of men according to marital status in Léo was radically different from the rest of the country. For the whole Belgian Congo, 24% of men aged sixteen years or over had never been married, while 3% were widowed and another 3% divorced. In Léo, 42% of adult men were unmarried, 1% widowed and 2% divorced.

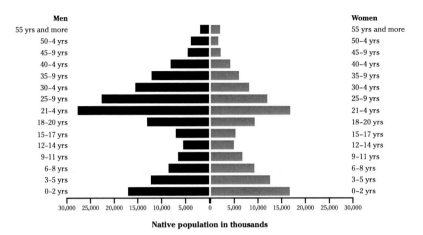

Figure 6 Age pyramids of Léopoldville in 1955.

Prostitution involved mostly unmarried or divorced men and women and the gender imbalance was even more marked if married people were excluded. In the unmarried/divorced category, there were 50,659 men and 9,344 women in Léo, for a 5.4 ratio. By comparison, in Elisabethville, the second largest city, there were 9,537 unmarried or divorced men, and 2,875 unmarried or divorced women, for a 3.3 ratio. In the early 1950s, Léopoldville was the city in central Africa with the highest proportion of adult men not living with a spouse, twice as high as in Usumbura, and three times higher than in Elisabethville. The stable overall male/female ratio in Léo in the 1950s, when the city's population was doubling every five years, masked a much higher ratio among the unmarried portion of the population and implied a dramatic increase in the absolute number of men not living with a female spouse, and thus of potential clients for sex workers.[60,62,63]

Furthermore, at the time it was generally considered unwise for a man to marry outside his own ethnic group, and the shortage of women was worse in some of the tribes, such as the Basuku and the Bayaka. These two ethnic groups were migrant workers who would walk all the way to Léo (two or three weeks to get there, two or three weeks to come back), where they spent six to nine months before returning to their villages where the women stayed. In 1955, there were 9.4 Bayaka men and 16 Basuku men in Léo for each woman of the same tribe. Conversely, the Baluba, Bapoto, Bakula, Batetela and Basonge had, against all odds, an excess of adult females and were certainly overrepresented among the free women. The differences between ethnic groups were even more extraordinary when looking only at the currently unmarried. There were 2.5, 1.9 and 1.2 unmarried women for each unmarried man among the Bapoto, Basonge and Batetela respectively. For the Baluba and Bakula, the situation was complicated: an excess of males among the bachelors, but 3 to 5 women for each man among the divorced or widowed. At the other extreme, 47 unmarried Bayaka men competed for each unmarried woman. For the Basuku, this ratio was infinite: there were 3,070 unmarried men, and not a single unmarried woman! There must have been a corresponding heterogeneity in the ethnic distribution of men and women involved in the sex trade.[64]

As a proxy for the cumulative incidence of STDs which often cause infertility, 35% of women aged forty-five years or over living in Léo in 1955 had never had a child, compared to 20% for the whole country. It is remarkable that the proportion of infertile women was lower among the younger cohorts: only 16% of those aged twenty-five to thirty-four had never given birth. This might reflect a higher incidence of STDs in the distant past, and perhaps a preferential migration towards Léopoldville of women repudiated by their husbands because they could not produce offspring. Prostitution was driving infertility but infertility was also driving prostitution.[60]

History then accelerated the urbanisation process. Around the time of independence, the number of jobless men in Léo increased dramatically. In 1955, only 6% of male adults were unemployed. In the years immediately before independence, in the context of strong nationalist fervour, Belgian authorities relaxed the previously stringent restrictions on the movements of individuals and the unemployment rate swelled to 19% in 1958 and 29% by the end of 1959, a process made worse by an economic recession. The Belgian government tried to repatriate the redundant workers to rural areas, especially after the anticolonial riots of January 1959. Cash bonuses were offered to the unemployed who chose to go back to their home villages. These measures did not work, as political events were unfolding much faster than anybody had predicted. Five days after the country became independent on 30 June 1960, a mutiny broke out among rank-and-file soldiers, which spread like wildfire. Chaos ensued. Following massive migrations to the capital, the closure of several companies and the departure of many Europeans, the unemployment rate shot up to 49% at the end of 1960.[45,60,62,65]

Throughout the post-independence troubles, Léopoldville remained rather peaceful and safe. The population of its peripheral areas increased eleven-fold over just two years, from 31,458 in 1959 to 358,308 in 1961. Many came from the Kwilu-Kwango region, east of Léo, where an insurrection led to much instability. After paying a token fee to the traditional land owners who had been dispossessed decades earlier by the government or private companies, they occupied large tracts of land near the recently inaugurated Ndjili international airport as well as in the Kisenso, Makala and Selembao districts. Squatting was encouraged by the emerging political parties as a way of repossessing tribal land. For tens of thousands of Congolese, this was a once-in-a-lifetime opportunity to get a free, or almost free, plot of land in the capital.[45,65,66]

Thus, from a city of wage earners, many of whom worked for large companies, Léo became a city of the unemployed, who out of necessity tried to make a living in the informal sector, or became 'parasites' of relatives with a regular income. Consumer goods of all kinds were retailed in very small quantities, and the modest benefits of petty trade became a major force in the redistribution of wealth. By 1963, 70% of the income of school teachers was spent on food, and it is likely that this percentage was even higher for those without a regular income. Léopoldville was renamed Kinshasa in 1966, after the name of one of the pre-colonial villages: 'Léo' became 'Kin'. Over the decade that followed independence, its population increased three-fold, to 1.3 million in 1970, when the unemployment rate reached 70%, and doubled again to 2.7 million in 1984. It is currently thought to be somewhere between 8 and 9 million.[67–69]

The gender imbalance progressively disappeared after independence. At the end of 1967, a census in Kinshasa showed that the male/female ratio was near unity for those under the age of thirty, while above this threshold there were 1.45 men for each woman. This normalisation of the sex ratio was related to two factors. First, more and more of the inhabitants of Kinshasa were born locally, attenuating the effect of the preferential migration of males. Second, many of the recent arrivals had fled their own region due to civil strife, and in such circumstances there was less of a difference between men and women, in contrast with the earlier economic migrations where the pull factor was stronger on men. These forces implied that eventually the sex ratio of the overall population of Kinshasa would get close to one, which it did. In Brazzaville, this

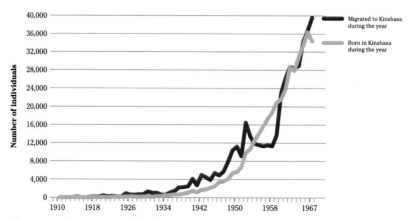

Figure 7 Migrations and births in Léopoldville–Kinshasa.

ratio reached unity in 1974, and remained close to equilibrium thereafter.[46,70–72]

The graphic in Figure 7 illustrates the fluctuating patterns of migration into Kinshasa as well as its relationship to the number of people born in the city. It was based on the 1967 survey, and therefore those migrants who did not stay or died were not counted (which means that the number of migrants in earlier years was substantially underestimated compared to more recent periods). It shows the strong migrations experienced during and after WWII, a temporary decrease during the recession of the late 1950s, and then a huge increase immediately after independence. During these same periods the number of births in Kinshasa increased steadily so that by the mid-1950s it was about equal to the number of migrations.

A short journey

The links between Brazzaville and Léopoldville have been so strong for such a long time that they are in essence two components of a single conurbation, and this should be taken into account when we assemble the puzzle at the end of this book. Their geographic proximity is illustrated in the satellite photograph shown in Figure 8. At this point, the Congo is six kilometres wide. Most of the intercity traffic was carried by a company called FIMA, from the names of its two Italian owners. FIMA operated a dozen boats of different sizes, including a

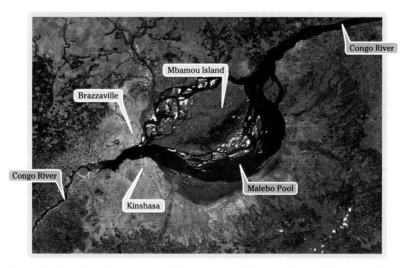

Figure 8 Satellite photograph of Kinshasa and Brazzaville, early twenty-first century.
From the NASA Visible Earth catalogue (http://visibleearth.nasa.gov).

large one that could take automobiles, built by the Léopoldville ship-yard. A regular ticket cost 25 francs, and there was a never-ending queue at the counter from early morning till mid-afternoon, with two or three departures each hour. In addition, it was possible to cross the Congo in dugout canoes to visit relatives, trade various goods, avoid payment of taxes or conscription, be forgotten for a while after a brush with the law, etc. One just had to hire a fisherman for an hour.[73,74]

During the post-war era, for a musician to be considered truly successful, he had to perform regularly on both sides of the river, and popular music, which was completely out of the control of the European colonists, became a further unifying factor between the twin cities. Starting in 1949, football games between sponsored teams of Léopoldville and Brazzaville were held regularly, and thousands of supporters could travel to the other side to cheer on their own team. Ideas were also exchanged, and the relative freedom and less blatant racism of Brazzaville led many visitors from Léo to realise that their own situation was no longer acceptable. Some of these migrations were more permanent, and already in the post-war years Léo had the largest population of Moyen-Congo nationals after Brazzaville. The extent of this interpenetration was revealed in times of crisis. In August 1964, in the midst of a dispute with the leftist government of Congo-Brazzaville, the Tshombe government of Congo-Léopoldville forcibly expelled from its capital all nationals of the former country. Over just a few days, 100,000 individuals crossed the river to the safety of Brazzaville. Later, as the economic situation of Zaire deteriorated during Mobutu's corrupt and incompetent dictatorship, mass migrations occurred mostly the other way. By the end of the 1980s 300,000 Zaireans were thought to be living in Brazzaville.[73]

Meanwhile in Cameroun

There, the largest city had always been the port of Douala. Possibly because it was a mandated territory, there was little attempt to limit the movement of women to the cities. Compared to Yaoundé, Douala's demographic boom occurred earlier, immediately after WWII. Its population stabilised around 40,000 in 1936–46, and then shot up to 100,000 in the early 1950s and to 120,000 in 1957. The male/female ratio varied between 1.2 and 1.35 during WWII, increasing to 1.7 during the post-war period when Douala attracted many male migrants, but quickly decreased to 1.2 in 1958.[75]

Yaoundé was established by the Germans in 1889 as a trading post. In 1916, it was the meeting point of the French and British armies that took Kamerun from the Germans. Five years later, Yaoundé rather than Douala was chosen as the political capital of Cameroun Français, because it was more central, cooler and more comfortable for Europeans, but also because it was deemed safer should the Germans try to return. While Douala remained the economic metropolis, Yaoundé became a quiet city of civil servants, with only 6,500 inhabitants in 1933. From 29,000 in 1952, its population increased more rapidly with the post-war economic boom, to 54,000 inhabitants five years later. There was a large influx of men, while the women followed a few years later. The male/female ratio was as high as 3.1 in 1955, quickly declining to 1.3 in 1957. After Cameroun became independent, the population of Yaoundé increased from 70,000 in 1960 to 300,000 twenty-five years later, while its male/female ratio remained around 1.2.[75–76]

Thus, in all urban centres located near the habitat of the *P.t. troglodytes* chimpanzee, a gender imbalance resulted from the population policies of the colonial powers, and from the very nature of these booming towns which attracted male migrants in search of a better life. This excess of males was more severe, for a longer period of time, in Léopoldville. In the next chapter we will see how various types of prostitution emerged to satisfy the sexual needs of these lonely men, the perfect breeding ground for the sexual amplification of HIV-1.

6 | *The oldest trade*

Prostitution facilitates the spread of all sexually transmitted microbial agents. There is no doubt that it played a crucial role in the dissemination of HIV-1 in many parts of the world, including during the first few decades of the emerging epidemic in central Africa. In this chapter, we will review what is known about the development of prostitution (or sex work, as some prefer to call it) in the burgeoning cities located close to the natural habitat of the *P.t. troglodytes* source of SIV$_{cpz}$/HIV-1, a process that was intimately related to the urbanisation we have just examined.

The core group

Immediately after the African HIV epidemic was recognised in the mid-1980s, prostitutes and their clients were identified in many countries as the core group within which the virus is exponentially transmitted in the early stages, a process facilitated by the extraordinary prevalence of STDs among these women, which increase the efficacy of heterosexual HIV transmission. Eventually, male clients infect their subsequent female partners not involved in the sex trade, enabling the virus to move out of the core group and into the general adult population. From a concentrated epidemic, it becomes a generalised one.

It is only recently, however, that the contribution of transactional sex to the overall dynamics of HIV transmission in large African cities has been quantified, following reliable assays for detecting anti-HIV antibodies in specimens obtained from clients having just paid for sex. In Accra and Cotonou, such measures revealed that roughly three-quarters of all cases of HIV infection among men had been acquired from prostitutes. In West Africa, HIV prevalence in the adult male population remains generally ≤ 3%, while it ranges between 5% and 15% among clients of sex workers and between 20% and 75% among the sex workers themselves. When HIV becomes highly prevalent, as in some

84

countries of southern Africa where 35% of adult women are HIV-infected, a lower fraction of cases of HIV in men are acquired from prostitutes because then any sexual activity becomes risky.[1–2]

The extraordinary rapidity with which HIV disseminated among sex workers was documented by chance in Nairobi, where several hundreds had been followed since 1980 for a study of chancroid, an STD which causes large and painful ulcerations of the genitalia. Specimens of serum had been kept frozen and were tested for HIV antibodies retrospectively. In 1981, only 4% of Nairobi prostitutes were HIV-infected. Just two years later, more than two-thirds of them were HIV-infected. Among men who consulted in an STD clinic, many of whom were clients of sex workers (from whom they had usually acquired their STDs), none was HIV-infected in 1980, 6% were in 1982 and 15% in 1985.[3]

What happened? The Nairobi sex workers had on average 1,400 paid intercourses per year, and condoms were rarely used. Once an initial HIV-infected client infected a first prostitute, this woman developed a high viraemia lasting a few weeks, corresponding to what is now called 'primary' HIV infection. During this period, she shed large amounts of HIV in her genital secretions, and the pathogen was transmitted to a few of her clients, who in turn developed a transient period of high viraemia. This augmented the number of HIV-infected clients who then transmitted the virus to other, previously uninfected, sex workers, further increasing the risk of transmitting HIV to subsequent clients. An extremely effective vicious circle was created.

Because of these findings, it has been long assumed that prostitution was the key determinant of the emergence of HIV in central Africa before 1981: the urbanisation and the social disruptions caused by colonisation led to urban prostitution, which then sexually amplified HIV once it had been introduced into this core group, from an initial cut hunter who had migrated to the city.

Before we review what might really have happened, I want to make a fundamental point: there are many levels of prostitution, loosely defined as the exchange of sex for money or gifts. The Nairobi prostitutes described above, as well as those studied in many other cities of Africa, from Kinshasa to Kigali and Abidjan to Accra, are at one end of the spectrum, and constitute the high-risk group. They have no income other than from prostitution. Because they are older and less attractive, they need to service several clients a day to make ends meet.

They live from day to day and are unable to save much. Each client pays as little as \$0.50–1.00 per intercourse and the transaction takes half an hour, sometimes less. They cannot afford to refuse any client. These women accept themselves as prostitutes, and do not care whether the rest of society sees them as such. Poverty aside, this is similar to the prostitution that has existed for a long time in the red light districts of Amsterdam and other European cities.

At the other end of the spectrum, in the low-risk group, is the college student who has sex with two older men each month, to help pay her tuition fees. These men have sex repeatedly with the same girl, once or twice a month, over a long period of time, a grey zone between concomitant partnerships and soft prostitution. The risk of that girl acquiring HIV from one of her sugar daddies is low. If the prevalence of HIV among men is 5–7%, as in mid-1980s Kinshasa, there is a high probability that none of her two regular and exclusive clients is actually HIV-infected, and the girl's risk would be zero, until she is exposed to other men.

Also in this low-risk category, which was the rule rather than the exception in central African cities from the 1930s to the 1950s, a 'free woman' would have, say, two or three regular patrons with whom she would spend several hours during each visit, not only having sex but also talking, washing their clothes and cooking. If HIV prevalence among clients of free women in colonial Léopoldville was 0.1%, and assuming that each free woman had on average three regular patrons, then for 99.7% of free women the risk of acquiring HIV would have been zero. The initial SIV_{cpz}-infected client may infect the free woman with whom he is regularly having sex, and she may then infect another of her regular patrons with whom she is having a concomitant relationship. But for the virus to spread outside this closed unit, the HIV-infected man must have sex with another free woman, or the infected free woman must develop a relationship with new clients. So the potential for some amplification of a sexually transmitted virus existed, but the vicious circle would have needed a long time to develop, or may not have developed at all.

In between these extremes, there is a heterogeneous group of mid-level prostitutes, whose risk of acquiring HIV is higher than the free women but much lower than the old sex workers from a Nairobi slum. This category includes the high-class prostitute who picks up one or two rich clients per week, with whom she will spend the whole night, or the woman who has another full-time occupation (say, as a bartender) but complements her meagre income with a few clients.

Hospitality and housekeeping

How much prostitution, loosely defined, was there in central Africa in the first half of the twentieth century? Information about prostitution in AEF, Cameroun and the Belgian Congo can be retrieved from the few books and articles published on the topic, from the annual reports of the health systems and, for Cameroun, from the annual reports sent to the League of Nations and the UN. The quality of the information varied. It is easy to find information about the regulations and laws concerning prostitution, but much less about how these rules were implemented in practice. Reports of the French colonial health systems contained a section on 'social diseases', which included STDs (syphilis, gonorrhoea and others). The authors sometimes added comments about prostitution, which must be viewed with caution given the overtly racist nature of these reports before WWII.

Did prostitution exist before colonisation? As might be expected from the diversity of ethnic groups and cultures, there was substantial heterogeneity in sexual customs. Observers writing about Cameroun and Gabon noted that the status of women was deplorable. Becoming a prostitute, as this concept is usually understood, implied a degree of freedom which simply did not exist initially. In some ethnic groups, a woman was considered property, for which a bridewealth payment had been made to her family. The husband, especially if polygamous, could dispose of his property as he wished. One of the wives could be asked to have sex with a friend, a relative or visitor, often for payment to the husband in cash or in kind but sometimes for free, in what corresponded more to 'sexual hospitality' than prostitution.[4–7]

In the Belgian Congo, early social scientists described traditional forms of prostitution among the Baluba of the Kasaï region. Among the Babunda and Bapende of the Kwango region, east of Léo, fifteen to twenty young men might get together to hire a prostitute (*mobanda*) for up to two months, and payment (in rolls of salt) was made to the girl's mother. The young woman would do this only once in her life; it was not considered dishonourable and would not decrease her chances of getting married later. In other areas, a polygamous man could 'rent' one of his wives to another man for a predetermined period of time, for a fee.

Among the Baholoholo of the western shore of Lake Tanganyika, some villages were specialised in prostitution. These practices were uncommon, but the concept of romantic love was the exception rather than the rule. Missionaries identified the development of Christian-type families as a top priority.[8–9]

A different type of prostitution emerged with the arrival of the white man. As early as 1884–5, during Brazza's second expedition to the pool, his own brother Giacomo and another Italian man took 'wives' within days of their arrival, paying five francs per month in local commodities. In the first decades of colonial rule, up to 95% of the European population in central Africa was male, and they could easily find concubines, in exchange for money or other material advantages for the women or their relatives. A well-known euphemism in the early history of the Belgian Congo was the *ménagère* (housekeeper), who in practice provided sexual services, in addition to cooking, doing the laundry, etc. In Brazzaville, many Europeans also sought comfort from their *ménagères*, mostly Gabonese women who had been in contact with Europeans for a longer period than those living in the interior and spoke a bit of French.[4,10–13]

Father Arthur Vermeersch, a Jesuit theologian, described the *ménagère* as 'the illegitimate companion, hired by the month at 25 francs, or for the whole term according to some pre-determined fee'. Europeans vacating their posts would provide newcomers with a *ménagère*, along with the house and furniture, while others were sent by the village chief, who got paid for it. Once this deal had been done, the woman kept the payments received from the white man, in cash or in kind. Some *ménagères* enjoyed this new-found power and relative wealth. Vermeersch observed: 'In the kingdom of the blind, the one-eyed man is king; in the country of the negresses, the *ménagère* is queen.' Some Europeans, in line with local customs, entertained more than one *ménagère*. Of course, the missionaries disapproved of such behaviour. Vermeersch, one of the few prominent Catholics who dared to criticise publicly the leopoldian system, saw this form of prostitution as one part of a larger process in which European colonists were suddenly freed from all the social and moral restrictions of the societies in which they had grown up, and which led to the atrocities of the EIC period. He probably had a valid point.[14]

A European colonist could easily recruit another *ménagère* if no longer satisfied by the current one. And a *ménagère* may, over the years, have sequential relationships with several Europeans, as they left the colony at the end of their term. Women in search of a patron would move temporarily to Boma and Matadi, where the boats arrived from Antwerp. It would have been very much against the *ménagère*'s interests to have concomitant sexual relationships with African men: giving birth to a black baby would bring her current lucrative relationship to an abrupt end.

This phase in the history of prostitution in central Africa probably played no direct role in the emergence of HIV-1. It would have been highly unlikely for any European man to have acquired SIV_{cpz} while hunting or butchering a chimpanzee and to start a chain of transmission. And even if HIV-1 had been introduced by one of the *ménagères*, who perhaps had cut up some chimpanzee meat, the rate of partner exchange was too low for a sexually driven epidemic to develop. However, this phenomenon played an indirect role, by setting an example. For many African women, it became apparent that instead of staying in their native areas and having unpaid intercourse with a husband they disliked, who had made a deal with their own relatives, they could move into these new cities and out of their traditional status of female subordination. While still having sex with men they did not like, they at least got some income out of it and lived freely once these paying partners had returned to Europe. Furthermore, despite vigorous attempts by Catholic and Protestant missionaries, the colonists could not in all conscience repress prostitution among the natives when large numbers of them entertained similar relationships.

Thousands of mulattoes were born of these loveless unions between Europeans and their *ménagères*. Their fate would depend upon recognition by their father. About 10% were recognised, in which case the fathers would take them back to Belgium at the end of their term, and they would never see their mothers again. The others stayed with their mothers who might have been given a small sum of money for that purpose. The poorest would end up in specialised orphanages set up by Catholic missions. Mulattoes were treated as Africans by the colonial segregationist system, while being rejected by the Congolese as foreigners.[15–17]

It was not until about 1910, when small cities were created in which the African male population was much larger than the female, that prostitution appeared in which African men were having sex with African women for money or gifts. These women were usually unmarried or divorced. For some of them, becoming a prostitute was a kind of liberation. They would move to the cities, away from family and societal constraints and values, free to behave as they wished. To this day, it is noteworthy that the Lingala word *ndumba* can mean either a prostitute, or simply an unmarried woman no longer dependent on her relatives. In Congolese French, this became *femme libre*, a free woman, who had broken away from the control of her guardians, whether husband or kin, and whose life depended on her own intelligence and resourcefulness.

How did soon-to-be-free women manage to reach the city, given the stringent regulations on female migrations described in the preceding chapter? Some convinced a man to marry them and ditched their husband as soon as they got their papers. In other cases, a fake marriage sufficed. The woman showed up at the district office and produced false documents attesting that a bridewealth had been paid. It was possible to get married without the husband being present.[18]

From these early days, the practice of prostitution in central Africa differed from what was commonplace in Europe. Apart from a few cases where husbands benefited from one of their wives selling sex (they showed up at the European customer's house, pretending to be angry and asking for compensation to avoid a scandal), free women had no pimps, either in the 1920s or at any subsequent time during the colonial era or after decolonisation. Until 1960, there were no brothels and clients were not picked up on the street. Male clients visited prostitutes where they lived, and the women provided more than sexual services. This was a low-risk type of prostitution, as defined earlier, or semi-prostitution as it was called by some authors.[4]

Venus's curse

Sexually transmitted diseases have long been recognised as a marker of sexual promiscuity, often associated with transactional sex. Much later, it was understood that these common infections greatly enhanced the efficacy of heterosexual transmission of HIV, and that prostitutes and their clients were at the centre of the transmission dynamics of both the traditional STD and the novel one, HIV/AIDS. Here we will see that prostitution and STDs were intricately related at the time that HIV-1 managed to emerge in central Africa.

In the early days of the colonial health system, STDs were the number two priority, after sleeping sickness. They represented a serious health hazard for Europeans, as the treatments for syphilis were not very effective. Furthermore, STDs were seen as a threat to the demographic stability of the colonies. Untreated gonorrhoea or chlamydia in women can lead to obstruction of the tubes and infertility. Syphilis among pregnant women often causes a spontaneous abortion, premature delivery or stillbirth. The colonisers needed to guarantee the long-term availability of the African manpower needed for public works and private companies, and were very concerned about the declining population of Gabon, parts of the Belgian Congo and other areas. Thus, although not very effective, efforts were made early on to control the spread of STDs.

In Léopoldville, Europeans drove prostitution in its early stages, especially the *petits Blancs* ('little Whites'): the mechanics, bakers, butchers and other small traders. As early as May 1909 and again in November 1913, edicts regulating prostitution were issued, aimed at protecting Europeans through the registration, regular medical examination and compulsory in-hospital treatment of prostitutes found to have a venereal disease. The approach used in Belgium was transplanted into its new colony but few if any of these regulations were actually implemented on a significant scale. In Boma, the hospital's 1909 report mentions that thirteen prostitutes came twice a week for STD screening (however, later reports noted that it was difficult to enforce this regulation and that very few prostitutes could be examined regularly). The same year, the medical officer in charge of the Hôpital des Blancs in Léopoldville complained about the deplorable moral situation, noting that more than half of the ninety European civil servants in Léo were currently being treated for syphilis. In 1921, an edict made the treatment of STDs compulsory, and the patients could be forced to remain in hospital until the end of treatment. This was reinforced ten years later, when another edict made the treatment and reporting of a number of infectious diseases (including STDs) not only compulsory but also free.[4,12,19–23]

In Cameroun, as early as 1921, it was recognised that prostitution was a major factor behind STD transmission. European-type prostitution was thought to exist only in the port city of Douala. The following year, perhaps more realistically, it was acknowledged that prostitution existed in other urban centres as well, often involving women who had paid back the bridewealth to their husbands, thus becoming free and independent. In 1923, the commissioner issued a decree regulating prostitution. Prostitutes had to be registered at the local police station and provide information about where sexual services were dispensed. A sanitary carnet was required, and check-ups were to be done at 14:00 every Saturday in designated dispensaries. Brothels needed to be author-ised by the administration, which was akin to legalising prostitution. Fines (1 to 50 francs) or jail terms (one to five days) were to be imposed on offenders. However, just a few years later, in a small book about the 'venereal danger' in Cameroun, a public health official noted that the regulation of prostitution was rather ill-advised and ineffective, given the large number of sex workers. In its first post-war report to the United Nations in 1947, France formally had to answer more than 200 questions, one of which concerned prostitution. The law of 1923 with its weekly check-ups was mentioned, but without any information about whether this was actually implemented. There was not a single brothel in Cameroun at that time.[5,24–27]

In 1909, sanitary check-ups were made compulsory for prostitutes in Brazzaville, and in 1912 about fifty showed up each week. The 1927 report for French overseas territories mentioned that in Brazzaville sex workers had to go for a weekly examination and those with an STD were to be hospitalised during treatment in order to limit transmission. Interestingly, the regulations were at least partially implemented: in 1931, serological surveillance of prostitutes showed that 52% had a positive 'syphilis' serology. As will be explained later, it is possible that some (or many) of these positive tests were caused by another disease, yaws, which is not sexually transmitted. In 1933, an STD clinic was opened in the Brazzaville hospital, and many of the patients were sex workers. By 1954, health officials were more pessimistic (or realistic?): prostitution was said to be flourishing so much in urban centres that any kind of control was futile.[28–33]

In 1932–3, in the Adoumas district of Gabon, the birth rate was measured at 16 per 1,000 while the overall death rate was 41 per 1,000, implying that the total population was shrinking by 2.5% each year. A similar decrease was observed in the Mimongo district next door. This was attributed to a high incidence of STDs. Antisyphilitic drugs made up half of the budget of Gabon's national pharmacy, which prompted a behavioural investigation by medical officers. A non-traditional form of prostitution was noted to have emerged during colonisation because the cost of bridewealth had increased so much that only older men could afford to marry, creating a demand from younger men for commercial sex. The cash needed to pay head taxes was also seen as a contributing factor.[34-35]

As early as 1928, as an explanation for the high incidence of syphilis and gonorrhoea, health officers in Oubangui-Chari reported that prostitution was very common in Bangui and other centres, and suggested that prostitutes should be registered and undergo weekly examinations. The 1945 report noted that prostitutes were moving between towns, following seasonal variations in demand, but that this trade was not tolerated in the villages. As a result, STDs were much less common in rural areas. Soldiers in urban centres and administrative posts were noted to be regular clients of sex workers.[36-37]

Construction of the CFCO railway became a major driver of prostitution in AEF. In Oubangui-Chari, between 1925 and 1932, 41,780 workers had been recruited, sent by boat to Brazzaville after walking all the way to Bangui. On the river boats, only 12% of the men were accompanied by their wives. In the railway workers' camps, there were eleven men for each woman. The consequence was utterly predictable: prostitution flourished in and around the many camps between Brazzaville and Pointe-Noire, and STDs became epidemic. On pay day, most of the money went to paying debts to sex workers incurred over the previous weeks.[38-41]

Prostitution in Léopoldville

Now let us get closer to the heart of the matter, the very area where HIV-1 managed to expand and diversify. Given the huge gender imbalance, large-scale prostitution appeared early in the history of Léo, and was already noted by colonial officers and Catholic missionaries as being a major problem in 1925. In 1928, out of 6,000 adult women in Léopoldville, only 358 were living with a husband. Starting in 1930 the Belgians levied a tax on the 'healthy women theoretically living alone' in what was certainly one of the most pragmatic actions ever taken with regard to prostitution. Adult women living with a spouse or with relatives were exempt from paying this tax, as were women with two or more children. In 1946, out of 28,000 adult women in Léo, around 5,000 (18%) paid the 50-franc tax, tripled to 150 francs ($3) the following year, equivalent to ten days of wages for the average worker. In Stanleyville, more than 30% of adult women paid this tax in 1945, which represented 20% of the city's total revenues.[4,11,42-47]

This fiscal category of free women not financially dependent on a man was a mixed bag and encompassed genuine prostitutes or semi-prostitutes, concubines, petty traders who made a living in the informal sector, as well as grey areas in between. The semi-prostitutes had small, changing sets of 'lovers' or clients who ordinarily gave them 'presents' in return for sexual favours granted regularly over a period of time rather than strictly cash payments in return for intermittent sexual encounters. These ongoing relationships were understood by both parties not to be exclusive, there was no intent to have children, and the parties lived in separate residences.[45]

The colonial administration was tolerant towards prostitution, because it facilitated its day-to-day operations. Initially, many men were brought to the cities as workers for a limited time, and it was easier to send them back to their villages after a year or two if they had remained alone and satisfied their sexual needs with a local free woman, than if they had a wife and kids established in the city. The gender imbalance described in the previous chapter, and the ensuing urban prostitution, were parts of a system which required a high degree of workforce mobility. The same mobility was expected of Europeans, typically hired for a renewable three-year term.

By the mid-1940s, Emmanuel Capelle, the territorial officer in charge of Léopoldville, described its moral situation as 'pathetic': given the huge surplus of males, the market for commercial sex clearly favoured the women, making it a sellers' market. In her research about the women of Léopoldville in 1945, Suzanne Comhaire-Sylvain, a Haitian anthropologist married to a Belgian, noted that prostitution was not limited to single women, and that some married women or teenagers still living with their parents sold sex on a part-time basis to supplement the family income. In Elisabethville, prostitution was also rampant; many recruits had been introduced to the trade by their own mothers, sisters and even grandmothers, all of whom benefited from the substantial income generated by this activity.[44,48,49]

Henri Bongolo, a former sergeant of the Force Publique who served in the medical unit that went all the way to Burma during the war, was one of the first Congolese administrators of Léopoldville. In 1947, he described how everything to be done in the capital was expected to be associated with some kind of remuneration: 'there is no longer anything which is sentimental or disinterested: commerce everywhere'. At the same time, Father Van Wing, a Jesuit scholar, noted that 'producing and earning money had become the main leitmotiv, in urban as well as rural areas' and that 'the importance given to spiritual matters decreased in proportion to the increase in the love of financial gain'. Reading this was a revelation, for I had long thought that this attitude, so widespread in the Kinshasa I had known for more than thirty years, was a by-product of the materialism of the Mobutu regime. Not at all![50,51]

Bongolo described how the customary institution of dowry, which in essence represented a pact between two families guaranteeing the stability of the union between a man and a woman, had been corrupted by money to the point where it often became a purely commercial transaction. Some families were asking up to 10,000 francs ($200) of bride-wealth to be paid in cash, a fortune for most potential candidates (a few years of wages). Why? Because such families were already getting a substantial income (600 francs per month) from their daughter selling sexual services to better-off men, including but not only Europeans, and they naturally asked for substantial compensation for a marriage that would cut off this source of income. Rather than being ashamed of their daughters selling sex, for many parents prostitution became a goal, a good way to increase the whole family's standard of living. Bongolo attributed this situation not just to women having freed themselves from their traditional customs but also to the huge surplus of men in Léopoldville, which gave women the upper hand. The status of prostitute was so attractive that married women often thought this would be a good idea for them as well. They became free women.

The development of prostitution in Léopoldville had followed tribal lines, through networking between free women in the capital and their upcountry relatives. The Baluba women were especially prominent. In 1958, a quarter of Baluba women in Léo were unmarried. In Elisabethville, at the other end of the country, Baluba made up 26% of the population but accounted for 43% of the free women. Thirty years later, university students in the same city were still calling prostitutes 'Mama Kasaï', from the region of origin of the Baluba.[52–53]

In the only document of the colonial era that attempted to quantify prostitution, public health physicians described a programme for the control of STDs in Léopoldville. Demand for transactional sex was driven by the gender imbalance, aggravated by the custom of observing a long period of marital abstinence after a woman gave birth (*walé*), a traditional family planning measure. The supply was driven by the income of sex workers being two to three times higher than that of other women. Clinics provided STD screening and treatment. A card was stamped to prove that the free woman had attended the regular mandatory screening. Since the clinic was located in the Barumbu district of eastern Léo, the card became known as the Carte de Barumbu.[54-55]

Through these registration and screening efforts, the medical officers estimated that there were 5,000 to 6,000 women in Léo for whom prostitution was the sole source of income, to which should be added an indeterminate number of part-time sex workers (married women, students living with their parents). In the first nine months of 1958, the two STD clinics registered 4,321 *femmes libres*, presumed to be prostitutes, so the 5,000–6,000 total estimate does not seem far-fetched. In other words, almost 10% of the 60,000 adult women in Léo were involved in the sex trade, and there were 50 sex workers per 1,000 adult men. By comparison, in the early 1990s there were between 10 and 20 prostitutes per 1,000 adult men in Cotonou, Yaoundé, Kisumu (Kenya) and Ndola (Zambia). In other words, in the late 1950s there were up to five times more sex workers *per capita* in Léopoldville than in other African cities today.[56,57]

The voice of Congo

In 1945 the monthly *La Voix du Congolais* was launched, the first publication in the country written by and for Congolese. It was heavily subsidised by and, according to many, subservient to colonial power. The opinions expressed were not representative of the general population, but only of the *évolués* who subscribed to the periodical. The *évolués* were the Congolese who had 'evolved' through education or assimilation and accepted European values and patterns of behaviour. They spoke French, held white-collar jobs and were primarily urban. Many articles were published concerning prostitution, which all of the (male) writers naturally abhorred. Apart from its immorality, the most deleterious impact of prostitution was a falling birth rate, which concerned not just the colonisers but the colonised as well. Traditional life had centred on the survival and prosperity of the clan rather than the individual; women who became infertile because of prostitution could no longer contribute to this important task.[18,58-62]

The writers for the *Voix du Congolais* identified multiple and interconnected causes of prostitution: the emancipation of women from their previous status as inferior human beings whose lives were controlled by their clan, a process that had been driven by conversions to Christianity; prior to this, all women were married off by their clan at a young age, even before puberty, and thus when deviant behaviour occurred it was by definition adultery rather than prostitution; migration to urban centres and the ensuing erosion of respect for ancestral customs; the behaviour of European men, many free women having started their careers with an affair with an expatriate and discovering that this type of life was far better than their traditional fate; materialism and greed, when the young women and/or their parents discovered the joy of having money to spend; the excessive price of bridewealth, which made it difficult for young men to marry and left many young women without a financially suitable husband; the proliferation of bars of all kinds; and the lack of employment opportunities for women, which was related to their illiteracy. From their discussions, it is clear that free women concentrated on two or three men, some of whom were married. They often confronted the legitimate wives, hoping that a divorce would ensue and that they would get a more regular income from the man. Having hurried intercourses with a large number of men never crossed their minds.

The solutions proposed varied considerably: increase the tax on unmarried women or eliminate it completely; make the mutation pass-port harder to get or, the opposite and probably wiser approach, allow all women into the cities to correct the male/female imbalance; fine parents who encouraged their daughters to get into prostitution; control the activities of bars where underage girls and boys should no longer be admitted; improve the educational status of women to make it easier for them to find jobs and other sources of income; and regulate the price of bridewealth. Some proposals were clearly impractical, such as expelling all unmarried women from urban centres, forcing them to take up farming, or stopping the rural exodus completely. Of course, none of their recommendations was ever implemented.

Across the river

Prostitution also developed early in the history of Brazzaville. In 1914, there were a few hundred prostitutes, mostly from the upper Congo, at least according to a Swedish missionary. Unless this estimate was exaggerated by an observer concerned with moral issues, it represented a substantial fraction of the city's population, then around 6,000. At the same time, Mgr Augouard, Brazzaville's powerful Catholic bishop, expressed concern that mulatto girls, themselves born of a peculiar form of prostitution, would end up practising the same trade as their mothers. Augouard complained that the debauchery of many colonial officers provided a terrible example for the Africans he was trying to convert to Catholicism.[12,63]

By a strange paradox, the work of Augouard and his fellow missionaries led to unexpected outcomes. Missionaries had fought to get rid of the internal domestic slavery, and they thought the fate of married women was not much better: they were some kind of marital commodity, which made it impossible for children to be raised in truly Christian families. Thus missionaries pushed hard for the emancipation of women and the abolition of polygamy, directly and through the colonial authorities, while nuns developed activities aimed at improving the status of women. Many of the traditional and repressive customs towards women were made illegal, but this new-found freedom apparently led to some degree of licentiousness. No longer forced to have sexual relations with a man selected by their kin, some women opted for something that was easier to attain than the proposed idealistic monogamous union based on love and the Ten Commandments: the trade of sexual services.[63–64]

By stepping up demand, the building of the CFCO railway fuelled prostitution in the AEF capital, while the economic depression of the 1930s increased the number of women who sought to supplement their family's income and pay their head taxes through transactional sex. Demographically, the surplus of males was more pronounced in Poto-Poto (1.68 men per woman) than in Bacongo (1.13), the other large African settlement of Brazza where, as in Léo, women were considered to have the upper hand. During the late 1940s in Poto-Poto, a district inhabited by migrants, 60% of men aged eighteen to forty were unmarried, a proportion similar to that of contemporary Léo, but only 4% of women lived alone or with other adult women, compared to 12% in Léo. As a percentage of the population, prostitutes were less numerous in Brazza, where urban prostitution was also seen to be both a cause and a consequence of infertility.[65–66]

The organisation of prostitution in Brazzaville did not differ much from that in Léo, and some of the sex workers moved back and forth between the two cities, according to which they considered the most lucrative market. Any sexually transmitted pathogen, including HIV, introduced on one side of the river would swiftly reach the other side. Higher-class prostitutes formed mutual aid associations, which conducted negotiations with bar owners and were known under various proper names: Lolita, Dollar, Élégance, Diamant. Similar associations existed in Léopoldville, under similar names: La Beauté, Les Diamants, etc. Free women were proud to show each other how much wealth, fancy clothes and jewellery they had acquired on their own from their trade. For some, it was a very lucrative business: they could bring their parents up to 5,000 francs ($100) per month, a huge amount of money at the time, and naturally fathers would not ask too many questions about the source of such a godsend.[12]

Official policies towards prostitution fluctuated over time. In 1940 it was decreed that prostitutes must not only be registered but also photographed and fingerprinted and have compulsory medical examinations. Prostitutes who refused to comply would be jailed for up to three months. Just a few years later, in the midst of WWII, officially authorised brothels were opened to cater to the soldiers waiting to be sent to the frontline (in this case, Libya). The best known was called La Visite and was owned by a Madame Rose from Cabinda. After the war, brothels were again made illegal and prostitution returned to the informal sector, but the proliferation of bars and dance halls provided new venues for a flourishing sex trade.[12,65–67]

In the Catholic newspaper *La Semaine de l'AEF*, prostitution in Brazzaville was scrutinised in articles published in 1955. The causes were the same as in Léo, and the proposed solutions also went along the same lines. There was more of an emphasis, however, on the associations of free women, which either operated small brothels or were closely associated with specific bars which used their presence in their advertisements aiming to attract clients. The correspondents proposed to disband such associations. A more stringent control of free women crossing the river from Léopoldville was advocated.[68]

Independence: for whom?

We have seen in the previous chapter that shortly after the Belgian Congo's independence in 1960, the population of Léopoldville expanded rapidly. Administrative controls over migrations were abandoned and the capital had to cope with a large influx of internal refugees

fleeing the country's civil wars. And a large number of Bakongo from
Angola took shelter in Léo when war broke out between liberation
movements and the Portuguese army.

In a study of Léopoldville sex workers in 1962–3, Jean La Fontaine
noted that the vast majority were still operating as they had done prior
to the country's political independence; namely, having long-term
simultaneous relationships with three or four men, with the free
woman providing a variety of services similar to those that would
have been expected of a wife and having some kind of friendship with
her patrons, who provided general and regular support rather than a
fixed fee for each intercourse. Their most important skill was to avoid
having two clients present in their compound at the same time. Free
women were considerably wealthier than married women. But La
Fontaine also noted a diversification of prostitutes: at one end, the
luxury prostitutes, called *vedettes* or *basi ya kilo* (the latter because
they could buy expensive goods by the kilogram, especially those who
had recycled their income from prostitution into the trade of other
goods); and at the other end, the *chambres d'hôtel* prostitutes, who
could have a quick half-hour session without much conversation being
exchanged. This is the first description of high-risk prostitutes for whom
sex was a purely commercial transaction. Anatole Romaniuk, a demog-
rapher who worked in Léopoldville before and after 1960, also
described a change in the character and volume of prostitution as a
consequence of the political disorders, as did sociologist Alf Schwarz,
who studied women working in the Léo factories, many of whom had
previously been involved in the sex trade.[11,52,69]

Paul Raymaekers, an observer of life in the surrounding squatter
areas of Léopoldville, noted the same phenomenon, which he attributed
to social changes and high unemployment rates, but he provided more
details. A new form of prostitution clearly emerged in Léo in 1960–1,
around brothels called 'flamingos', from the name of the first bar where
this began. Initially the flamingos were clandestine bars where alcohol
could be bought after hours, but soon their activities were expanded to
include the sex trade, by setting up discreet annexes for this purpose. In
the Matete area, of 708 houses enumerated, there were no less than
twenty-seven flamingos. Similar concentrations of flamingos were
found in many other parts of Léo, including Ngiri-Ngiri, Barumbu, in
front of the Makala sanatorium, etc. The downmarket brothels, called
londone, were small shacks with one or two rooms, quickly set up on

some unoccupied piece of land, often near the street markets. Outside, men could be seen patiently queuing for their twenty minutes of pleasure. At the opposite end of the spectrum were the flamingos frequented by the Congolese elite and UN military. The law of supply and demand dictated lower prices if the client was unemployed and higher prices after pay day or if the UN soldiers came from an industrialised country. Among an admittedly small sample of twenty young men interviewed, all knew at least five flamingos and thirteen admitted to having bought sex on at least one occasion. Also reflecting the extent of this new phenomenon, a wide diversity of Lingala or Kikongo terms appeared describing sex workers: *londoniennes, boma l'heure* (kills time), *molaso* (rubber band), *katula kiadi* (removes sadness), *mobikisi* (helper), Good Year or Caterpillar (good for all conditions ...).[55,70–72]

In a study of women in Léopoldville conducted in 1965, Suzanne Comhaire-Sylvain also noted the extraordinary proliferation of flamingos: just in the Matete district, out of about a hundred bars where alcohol was sold, sex could also be bought in eighty. In the Bandalungwa district, there were at least twenty such dance halls/brothels, usually well located at crossroads or near open air markets or gas stations. Others were situated in residential streets, and it was just too bad for the neighbours. Comhaire-Sylvain described a diversification in the patterns of sex trade and identified four categories. First were the full-time sex workers, unmarried or divorced women who would spend many hours each day picking up clients in a flamingo or bar or on the street. Although she did not provide estimates of their average number of clients per day or per week, this type of practice implies quite a high volume (and high risk). Second were the part-time sex workers: unmarried or divorced women who had another occupation but sold sexual services once in a while to supplement their income. Third were the clandestine sex workers: teenagers or married women who sold sex occasionally without their parents or husbands being aware of this lucrative part-time activity. The latter two categories implied a low volume of clients, and a different client each time. Fourth were the free women, corresponding to the lowest risk for HIV: these upmarket semi-prostitutes had just a few paying partners, whom they had the luxury of selecting and who would enjoy their company regularly.[73]

Thus in the early 1960s there appeared for the first time in Léopoldville a group of women having not three or four different sex partners per year but three or four per day, a pattern of prostitution similar to the one in Nairobi which led to the exponential amplification of HIV-1 twenty years later. Once a first high-risk sex worker got HIV-1 from a client, in the ensuing months she would have the opportunity to infect a few other men, some of whom would then infect other prostitutes they had sex with. The conditions of a sexual amplification of HIV were ripe, possibly the turning point in the sexual spread of HIV-1 in Léopoldville.

This evolution was a consequence of the enormous social changes that occurred after 1960, with a massive influx of refugees and migrants who settled in the capital, and a staggering rise in unemployment. The resulting pauperisation had a profound impact on the sex trade. Potential clients did not have enough money to provide gifts or regular support to a free woman whom they would visit time and again; they barely had a few pennies for a brief session. And poverty among young women had grown so much that some had no option but to accept those few pennies which, multiplied by the number of clients they could fetch in a day, allowed them to satisfy their basic needs. Unlike the free women, this new class of high-volume, low-price sex workers did not have the luxury of turning down a client they disliked.

In July 1968, the Zairean minister of justice ordered all brothels to be closed. This did not impact on the volume of the sex trade, as the owners simply modified their premises. They added a bar and dance floor, where the clients could select their sex worker over a few beers. Or they pretended they operated a small hotel, where rooms could be rented by the hour. Again, there were no pimps: the owners made their profit on the alcohol or from renting the rooms, and the sex workers kept the money paid by the clients. By the end of the 1960s, the system of health cards for sex workers was still in place, theoretically requiring a monthly visit and syphilis serology twice a year. Prostitutes had to show up at the Centre de Prophylaxie in the compound of the central hospital, and about 7,000 women attended more or less regularly. Health surveillance of prostitutes vanished in the 1970s, as the resources of the Zairean state were eroded by an ever-increasing percentage of national revenues being diverted into the numerous bank accounts of the president and his cronies. But the diversified patterns of prostitution did not change much until the early 1990s, when poverty became so great that few men could afford to buy sex. Hunger and libido are mutually exclusive.[74–75]

7 | *Injections and the transmission of viruses*

Ten years ago, a group of scientists argued that unsterile injections played a role in the emergence of HIV in Africa (and that serial passage of the virus within syringes altered it in a way that made it more virulent and/or more transmissible, something which remains debated among virologists until now).[1] As mentioned in the introduction, after studying this question for some time I came to the conclusion that they were right, that a substantial part of the early amplification of HIV-1 in central Africa occurred through the re-use of improperly sterilised syringes and needles, and that this mechanism was probably as important as the sexual amplification which we just reviewed. It will be impossible to prove this directly. But like a crown prosecutor who has not found the exact gun used in a crime, in the next three chapters we will assemble circumstantial evidence that would ultimately convince any jury. We will first examine how HIV but also HBV and HCV can be transmitted through injections.

Parenteral or iatrogenic

Parenteral is synonymous with injectable; it literally means to bypass the gut, by administering a drug (therapeutic or recreational) or blood product as an injection, either into a vein (IV), muscle (IM), the tissues underneath the skin (SC) or the skin itself (intradermal (ID)). *Iatrogenic* means during health care; the transmission of pathogens between intravenous drug users is not included in this latter definition, but non-injection modes of healthcare transmission are (for example, during an organ transplant or some other invasive procedure). In sub-Saharan Africa, there is much overlap between these two terms, parenteral and iatrogenic, because the continent has few drug addicts (such a habit is far too expensive) and few patients undergo invasive medical procedures during which a virus could be transmitted.

The parenteral transmission of HIV-1 has wiped out a generation of haemophiliacs, infected tens of thousands of recipients of blood transfusions in the late 1970s and early 1980s and continues to be an important mode of transmission among injectable drug users (IDUs) throughout the world. In developed countries that have implemented a universal programme of immunisation against HBV, the parenteral transmission of the latter is now uncommon, except among older unvaccinated drug addicts. However, the iatrogenic transmission of HBV continues in developing countries where the vaccine has only recently been incorporated into the national immunisation programme. And transmission of HCV, for which there is no vaccine, continues among IDUs in industrialised societies, as well as in the general population of the developing world. Other viruses can be transmitted parenterally but this occurs infrequently and can be ignored for the sake of our discussion.

The main difficulty in studying the potential contribution of the iatrogenic or parenteral transmission of HIV-1 in its emergence in the first half of the twentieth century is the high mortality among infected individuals, nearly all of whom die within fifteen years of primary infection. They are no longer available for epidemiological studies trying to correlate HIV-1 infection with ancient exposures to injectable treatments of tropical and other infectious diseases. The only option is to use other infectious agents, which are compatible with prolonged survival, as a proof of concept: if these other viruses were transmitted iatrogenically, then presumably the same could have happened with SIV_{cpz}/HIV-1.[2]

HIV-2 infection is an interesting candidate for such studies because of its lower pathogenicity: a substantial percentage of individuals infected with this other simian-turned-human retrovirus, which originated from the sooty mangabey rather than the central chimpanzee, and in West Africa rather than central Africa, never develop AIDS. We carried out an epidemiological study in Guinea-Bissau which revealed that among elderly individuals living in Bissau in 2005, HIV-2 infection was correlated with three distinct parenteral exposures: past treatment with IV or IM drugs for sleeping sickness (before 1974), past treatment of tuberculosis with IM streptomycin (before 1992) and the ritual excision of the clitoris. However, HIV-2 is not present in central Africa and cannot be used as a model for transmission of blood-borne viruses in the very countries where HIV-1 emerged.[3–4]

The other pathogen that can be used for such proof of concept studies is HCV. HCV is compatible with prolonged survival, as less than 25%

of infected individuals go on to develop cirrhosis or cancer of the liver. Furthermore, its sexual transmission and mother-to-child transmission are rather ineffective, so that the parenteral route accounts for the overwhelming majority of cases. In industrialised societies, HCV transmission during blood transfusions has been eliminated through screening, so that most new cases of HCV infection are acquired during intravenous injections of recreational drugs. In sub-Saharan Africa, some transmission still arises during the administration of unscreened transfusions, but most cases are thought to be acquired via injections during health or dental care.[5–6]

In contrast, HBV is not a good marker for the parenteral transmission of viruses in sub-Saharan Africa because it is more infectious and transmitted effectively through several other mechanisms. There, a large number of children get infected with HBV: some from their mothers but the majority from other children, possibly through chronic skin wounds which are extremely common in underprivileged populations. Very few of these children develop acute hepatitis with jaundice when they acquire HBV, but 10–15% remain chronic (and infectious) carriers and can develop long-term complications, while the remaining 85–90% becomes immune. Those who managed to avoid HBV during childhood acquire it sexually at adolescence, and in central Africa around 95% of adults have antibodies against HBV. There is little room for the parenteral transmission of HBV in adults, and for that reason HCV is a much better marker of the parenteral/iatrogenic transmission of viruses. In industrialised countries there was never much transmission of HBV during childhood with the result that, until the vaccine became widely used, most adults were immunologically naive with regard to HBV and could be infected parenterally, either during health care or while using injectable recreational drugs.

HIV among drug addicts

The high efficacy of the parenteral transmission of HIV-1 has been documented time and again in studies of IDUs conducted during the early part of the epidemic, before this risk was understood and before partially effective prevention measures could be implemented in this hard-to-reach target group. Along with outbreaks that occurred during health care, this constitutes the best proof of concept for the potential transmission of HIV-1 during medical injections with improperly sterilised syringes and needles, because the quantity of blood (and thus the number of viruses) left in a syringe after an IV injection of cocaine or heroin is approximately the same as after similar equipment has been used for the IV administration of a pharmaceutical agent. This is in stark contrast to transfusion-related HIV infection, where the amount of infectious blood is much larger. Among IDUs the transmission of HIV-1 occurred from a first to a second addict, from this second to a third one, and so on, unlike what happened to haemophiliacs, many of whom could be infected via the same lot of a coagulation factor, which had been prepared through a pooling process from thousands of donors.

Collections of samples obtained before HIV assays were marketed allowed a retrospective description of the spread of the virus among IDUs. In New York, where the virus was introduced in the mid-1970s, more than half of addicts were infected by 1982. In Edinburgh, HIV prevalence rose rapidly to 51% in the early 1980s, with most seroconversions occurring within a two-year period. In Bari, Italy, HIV seroprevalence among IDUs increased from 0% in 1979 to 76% in 1985 while in Valencia, Spain, it increased from 11% in 1983 to 48% two years later. In Geneva, prevalence increased from 6% in 1981 to 38% in 1983. Among the drug addicts of Milan, HIV prevalence was 8% in 1981, 35% in 1983 and 60% in 1985. In Bangkok, HIV prevalence among IDUs increased from 1% at the end of 1987 to 43% by the end of the following year.[7–13]

Transmission among IDUs continued even where comprehensive interventions, including needle exchange programmes, were put in place. In Vancouver, at the very time and place of an international conference heralding the development of effective antiretroviral therapies, 23% and 88% of IDUs tested in 1996 were infected with HIV and HCV respectively. And such outbreaks continue to occur today, nearly thirty years after the identification of HIV as the cause of AIDS. In Sargodha, in the Punjab province of Pakistan, HIV prevalence among IDUs increased from 9% in 2005–6 to 51% the following year.[14,15]

These are all good examples of the exponential transmission of HIV from blood to blood through the sharing of syringes and needles. The probability of transmission per act when an HIV-negative addict uses a syringe or needle recently used by an HIV-infected drug user is somewhere between 0.7% and 1.1%, an order of magnitude higher than when a seronegative individual has sex with an HIV-infected partner (the risk of transmission per intercourse is 0.1%). These are summary estimates and the risk of parenteral (or heterosexual) transmission must be substantially higher when the index HIV-infected person is experiencing the high viraemia that characterises primary HIV infection. This creates a vicious circle in which the HIV-negative addicts are, month after month, increasingly likely to share their injection paraphenalia with someone who is HIV-infected. The result is that today HIV prevalence nationwide among drug addicts is 37% in Russia, 40% in Spain, 43% in Indonesia and Thailand and 72% in Estonia. Worldwide, out of 16 million intravenous drug users, about 3 million are HIV-infected.[16–18]

Iatrogenic epidemics of HIV

Several small outbreaks of HIV transmission through health care have been reported. As these generally involved just a few patients, it is difficult to use this information to infer what could have occurred on a much larger scale in sub-Saharan Africa. However, more to the point of this discussion, two epidemics (by definition, an epidemic corresponds to a much larger number of patients than an outbreak), both of which involved children, can be used as a further proof of concept for a large-scale transmission of HIV-1 during health care.

Shortly after the fall of Ceausescu in 1989, a medical journal reported that 367 children in Romanian hospitals and orphanages had tested positive for HIV. Of the 1,168 cases of AIDS reported to the Romanian ministry of health by December 1990, 94% had been documented among children less than four years of age. This age distribution was extraordinary. Two-thirds of paediatric cases occurred among children abandoned by their parents and living in orphanages or long-term care facilities. Less than 10% of the mothers who could be located were found to be HIV-infected, implying an unusual mode of infection of the children.[19,20]

At the time in Romania, transfusions were given to malnourished children as a way to provide them with many nutrients. Because the recipients needed small volumes of blood, a unit was generally split and administered to two or three children. One third of cases occurred in children who received transfusions of unscreened blood, and the others were attributed to multiple therapeutic injections with syringes and needles used over and over again without proper sterilisation. Many children with AIDS had received 300 or more lifetime IM injections, an extraordinary number.[20]

Cases were distributed unevenly throughout the country. The largest numbers, about half of the total, were seen in the Constanta district, east of Bucharest. A nationwide survey of 12,000 institutionalised children under four years of age revealed that 10% were HIV-infected. Among institutionalised children in Constanta, HIV prevalence was 48% in those aged less than four years, but 0% in those aged four or more. This reflected a much more intensive use of medical injections and transfusions in the first years of life, as well as a cohort effect: nosocomial transmission occurred only after HIV-1 had been introduced into Romania in the 1980s.

Further studies suggested that injections rather than transfusions were the mode of infection for most children, even those who had received transfusions. The testing of more than 400,000 units of blood in 1990–1 documented that the HIV prevalence among donors was only 0.007% for the whole country and 0.025% in Constanta. This implied a low risk for the recipients, even if the children were transfused ten times during their lives. A case-control study documented an association between HIV and multiple injections: the HIV-infected children, only a few years old, had received 280 injections on average, compared to 187 for the HIV-negative controls. These injections consisted of vitamins, antibiotics and vaccines.[21,22]

More than 5,000 children had been iatrogenically infected with HIV before this came to an end. When typing became available, it was shown that almost all HIV-infected children born of a seronegative mother were infected with HIV-1 subtype F. Among HIV-infected adults, subtype F accounted for 68% of infections, but subtypes A, B, C, D and CRF02_AG were also detected. Thus, multiple subtypes were introduced by Romanians who travelled to Africa or by foreigners who lived in Romania. Then subtype F was exponentially amplified, from child to child, by unsafe medical practices within the vulnerable subgroup of institutionalised infants and children. Subtype F isolates from Romania are similar to those from Angola, another communist country at the time, where the source of this tragic epidemic may lie. The other subtypes disseminated slowly in the adult Romanian population as they did in other European countries, mostly through sexual intercourse.[21,23–25]

A second dramatic epidemic occurred among children attending the Al-Fateh Pediatric Hospital in Benghazi, Libya, and attracted media attention because five unlucky Bulgarian nurses and one Palestinian doctor were sentenced to death for their alleged role in this tragedy. They were released after spending nine years in Libyan prisons. The problem was first recognised in 1998, when serological analyses showed evidence of a recent HIV infection in several children. Eventually, about 450 children (mean age: four years) were found to be HIV-infected. Many of them subsequently received health care in Swiss and Italian institutions, from where some of the details emerged. By 2007, fifty-two children had died.[26–28]

Two-thirds of the HIV-infected children had been hospitalised at the Benghazi hospital, while the others had received outpatient care; 46% of the HIV-infected children were also infected with HCV. Of twenty-five mothers initially tested, only one was HIV-infected, implying that the other children had certainly not been infected from mother-to-child. Later, eighteen additional mothers were found to be HIV-infected, but it seems that most were infected from their child (presumably during breast feeding) rather than the other way around, because none of the fathers was HIV-infected. All children were infected with the same recombinant CRF02_AG strain, with little genetic variation between isolates, implying a common source for the HIV-1 epidemic and rapid transmission of the virus.[26–27]

Unfortunately, foreign investigators had little direct access to epidemiological information from Libya, and of course Libyan investigators could not talk since colonel al-Gadhafi's dictatorial regime had already decided who to blame: the foreigners, who they said had deliberately infected the children as part of a Central Intelligence Agency (CIA)- or Mossad-inspired plot. So we do not know for sure exactly which procedure(s) led to nosocomial transmission of HIV-1 and HCV. All the victims had had blood drawn at the hospital, most had received some form of IV therapy, but few had received transfusions. Many children had spent some time in the 'semi-intensive care unit' of the hospital. Infection control practices were so deplorable that it seems likely that transmission occurred through more than one type of procedure.[26–27]

Molecular clock analyses showed that the most recent common ancestors for the HIV-1 and HCV isolates predated 1998 by a few years, implying that the two viruses were already spreading in the hospital before the expatriate healthcare workers arrived in Benghazi, a conclusion confirmed by the finding that some of the infected children had not received care at the hospital after 1997. Given that the CRF02_AG strain is found mainly in central and West Africa, it seems likely that the original case, the Benghazi patient zero, was one of the 1.5 million African migrant workers who lived in Libya.[29]

It is of course a scandal and a tragedy that so many children got infected with HIV through the re-use of needles and other medical devices in a country so rich with oil money, and that scapegoats were jailed for so long as a public relations diversion from the real culprit: the Libyan regime. But this epidemic, the previous one in Romania and two smaller outbreaks in the former Soviet Union illustrate how HIV-1 can be exponentially amplified through unsafe injections, much like what happens among IDUs. If such epidemics could arise after the existence of HIV-1 was known, they must certainly have occurred before the new disease and its aetiological agent were identified.[30]

The largest ever iatrogenic epidemic

At the turn of the century, studies in Egypt demonstrated that the iatrogenic transmission of another blood-borne virus, HCV, could reach a massive scale. Of course Egypt is not inhabited by *P.t. troglodytes*, so HIV-1 could not possibly have emerged in the Middle East. But as an example of the potential for well-intentioned disease control interventions to transmit blood-borne viruses, the Egyptian experience is hard to beat.[31]

Schistosomiasis is caused by a parasite with a complex life cycle, which is acquired during exposure to water inhabited by the snails that constitute its intermediate host. In the most common form of schistosomiasis, adult worms live in the blood vessels around the rectum, causing bloody diarrhoea, or liver fibrosis when their eggs manage to travel up to the liver. There is also a variety in which the adult worms live around the bladder, with the eggs excreted into the urine rather than the stools; such patients pass blood in their urine.

Schistosomiasis used to be highly endemic in the Nile delta, where mass treatment campaigns with parenteral drugs led to the HCV infection of millions of individuals. The use of tartar emetic, a very old drug against schistosomiasis, had begun in 1921, and the ministry of health started organising large-scale campaigns in the early 1950s. Between 1964 and 1982, more than two million injections of tartar emetic were administered each year to 250,000 patients. On average they received ten to twelve weekly IV injections through hastily sterilised syringes and needles, boiled for only one or two minutes or not at all. In specialised centres, more than 500 patients could be treated in an hour. Tartar emetic was not very effective: many patients relapsed or were re-infected, and had to receive further cycles of the drug. The historical information is congruent with what was calculated using the same molecular approaches as we reviewed for HIV-1, which indicated an exponential growth in the number of HCV-infected individuals between 1940 and 1980.[32–33]

For the whole country, 22% of individuals aged ten to fifty years became infected with HCV. HCV prevalence is lower (6–8%) in residents of Cairo and Alexandria, but reaches 19% to 28% in Upper, Middle and Lower Egypt. Prevalence is higher among the older age groups, who were exposed repeatedly to schistosomiasis treatments. In Lower and Middle Egypt, more than 50% of individuals aged forty or more are HCV-seropositive. In all these regions, there was a correlation between exposure to schistosomiasis treatment and HCV infection. The same interventions also led to the iatrogenic transmission of HBV, but in this case the relationship was blurred by the other modes of transmission of HBV.[31]

HCV infection in central Africa

Now let us get geographically closer to the heart of the story. After Egypt, central Africa has the highest HCV prevalence in the world: 6.0% of adults overall and 13.8% in Cameroon. In several areas of Cameroon, more than 40% of elderly individuals became HCV-seropositive. What epidemiologists call a cohort effect (the exposure to a given pathogen varying according to the year of birth) was demonstrated, with HCV prevalence reaching 40–50% among people born before 1945, about 15% for those born in 1960, and 3–4% for younger individuals born after 1970. In several studies, HCV prevalence plateaued at the same point, corresponding to a year of birth around 1930–5 (Figure 9). So most of the parenteral transmission of HCV must have occurred between 1930 and 1970.[34–42]

Molecular clock analyses confirmed this conclusion and revealed that in Cameroon, Gabon and the Central African Republic, the number of HCV-infected individuals started increasing exponentially between 1920 and 1940, continuing for two or three decades. Since the heterosexual transmission of HCV is relatively ineffective, this indicates massive parenteral transmission of at least one blood-borne virus in the very areas inhabited by the *P.t. troglodytes* source of HIV-1. This parenteral transmission took place during the colonial era, starting at the same time, give or take a few years, as SIV_{cpz} successfully emerged into human populations to become HIV-1. It is hard to believe that this represents merely a strange coincidence.[42,43]

In Cameroon, populations with a high HCV prevalence come from Yaoundé or villages in the southern rain forest (Figure 9 and Map 5), and prevalence is much lower in the north. A similar north–south gradient in HCV prevalence was observed in territories that used to be part of AEF, with a low prevalence in Tchad and the Central African Republic and a high prevalence in Gabon. This means that the diseases during the treatment of which transmission of HCV occurred were more common in the southern rain forests than in the arid north.[42–45]

It seems plausible that not all medical injections carried the same risk of HCV transmission. Again, data gathered during studies of healthcare workers occupationally exposed to their patients' blood can be informative. Healthcare workers exposed to HCV experience a higher risk of infection when a hollow-bore needle had been placed in the index patient's vein and when they sustain a deeper injury; these risk factors

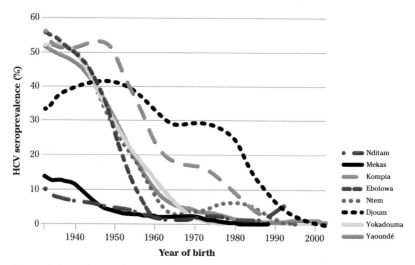

Figure 9 Prevalence of HCV infection at various sites in Cameroon by year of birth.

Adapted from Pepin.[46]

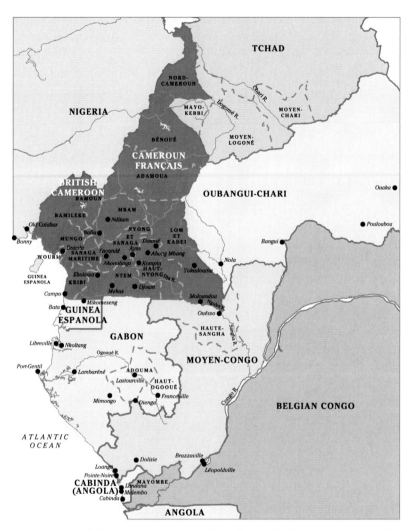

Map 5 Map of Cameroun Français and the four colonies that comprised the Afrique Équatoriale Française federation.

presumably reflect the higher number of viral particles accidentally inoculated. Extrapolating to the potential iatrogenic transmission between patients, the risk must have been higher with IV, intermediate with IM, and lower with SC or ID injections. And obviously the risk must have been proportional to the total number of injections received. The same conclusions can be extended to the transmission of HIV.

In Cameroon, researchers looked for HIV-1 nucleic acids in discarded needles and syringes that had been used on HIV-infected patients less than six hours earlier. One third of the syringes used for IV injections contained detectable virus, versus only 2% of those used for IM injections.[47–49]

Inoculation hepatitis

Now we will go back in time to try to assess what medical doctors and nurses working in central Africa in the first half of the twentieth century could have known concerning the potential transmission of viruses during medical care. Presumably, understanding these risks might have made them more careful. We can assume that the level of understanding among these pioneers of tropical medicine was no higher than among their counterparts working in Europe. Most of the knowledge about blood-borne viruses that eventually trickled down to medical practitioners in Africa originated from Europe.

During this period of interest, little was known about viruses in general and even less about putative viruses potentially causing hepatitis. Unlike bacteria and parasites, viruses were too small to be seen during direct or stained microscopic examinations of specimens. Their culture required the support of cells, while for bacteria an agar plate with the right nutrients would suffice. Nor were clinicians at the time able to measure liver enzymes in the blood, which is essential to the diagnosis of hepatitis, whatever its aetiology. These enzymes are released when there is inflammation in the liver.

In practice, 'hepatitis' was diagnosed when a patient developed jaundice for which there was no other apparent explanation (in the tropics, this investigation would include negative smears for malaria). Cases of hepatitis not severe enough to cause jaundice would be missed, while some patients with other conditions associated with jaundice were misdiagnosed as having hepatitis. The diagnoses were pretty reliable, however, when outbreaks occurred: if dozens or hundreds of somehow-related patients developed jaundice within a limited time frame, there was no doubt that this corresponded to hepatitis caused by an infectious agent.

'Inoculation hepatitis' or 'serum hepatitis' began to be described in textbooks from the 1940s as appearing after various medical interventions including, in Europe, the treatment of syphilis with arsenic-based drugs, usually administered as a series of weekly IV injections. Clinicians distinguished between early arsenical hepatitis, occurring around day 9 and presumed to be drug-related, and late hepatitis, occurring after about 100 days, which was thought to be infectious.[50–55]

Before WWII, only 1% of syphilitics treated with IV arsenical drugs developed jaundice, but wartime conditions and shortages led to a quicker turnaround of syringes and needles. In several military clinics in Britain, between 50% and 75% of men treated for syphilis developed jaundice! Similar epidemics occurred in civilian hospitals after the virus had been introduced by returning soldiers who had received initial doses of some IV drug in a military clinic. This was attributed to the re-use of glass syringes, which were in short supply, so they could not be boiled between patients (it would have taken too long for the syringes to cool down before they could be handled again); they were put into a disinfectant briefly or they were merely rinsed with water. Before a drug was injected IV, the nurse had to aspirate a small quantity of blood to make sure that the needle was properly located within a vein. When the drug was pushed into the vein, a minute quantity of blood remained in the syringe and the needle, some of which ended up being injected into the vein of the next patient(s).[54–57]

When outbreaks of jaundice were described after the treatment of syphilis and other infections with penicillin, then a revolutionary drug, it became more and more difficult to attribute these cases to anything other than a transmissible agent. Furthermore, a viral cause was suspected when it became apparent that the nurses who administered the IV injections, as well as the laboratory technicians who handled the blood samples sent for testing, were themselves at risk of developing jaundice. These outbreaks certainly corresponded to infection with HBV, since most cases of acute infection with HCV do not develop overt jaundice. Obviously, to reach a risk of hepatitis of 50–75%, a vicious circle with exponential amplification of HBV was created. A first HBV-infected patient transmitted the virus to a few more; each of these second-generation cases infected a few additional patients, and so on.[58]

Around 1942, batches of a yellow fever vaccine which had been suspended in human serum (obtained from medical students) during its production caused 50,000 cases of jaundice among American civilians and soldiers. With this massive epidemic, the second major form of viral hepatitis was given its current name. Strongly associated with injections and not displaying any seasonality, it became known as hepatitis B, to distinguish it from the other form of infectious hepatitis, hepatitis A, which was not associated with injections but displayed marked seasonal variations in incidence. When US army veterans who had developed hepatitis in 1942 after receiving the yellow fever vaccine were tested in 1985, four decades later, 97% of them had antibodies against HBV, as did 73% of those who had been vaccinated without developing overt hepatitis, compared to only 13% of those not vaccinated. If those who were infected but did not develop jaundice are added to the symptomatic cases, it can be estimated that 330,000 vaccine recipients were iatrogenically infected with HBV. Other vaccines, blood sampling through a common syringe (in clinics for diabetics or in a sanatorium), transfusions and administration of convalescent sera, plasma or injectable drugs were in turn all recognised as causing hepatitis B.[59–60]

There is no evidence that medical officers working in central Africa in colonial times became aware of these risks. The risk of inoculation hepatitis was not mentioned in any of the reports of the health systems of AEF and Cameroun that will be reviewed in the next chapter, while in the Belgian Congo its first description was published in 1953. Acute HCV infection is often asymptomatic or causes non-specific symptoms, without overt jaundice, and could not possibly have been recognised by the colonial clinicians. Infection with HBV is nearly universal in central Africa and generally acquired during childhood (when it rarely causes jaundice), which leaves little potential for its iatrogenic transmission to adults, in contrast to Britain, where most adults treated for syphilis had hitherto not been infected with HBV and were susceptible to an iatrogenic infection. Furthermore, when iatrogenic HBV infection did occur in sub-Saharan Africa, symptoms would have developed after a one- to four-month incubation period, making it difficult for doctors to recognise that this was related to a previous episode of medical care.

Reports of health services in Cameroun and AEF give no indication regarding how re-usable syringes and needles were sterilised between patients or how many times a syringe/needle might be used on any given day. A textbook for nurses, written by the chief medical officer of Gabon in 1931, gave instructions regarding how syringes and needles were to be sterilised, but these required an autoclave or a dry heat incubator, available only in hospitals and large health centres. What mobile teams and nurses working in small facilities without electricity were expected to do was unclear. Most injections were given by practical nurses with limited scientific training. Given the huge caseloads, the sterilisation process may have been shortcut or bypassed, as in Egypt. We will see later that, at least in the Belgian Congo, syringes and needles were not even boiled between patients. It seems likely that this was the rule rather than the exception.[61]

With this in mind, to estimate their potential role in the transmission of blood-borne viruses and particularly SIV_{cpz}/HIV-1 and HCV, we will review the major disease control programmes implemented in central Africa from 1921 to 1959, the topic of the next two chapters.

8 | *The legacies of colonial medicine I: French Equatorial Africa and Cameroun*

We have just seen how HIV and other blood-borne viruses can be transmitted through injections. Here we will examine the history of colonial medicine in the French territories of central Africa, where remarkable public health interventions ultimately proved successful in reducing the burden of tropical diseases, but at the same time caused the parenteral transmission of HCV, the HTLV-1 retrovirus and presumably SIV_{cpz}/HIV-1 as well. The core of the problem was that since the early drugs against infectious diseases were not very effective, they all had to be administered by injections, often IV, so as to maximise the drug concentration in the blood and in other tissues. As we will see now, tens of millions of IV injections were administered within the crucible of HIV-1, at exactly the right time.

The system

A remarkable peculiarity of French colonial history is the way medicine was organised: as part of the military. Young Frenchmen interested in a medical career in the colonies would usually get their degree at a medical school run by the armed forces in Bordeaux, before moving on to the tropical medicine institute in Marseilles, known as Le Pharo, after the name of the park where it is located near the old port. Overseas, they would start as a *médecin-lieutenant* and progressively, for the more talented, patient or motivated, move up the ladder to become perhaps a *médecin-colonel* or *médecin-général* at the end of their careers. Very few of them would be posted to the barracks to provide care for the colonial armed forces. Instead, they were posted to the hospitals and disease control units, working among civilians but remaining military doctors so that a strict hierarchy was maintained.

Disease control interventions and modes of healthcare delivery would be decided at the top of the pyramid, by the *médecin-général*, and implemented in a similar fashion throughout the colony following detailed protocols. There were precise definitions of what had to be reported and in what form, and the reports from each hospital or district would be merged into an annual report for the colony, containing an extraordinary number of tables, maps and graphs about the diseases of interest, their distribution, the treatments administered, the exact number of injections for each drug, and so on. Some of these annual reports contained 800 pages. Their format was the same for all colonies, so that they could be consolidated into an annual summary of the health status of overseas France.[1]

The other important feature of French colonial medicine was its population-based approach. While elsewhere in Africa colonial doctors were satisfied with providing care to whoever managed to show up at the local hospital or dispensary, the French wanted to provide basic health care to everybody, through the treatment of common and chronic tropical diseases. They kept reliable medical censuses of the population (their target), and their intent was to detect and treat all cases of a few selected diseases among this entire population. To do so, they funded and staffed mobile disease control teams who would roam through the bush, day after day, village after village, to examine everyone, find the cases and treat them in order to reduce the human reservoir of these infections and decrease transmission to the point where the disease would eventually disappear. Attending case-finding sessions was compulsory, and a medical certificate was issued for each person. This public health approach, with massive numbers of individuals treated in their own villages with injectable drugs against a few diseases, offered a unique opportunity for the transmission of blood-borne viruses, whose existence was unknown at the time, to a degree much higher than could have occurred in British and Portuguese colonies.

Fixed health care in hospitals and health centres was fairly limited initially, and it was just too bad for patients who developed an acute illness between the biannual visits of the mobile teams. Eventually, tensions arose between the champions of the 'vertical' approach (disease-specific mobile teams) and those who wanted to develop multipurpose fixed centres providing basic care available year round (the 'horizontal' approach, later renamed primary health care). The latter, of course, was necessary to provide care for acute and treatable conditions such as malaria, pneumonia, gastroenteritis, women with obstructed labour, and so on.

The mother of all tropical diseases

Eugène Jamot became the most famous French colonial doctor in Africa, and his biography illustrates the colonial medicine system as well as the development of the disease control interventions. Born in 1879, the first in his family to go to college, he studied natural sciences, taught for a few years in high schools in Algeria and Montpellier to accumulate some savings and then obtained his medical degree from Montpellier in 1908. After practising in France for two years, he decided he had other ambitions, partially prompted by an unhappy marriage, a difficult relationship with his mother and some problems with the justice system following a violent argument with his stepfather.[2–5]

After the tropical medicine course in Marseilles, his first posting was to Tchad, following which he received further training in Paris, and became deputy director of the nascent Institut Pasteur in Brazzaville. Two weeks after his arrival, WWI broke out and he was designated to serve as the medical officer of a column that invaded Kamerun from the AEF. After the successful conclusion of this campaign, he returned to Brazzaville from 1917 to 1921. By then a *médecin-capitaine*, he developed the overriding interest of his professional life: the control of sleeping sickness, which he conceived around specialised mobile teams. He led the first one which operated in Oubangui-Chari.[6]

Sleeping sickness (African trypanosomiasis), caused by a parasite called *Trypanosoma brucei gambiense*, was the first communicable disease for which large-scale control interventions were implemented in central Africa. The disease was first described in a European text in 1803 by Thomas Winterbottom, a British physician in Sierra Leone. One of its clinical signs, the presence of enlarged lymph nodes in the neck, was known to slave traders as an adverse prognostic sign, and the price of such slaves was reduced accordingly. After weeks or months of intermittent fever, patients develop chronic meningo-encephalitis characterised by profound daytime somnolence, hence its name, which would last for several months until the fatal outcome, which was universal if untreated.

Sleeping sickness did not spread to the Americas with the slaves due to the absence of its tsetse fly vector in the New World. It is thought that the massive displacements of populations that accompanied the European colonisation of central Africa in the late nineteenth century facilitated the dissemination of the parasite. Trypanosomes were imported into regions where the disease had hitherto been absent or uncommon, and spread rapidly in such immunologically naive populations. The high incidence of sleeping sickness preoccupied French and Belgian colonial authorities who, in some regions because of the morbidity and mortality caused by this disease, were running out of their labour force. Furthermore, a high incidence among Africans implied a high risk of transmission to Europeans, who often developed this lethal disease.

Indeed, the aim of many of the disease control initiatives implemented during the early colonial era was to protect the Europeans by decreasing the reservoir of the pathogen in the African population around them. Institutes of tropical medicine were established in Marseilles, London, Liverpool and Brussels to find technological solutions that would lower the mortality of Europeans in Africa, which was even higher in the centre of the continent than on the coast. A British government publication stated that 'in the days when the west coast was the white man's grave, the Congo forest would have been his purgatory'. The annual medical reports of each French colony started with a detailed section on health problems of the Europeans, with a list of all those who had died during the previous year, along with the cause of death: it was just too bad for your reputation if you had died from alcoholic cirrhosis or complications of syphilis.[7]

Substantial resources were allocated to the control of sleeping sickness, organised around what became known as the Jamot doctrine. The idea was simple: mobile teams would visit each village, examine everyone, detect as many cases as possible using simple methods (microscopic examination of blood or lymph node aspirate) and treat them on the spot with whatever drugs were available. Initially, drugs were not very effective for the patients themselves, who often died despite treatments which could not get rid of the parasites in the brain. However, the drugs reduced the patients' infectiousness by suppressing the presence of trypanosomes in the blood. For a long time trypanosomiasis treatment was geared more towards a collective benefit than improving the individual fate of the patient receiving these toxic arsenical drugs.

In these early days, members of the case-finding mobile teams did heroic work under harsh conditions. For instance, in the space of eighteen months in 1917–19, Jamot examined 89,743 individuals in Oubangui-Chari, diagnosing and treating (mostly with SC drugs) 5,347 trypanosomiasis cases, and did all this with only three microscopes and six syringes. They would spend twenty days per month in villages, sleeping in huts provided by the local population, with no facilities whatsoever. Much of the travelling between villages, many of which were inaccessible by road, was done by foot. They were taking a substantial risk themselves as they spent two-thirds of their lives in locations harbouring a lot of tsetse flies infected with trypanosomes. Several healthcare workers developed trypanosomiasis and died from the disease or its treatment. As a contribution to medical knowledge, some published their own cases, describing the progression of their symptoms in a type of scientific paper which has fortunately disappeared: the *auto-observation*. By shortening the period during which a patient was infectious, their interventions quickly proved effective, reducing the incidence of and mortality from trypanosomiasis by more than 65%. In 1922, Jamot was transferred to Cameroun Français, recently acquired by the French during WWI, where the authorities were discovering the extent of the trypanosomiasis problem inherited from the Germans.[6,8–9]

Jamot had a strong personality, was highly motivated and worked hard. He quickly became known for his favourite slogan: 'I will wake up the black race.' He obtained very substantial resources, to the point where his specialised and autonomous sleeping sickness organisation, created in 1926 and based in Ayos, east of Yaoundé, was seen by many in the administration as a state within a state. Jamot answered directly to the governor, and was independent of the chief medical officer of the colony and local administrative authorities. Several egos were bruised in the process. At one point, half of the medical doctors in Cameroun were working under Jamot, who coordinated twenty-eight mobile teams operating throughout the country, with a staff of 17 physicians and 400 healthcare workers.

He was revered by his subordinates, known as the *jamotains*, while his approach became the *jamotique*. In the communities visited, roughly 500 villagers were seen each day. The work was organised like a production line with each member of the team having well-defined roles: bureaucrats took care of the paper work (registries, individual certificates), nurses palpated the necks and marked with a cross the foreheads of those who needed microscopic examinations, a small army of microscopists would examine the blood and lymph node aspirates, yelling when a trypanosome was detected so it could be corroborated by the doctor, while other nurses performed the lumbar punctures for disease-staging on those found to be infected. Eventually, the doctor would prescribe the treatment to be administered by nurses, who would stay behind after the rest of the team had left for the next village. During Jamot's tenure in Cameroun, 150,000 cases of sleeping sickness were diagnosed and treated. However, when the incidence decreased, some of his medical colleagues wondered whether it was reasonable to spend so much on trypanosomiasis and so little on the fixed health facilities which would provide basic care all year round.

Jamot published forty scientific papers during his career, a large number for an African-based non-academic doctor. Some contain extremely detailed descriptions of the distribution of trypanosomiasis in Cameroun and of the treatments used. A free thinker, he repeatedly and publicly said that the dramatic epidemics of trypanosomiasis in Cameroun and AEF had been triggered by European colonisation and the forcible displacement of large populations. This freedom of speech did not sit well with his military status. Other conservatives did not appreciate that while remaining legally married to his French wife, who never went to Africa, Jamot lived for many years with a Fulani from north Cameroon whom he married according to tribal customs and with whom he had three children.

A forceful advocate of disease control in the African colonies, Jamot became well known in France, especially during the Paris colonial exposition of 1931, as the man who conquered sleeping sickness. He was honoured by scientific bodies, received the *Légion d'Honneur*, and was even nominated for the Nobel. He took advantage of his notoriety to obtain ever-increasing resources for trypanosomiasis control in Cameroun. Even though the incidence was now 90% lower than when he arrived, Jamot had a more ambitious goal: its eradication, which seemed possible given that there was no significant animal reservoir of the parasite.

His high profile would eventually cost him his job. His many enemies found a good pretext to get rid of him when one of his subordinates decided, apparently on his own, to double or triple the dose of a new arsenical drug, tryparsamide. This went on for more than a year with the result that hundreds of unfortunate patients in the Bafia area became blind, as the drug was toxic to the optic nerve. Jamot's implication in this disaster remained unclear. The young Bafia doctor was sacked but he protested and an inquiry was held. Jamot, who was then in France, did not show up at the ministry of colonies as requested. This was not appreciated. While on a stopover in Dakar on his way back, colonel Jamot received a telegram. He too had been fired from his post in Cameroun.[2–5]

He was sent to organise sleeping sickness control in French West Africa, from a base in Ouagadougou. Jamot spent the next three years crisscrossing this vast territory, finding 70,000 new cases. However, he was caught up in similar disputes with the medical and administrative authorities concerning the importance and degree of autonomy given to the sleeping sickness control organisation. Discouraged by what he viewed as a lack of understanding of the seriousness of the problem, in 1935 Jamot retired from the military and went back to his village in France to work as a general practitioner. A broken man, he died of a stroke a year later.

There is no doubt that Jamot and his teams saved entire communities from extinction. In some villages in the upper Nyong region east of Yaoundé, up to 97% of the inhabitants were found to have trypanosomiasis during successive surveys, and sleeping sickness was causing more fatalities than all other diseases combined. Other villages, which could not be visited in time by the mobile teams, had been entirely wiped out by the disease: a large part of the population had died, and others had left the area looking for a more secure location. After Jamot's departure from Cameroon, the concept of disease-specific mobile teams roaming the countryside was adapted for the fight against other tropical diseases, especially yaws and syphilis. But this very dedication and efficacy created tremendous opportunities for the iatrogenic transmission of blood-borne viruses.

To evaluate the potential contribution of tropical disease control interventions in the spread of viruses, a detailed review was necessary. Fortunately, good archives have survived to this day. Most of these reports were kept at the tropical medicine institute of Marseilles (located, quite appropriately, on the Allée du Médecin-Colonel Jamot): annual reports of the health services for Cameroun Français, Moyen-Congo, Oubangui-Chari, Gabon and AEF. The AEF included Oubangui-Chari, Moyen-Congo, Gabon and Tchad. As the latter is not inhabited by *P.t. troglodytes*, I collected data for the first three territories (from now on called AEF-3). For Cameroun, the annual reports sent to the League of Nations and United Nations were available at the UN library in Geneva. Additional information was found in annual reviews of communicable diseases in French overseas territories. For each disease of interest except malaria, it was possible to calculate the annual incidence (number of cases per 1,000 inhabitants), which is important for inferring which ones were the most likely factors behind the high prevalence of HCV described in the previous chapter and potentially the emergence of SIV_{cpz}/HIV-1. Denominators used to calculate incidence rates took into account the changes in boundaries between AEF territories and natural growth of these populations (Figure 4). At the time, few diseases were treated with orally administered drugs, so in practice an annual incidence of, say, 10 per 1,000 meant that during this year 1% of the population received a series of injections for the treatment of this specific disease.[10–23]

For a long time, treatment of sleeping sickness was based on drugs that contained arsenic, hence their general designation as arsenicals. The same arsenical drugs, or similar compounds, were also used to treat yaws and syphilis, among other infectious diseases. For most of the 1920s, SC atoxyl was widely prescribed, often combined with a second drug given IV, for instance tartar emetic (the drug used in Egypt to treat schistosomiasis). In the 1920s, the introduction of tryparsamide, a drug developed at the Rockefeller Institute, resulted in a dramatic improvement: patients with involvement of the brain could now be cured. Just for 1927–8, 900 kg of atoxyl (about one million injections) and 600 kg of tryparsamide (135,186 SC and 71,903 IV injections) were used in Cameroun by Jamot's teams. The number of injections declined thereafter (Figure 10), as the control efforts proved effective. After 1928, tryparsamide was usually administered IV while another arsenical drug, orsanine, given SC or IV, was used for early stage cases. In AEF, treatments were standardised through instructions of the *médecin-général*: twelve weekly SC or IV injections of orsanine if the cerebrospinal fluid was normal, or twelve weekly IV injections of tryparsamide if cerebrospinal fluid was abnormal, to be repeated annually for two more years to 'consolidate' the initial treatment. On average, tryparsamide-treated patients received thirty-six IV injections.[24–27]

Such once-a-week regimens were quite manageable as nurses left behind by the mobile teams could rotate between villages, treating all cases in a given village on Mondays, all cases in a second village on Tuesdays and so on, repeating this circuit twelve times. This mobility of

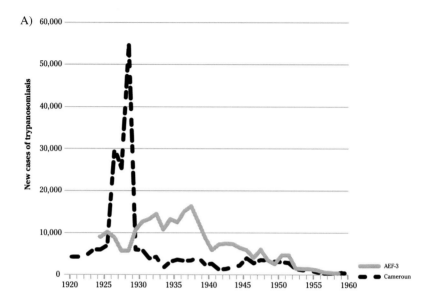

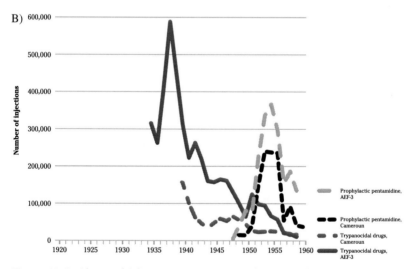

Figure 10 Incidence of African trypanosomiasis (sleeping sickness) in Cameroun Français and AEF-3, and use of trypanocidal drugs.
    Adapted from Pepin.[10]

practical nurses implied that the procedures for sterilising syringes and needles were minimal. However, they became extremely skilled at giving IV injections, as is evident in a movie about Jamot made in 1932, which can be downloaded from www.creuse-jamot.org/html/1931-1935.html. This film provides an extraordinary illustration of the scope of the sleeping sickness problem in Cameroun and of the methods used for its control.

Some trypanosomiasis patients who relapsed after standard therapy also received *hétérohémothérapie*: the repeated IM administration of 10–20 cc of whole blood from convalescent patients. The idea was that this blood contained high levels of antibodies against trypanosomes, which would be useful to patients who had difficulty getting rid of the parasite. Although this was certainly a good method for transmitting viral infectious agents (because the quantity of blood deliberately administered was much larger than whatever was inadvertently left in a syringe after it was flushed), it was probably not used on more than 1,000 patients.[13,28]

Data on the incidence of various diseases must be viewed with caution from a purely epidemiological perspective because year-to-year variations may reflect the more or less intense efforts made to find cases rather than true changes. For instance, the rising incidence of sleeping sickness in Cameroun around 1928 reflected the increasing resources devoted to its control: mobile teams explored areas where hitherto most cases had remained undiagnosed, unreported and untreated. However, even if imperfect for reconstructing disease dynamics, these data reflect accurately the numbers of patients treated with injectable drugs given for specific diseases.

In Cameroun, the incidence of sleeping sickness peaked at 54,712 new cases in 1928 (Figure 10). The disease was concentrated in a triangle east of Yaoundé (Akonolinga, Abomg-Mbang and Doumé) where in some communities almost everyone had to be treated. The incidence then decreased and stabilised at around 3,000 cases per year until 1952. The decline during WWII reflected reduced human and material resources for case-finding, as several of the medical officers were mobilised into general Leclerc's Free French Forces.[24,25,29,30]

In AEF-3, incidence of trypanosomiasis peaked in 1937 and the number of injections of trypanocidal drugs followed the same course, peaking at a staggering 588,086 injections. During the years for which detailed information is available, 74% of the 3.9 million injections used in the treatment of sleeping sickness were given IV (tartar emetic, suramin, tryparsamide, melarsoprol), 3% IM (pentamidine), 13% SC (atoxyl, trypoxyl) and for 10% the route is uncertain (orsanine). As discussed in the previous chapter, the IV injections provided the best opportunities for the transmission of blood-borne viruses.[10]

Apart from the short epidemic period in Cameroun, the annual incidence rates of trypanosomiasis were lower than 10 per 1,000 inhabitants (Figure 11). Thus the number of individuals who could have been iatrogenically infected with blood-borne viruses during trypanosomiasis treatment in colonial Cameroun was substantial (about 222,000), but not high enough by itself to result in the extremely high prevalence of hepatitis C (more than 40%) described much later throughout southern Cameroon, which must have resulted from a combination of interventions rather than from a single one.

However, we need just one of the trypanosomiasis patients to have been infected with SIV_{cpz}, acquired while manipulating chimpanzee carcasses, to initiate a chain of transmission that could have exponentially amplified the number of infected individuals. And the peak period for trypanosomiasis incidence and its injectable treatments, the late 1920s, corresponded closely, give or take a few years, to the dating of the most recent common ancestors of HIV-1 group M.

A new intervention, *pentamidinisation*, was launched in 1948. IM pentamidine, then a novel drug, was administered to the whole population of endemic areas as a preventive measure. Pentamidine was later used in the treatment of *Pneumocystis* pneumonia and, as seen in the introduction, an abnormal blip in its use played a role in the recognition of AIDS as a new disease in the US in 1981. Scientists of the colonial era mistakenly thought that pentamidine persisted long enough in the blood for a single injection to provide levels sufficient to abort infections with trypanosomes that might ensue over the following semester. In reality, there was little pentamidine remaining in the body two weeks later. In the early 1950s, more than half a million injections of pentamidine were given annually in French territories of central Africa (Figure 10). *Pentamidinisation* contributed to a further reduction in the incidence of sleeping sickness, not because it was truly preventive, but because single-dose pentamidine was curative for patients with recently acquired, often asymptomatic, trypanosomiasis.[31]

A description of the *pentamidinisation* procedures gives an idea of the potential for transmission of blood-borne pathogens:

A)

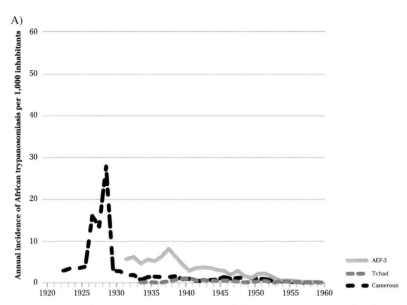

Figure 11 Incidence rates (per 1,000 inhabitants per year) of African trypanosomiasis, yaws and syphilis in Cameroun Français, AEF-3 and Tchad. Adapted from Pepin.[10]

The principles of mass production and time and motion study should be applied to ensure the maximum speed and efficiency in getting through, say, 250 injections in a morning. The man actually giving the injection should merely have to turn around in order to hand over his used syringe and take a freshly charged one. As he turns back again, a freshly iodined buttock, and the appropriate dose, should present themselves before him.[32]

Pentamidinisation was discontinued as endemic countries approached their independence. The injections were extremely painful, unpopular and associated with colonial rule. And as the incidence of trypanosomiasis declined further, priority was given to more pressing health needs, such as leprosy which had hitherto been neglected. Furthermore, outbreaks of gas gangrene (an infection that causes necrosis of the muscles, with a very high mortality rate) occurred in Gabon, Cameroun and Oubangui-Chari. Pentamidine bulk powder was diluted with locally procured water, some of which had been contaminated with *Clostridium* spores, which are very hard to kill. Dozens of deaths among healthy individuals as a consequence of a preventive intervention were unacceptable to local populations.

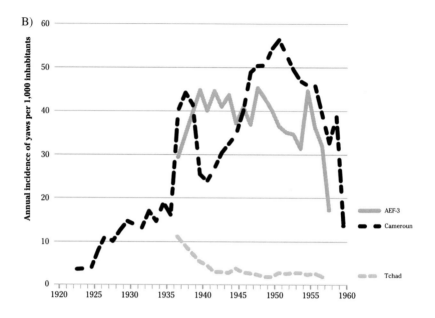

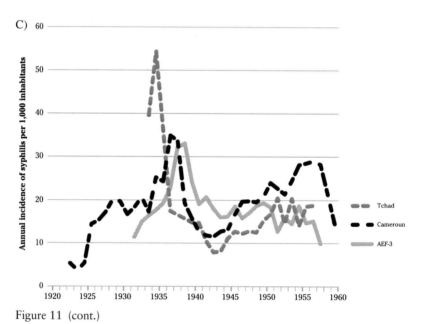

Figure 11 (cont.)

One of these iatrogenic tragedies, in Nkoltang, Gabon, where four-teen pentamidine recipients died of gas gangrene in 1952, provided an extraordinary example of the work of colonial spin doctors. While the inquiry revealed in confidential documents that the fault lay with the French nurse who did not properly sterilise the water that he had secured from a local source, which was itself contaminated with surface water, the official reports blamed the unfortunate recipients who were alleged to have applied some mud at the site of the injection as a pain-relieving method. This makes us wonder whether other iatrogenic complications, for instance outbreaks of 'inoculation hepatitis', would have been reported.[33–34]

Treponemes and metallic drugs

Chronologically, after trypanosomiasis, yaws and syphilis were the next diseases for the treatment of which huge numbers of injections were administered. They are caused by two subspecies of the same bacterium, *Treponema pallidum*, and are referred to as treponemal diseases, treated with antitreponemal drugs. Yaws, caused by *Treponema pallidum perte-nue*, is transmitted by non-sexual direct contacts. Its principal manifes-tation, skin lesions, can be spectacular, but there are few long-term complications. Its incidence was highest in children living in the forested areas of central Africa. In some populations mothers were deliberately infecting their children by inducing contacts with obvious cases so that their kids would develop immunity to yaws. On the other hand, sexually transmitted syphilis is caused by *Treponema pallidum pallidum*. It causes ulceration of the genitalia, after which it disseminates via the blood-stream, also causing skin lesions and later involvement of other organs including the aorta and the brain. Both infections were treated with arsenic-, bismuth- or mercury-based compounds and, since the mid-1950s, penicillin. Diagnoses of yaws were reasonably accurate because of the prominence of cutaneous signs. Although many diagnoses of syphilis, made without testing by nurses with only basic training, were doubtful (according to the health officials who wrote the reports), these patients were treated as if they indeed had syphilis.[35–36]

In Cameroun, the incidence of yaws increased dramatically in 1936, decreased transiently during WWII, peaked at 172,693 new cases in 1950 and slowly declined thereafter (Figure 12). For syphilis, a less marked biphasic pattern was seen. Throughout this period, annual

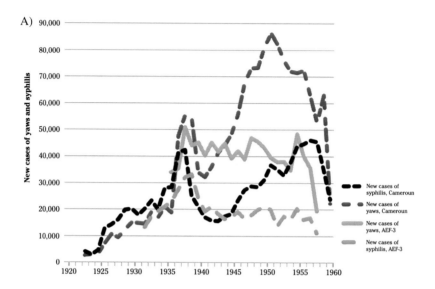

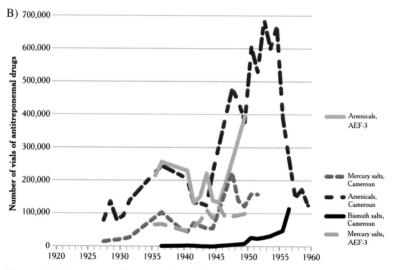

Figure 12 New cases of yaws and syphilis and consumption of antitreponemal drugs in Cameroun Français and AEF-3.
    Adapted from Pepin.[10]

incidence rates of yaws varied between 24 and 56 per 1,000 inhabitants; incidence of syphilis was lower, between 12 and 35 per 1,000 (Figure 11). In AEF-3, yaws peaked at 96,898 cases in 1954, while syphilis peaked earlier. Incidence rates of yaws were much lower in

Tchad than in AEF-3 or Cameroun, while there was little geographic variation for syphilis (Figure 11). Incidence rates of yaws and syphilis were highest in Gabon, where the ecological conditions facilitated the transmission of the former disease, while behaviours facilitated the latter.

Within Cameroun, there was little regional variation in the incidence rates of syphilis, but dramatic variations in the incidence of yaws, sometimes measured at over 200 per 1,000 inhabitants per year in the southern regions (where almost the whole population would be treated, mostly with injectable drugs, over just a few years) compared to less than 1 per 1,000 in the north. Coincidentally, the regions hyperendemic for yaws corresponded to the habitat of *P.t. troglodytes*.

Several therapeutic regimens with three to fifteen injections of metallic drugs were used: (i) arsenicals: IV novarsenobenzol, IV fontarsol, IM acetylarsan, IM sulpharsenol or oral stovarsol (children only); (ii) IM bismuth salts; or (iii) IV or IM mercury salts. Combination therapies made it possible to shorten the duration of treatment. Overall, patients received fewer injections than planned as some did not return when their skin lesions improved (in contrast with trypanosomiasis for which patients felt the need to receive all intended injections to improve their chances of survival).[37-40]

Data on consumption of antitreponemal drugs were more exhaustive for Cameroun, where the use of parenteral arsenicals increased dramatically, up to 688,750 vials in 1952 (Figure 12), in parallel with a rising incidence and better funding after the war. Overall, 51% of parenteral arsenicals used against yaws were administered IV. For bismuth salts, Figure 12 shows the numbers of vials. However, most of the bismuth came as bulk powder, which was then diluted locally with water. For 1952–4, it can be calculated that some 500,000 additional injections of bismuth were made each year. In AEF-3, use of parenteral arsenicals doubled to 394,189 vials in 1949; there is little information about bismuth. Mercury salts, cheaper but much more toxic, were abandoned in 1951.

When penicillin became available, older drugs were not abandoned immediately because the supply of the revolutionary drug was limited (and one can imagine that African colonies were not at the top of the list). In 1957, of 91,032 syphilis cases in Cameroun, 6% were treated with IM penicillin alone; others received metallic drugs alone (72%) or in combination with penicillin (23%). For yaws (105,513 cases) corresponding proportions were 43%, 46% and 11%.

It is remarkable that such a high incidence of yaws persisted despite millions of injections of metallic drugs, decreasing only after the introduction of penicillin, which was more effective, less toxic and easier to administer. The development of a depot form of penicillin, slowly absorbed from the muscle, made it possible to treat with a single IM injection the patients, their asymptomatic family contacts and, in some communities, all children. This eventually interrupted the chain of transmission but the disease was never eradicated. When incidence of yaws dropped to a low level, control programmes were discontinued, as this intervention now seemed far too costly compared to its limited health impacts.

From segregation to cure

Leprosy is a disease of skin and nerves caused by *Mycobacterium leprae*, a bacterium which reproduces extremely slowly (one division every twelve days, instead of every half-hour for many other bacteria), hence its sluggish progression. Apart from the all too evident disfiguring lesions of the face (and elsewhere), known since biblical times, leprosy alters sensory perception, which in turn leads to auto-amputation of the extremities. For a long time, many leprosy patients did not receive any pharmacological treatment and were segregated into leprosaria, euphemistically called 'agricultural colonies' in French Africa.

Figure 13 summarises the numbers of leprosy patients who did receive treatment. They were far fewer than cases of yaws or syphilis, but would ultimately receive the highest number of injections. Treatments were administered over several years, so these figures are a combination of new incident cases and prevalent cases diagnosed in the previous years. In Cameroun, from the late 1930s, a serious therapeutic effort was made. In AEF-3, which had fewer human and financial resources, the policy was not to bother with leprosy until modern therapeutic agents were introduced in the early 1950s. The extraordinary number of patients then treated included the cases that had been accumulating for decades because the disease was not lethal.

Initially, extracts of chaulmoogra, an Indian medicinal plant, were the main agents, given mostly IM (two to three times a week for the first year, then weekly for several years) but also orally, rectally, IV or directly in the lesions. Chaulmoogra was provided as bulk oil locally diluted or as vials. From the early 1930s to the late 1940s, following

A)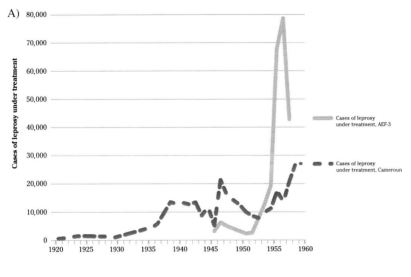

B)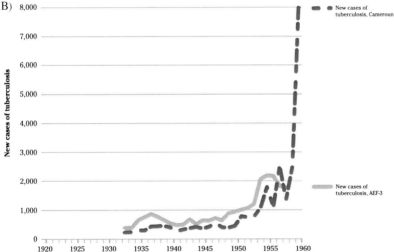

Figure 13 Cases of leprosy under treatment, and new cases of tuberculosis diagnosed in Cameroun Français and AEF-3.
Adapted from Pepin.[10]

enthusiastic reports by a renowned Saigon dermatologist, many lepers in Cameroun received IV methylene blue (a dye, resulting in greenish urine) concomitantly with IM chaulmoogra. The intended regimen of thirty to sixty IV injections over one year was often stopped prematurely due to adverse effects. Another medicinal product, aqueous *Caloncoba*, was given IV as an adjuvant to chaulmoogra. In 1939, 20% of Cameroonian lepers received chaulmoogra monotherapy, 24% *Caloncoba* monotherapy, 13% methylene blue monotherapy while others received various combinations of these. This wide variety of regimens indicated that none had a clear-cut beneficial effect. *Caloncoba* and methylene blue progressively lost favour.[38–39]

A new class of antimicrobial drugs, the sulphones, was introduced in the 1950s and proved dramatically superior. At last there was an effective treatment. Non-compliant patients received a depot sulphone solution, administered fortnightly by visiting nurses to patients queuing by the side of the road, while those thought to be more reliable were given an oral sulphone which they took every day at home. By 1957, all Cameroonian lepers received sulphones, 80% orally and 20% IM. In AEF-3, the proportion treated with IM sulphones varied from 15% in Oubangui-Chari to 60% in Moyen-Congo. These treatments were continued for a few years in patients with less severe leprosy and longer in cases of lepromatous leprosy where the bacterial load in infected tissues is higher.[41]

Quinimax

The other extremely common tropical disease for which injectable drugs were used on a large scale was malaria. Malaria can be caused by five different species of the *Plasmodium* parasites. *Plasmodium falciparum* is the most important by far, the one that kills. It causes fever with other non-specific symptoms such as muscle aches. In the severe form, the parasites destroy a large number of red blood cells (necessitating a transfusion), or lead to the occlusion of small blood vessels within the brain (the patient becomes comatose). In highly endemic areas of Africa, children develop some immunity against the parasite so that the severe forms are rarely seen above five years of age.

This disease received little attention in the annual reports of the colonial health systems because it was not a specific target of disease control interventions. Malaria was so common that its control was seen as being beyond the reach of even the most enthusiastic health planners. Counting cases was pointless in countries where half of the children carried a small number of malaria parasites in their blood year round. Furthermore, malaria was fatal almost exclusively among children, and the authorities were interested mainly in short-term investments in the health of adults who paid taxes, produced cash crops and could be conscripted into the colonial army.

Thus the treatment of malaria was left to the discretion of each hospital and health centre, and no statistics were tabulated. It is hard to estimate the proportion of cases treated parenterally, but various preparations of quinine were available. In francophone Africa, for a long time the most popular product was called Quinimax. Parenteral quinine was generally administered IV rather than IM because the latter route caused abscesses or even gangrene at the injection site. Quinine tablets were available, and the injectable forms were given mostly to patients when a rapid effect was deemed necessary (cerebral malaria, severe anaemia), or to those presenting with nausea or vomiting who would not tolerate oral administration. Injections became very popular among the Africans, who thought this route had to be more powerful than any oral medication, so that in practice the indications for the parenteral treatment of malaria were broader than those mentioned in the textbooks. Another antimalarial drug, quinacrine, could also be administered SC, IM or IV. Its use increased during WWII, when allied countries were cut off from their Asian sources of quinine. Chloroquine, which first appeared after the war, was almost always given orally.[37–39]

And the rest

In the 1930s and 1940s, only 1,000 cases of schistosomiasis were reported annually in Cameroun, and around 2,000 in AEF-3. Most patients were left untreated as the adverse effects of IM antimonials or IV emetine seemed worse than the symptoms of the infection. Clearly, the control of schistosomiasis did not play in central Africa the same role as in Egypt in the dissemination of blood-borne viruses.[42]

No parenteral drug was used against filariasis, another group of tropical diseases. Most cases corresponded to *Loa loa* or *Mansonella perstans* found incidentally creeping in the blood during examinations for malaria or trypanosomiasis. These infections brought about little symptoms and were left untreated. River blindness was uncommon in central Africa, in contrast with its disastrous impact in West Africa. The only short-lived attempt for its mass treatment with IV suramin took place in the Mayo Kebbi district of Tchad, which is outside our region of interest. This strategy was quickly abandoned because of the severe adverse effects induced by the destruction of the parasite.

Tuberculosis was remarkably uncommon until 1950, with fewer than 500 cases annually in Cameroun and less than 1,000 in AEF-3 (Figure 13). No treatment was offered and there was no attempt to segregate patients in sanatoria. Later, incidence increased dramatically, coinciding with the introduction of chemotherapy. Most patients received IM streptomycin daily for the first month, then two to three times per week for eighteen to twenty-four months, along with oral drugs. In Cameroun, annual streptomycin consumption increased from 100 (1949) to 511,941 grams (1959). The huge rise in incidence is troubling, and one wonders whether this may to some extent have reflected the early emergence of HIV-1, which substantially enhances the risk of developing tuberculosis. However, the introduction of effective treatments may have increased the number of patients seeking a diagnosis, the supply of diagnostic tests or the aggressiveness of case-finding activities, as will be reviewed in the next chapter for the Belgian Congo.[43]

Vaccines administered on a large scale were those against smallpox (since the early 1920s) and yellow fever (mid-1940s). The latter was a 'scratch vaccine' administered ID, simultaneously with the former. The policy was to re-immunise everyone every four to six years. Year-to-year variations (Figure 14) depended on vaccine availability, perceived threats and opportunities for immunisation by mobile teams. Other vaccines of unproven efficacy were given selectively and are unlikely to have played a part in the spread of blood-borne viruses.[44]

An accident of history

Spain owned a tiny colony in central Africa, Guinea Espanola (now Guinea Ecuatorial), which is also inhabited by the *P.t. troglodytes*. It consisted of a continental part, Rio Muni, squeezed between Gabon and Cameroun, and the Atlantic islands of Fernando Poo (now Bioko) and Annabon (the islands were part of a deal between Spain and Portugal, exchanged for the Sacramento colony in South America in the late eighteenth century). Reports of the health system suggest that the epidemiological situation of this small population was similar to that of Gabon and Cameroun, as were the health interventions. During the 1940s and 1950s, incidence rates of yaws varied between 37 and 50 per 1,000, syphilis between 3 and 4 per 1,000, and trypanosomiasis

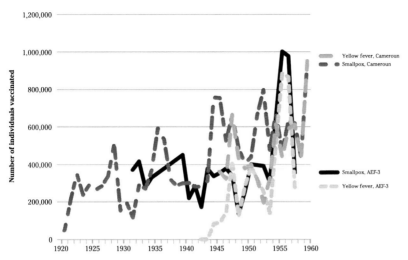

Figure 14 Number of individuals vaccinated against smallpox and yellow fever in Cameroun Français and AEF-3.
Adapted from Pepin.[10]

between 0.3 and 2.1 per 1,000. Pentamidinisation was used in some areas. It is thus possible that blood-borne viruses were transmitted in Guinea Espanola as well.[45–48]

From tropical diseases to blood-borne viruses

So the opportunities for the parenteral transmission of viruses throughout central Africa were numerous. Now we will try to understand how more than 40% of the elderly population of southern Cameroon got infected with HCV, as a model for the putative parenteral transmission of HIV-1. Given that HCV is transmitted more efficiently through IV rather than other types of injections, for any given patient the highest risk must have been for sleeping sickness cases treated with IV tryparsamide (around thirty-six injections) or leprosy patients given IV methylene blue or *Caloncoba* plus IM chaulmoogra over a period of years, followed by patients who received just a few IV injections, for instance to treat malaria, then those who received the biannual pentamidine IM injections and finally, at the other end of the spectrum, individuals given only intradermal immunisations every five years.[49]

Indeed, in Africa, Brazil and Asia, leprosy patients treated in the distant past are more likely than others to be infected not just with HCV but also with HBV and the HTLV-1 retrovirus. However, the proportion of Cameroonians ever treated for trypanosomiasis or leprosy was lower than the 40–50% who became HCV-infected in some areas, implying that other interventions must have played a role as well.[50–54]

In Cameroon, populations with a high HCV prevalence live in Yaoundé or communities in the southern rain forest (Figure 9 and Map 5). I initially believed that the HCV epidemic could have been driven by campaigns against yaws, for several reasons. First, the sheer numbers: from the mid-1930s till the late 1950s, in some regions, the whole population developed yaws within a few years and received antitreponemal drugs. Second, the age distribution: yaws was more common among children who had the opportunity to survive until the mid-1990s when HCV surveys were carried out. Third, the rise in incidence of yaws in Cameroun after 1935 corresponds chronologically to what can be inferred to be the period of highest HCV transmission. Fourth, the geographic distribution of HCV coincides with that of yaws, whose incidence was much higher in coastal and forested regions than in northern savannahs.[10]

The same north–south gradient in yaws incidence was observed in the AEF, now mirrored by a higher HCV prevalence in southern areas. In these countries, HCV prevalence is three to six times lower in Pygmies than Bantus, perhaps reflecting less intensive uptake of medical interventions among the former. There is also a north–south gradient in HTLV-1 prevalence, suggesting that this retrovirus may have been transmitted iatrogenically during the same interventions.[7,55–58]

But there was another common tropical disease with a marked north–south gradient in incidence: malaria. While malaria occurs throughout tropical Africa, its distribution is heterogeneous, in line with that of its vector, the female anopheline mosquito. The risk of malaria is quantified by the number of infective mosquito bites sustained each year by each person. In tropical Africa, the median number of infective bites is 77 per year, but in the rural and rainy areas of central Africa this number is generally ≥200. The record belongs to a village of Equatorial Guinea, where humans sustain 1,030 infective bites per year, three per day! In large cities such as Kinshasa and Brazzaville, the risk is lower (3–30 bites) because there is less stagnant water where the vectors can breed and many more humans in relation to the population of mosquitoes. But one just has to drive fifteen kilometres to the semi-rural areas around Kinshasa and the risk goes up to 620 bites per year.[59–61]

In the southern and forested areas of Cameroon, there is up to 4,000 mm of rain each year, compared to only 800 mm in the extreme north. The number of infective bites varies accordingly, with high values in the south-west of the country, and low values in the arid north. The risk of developing malaria, and of eventually needing to receive IV quinine, varies along the same patterns. Thus malaria also correlated nicely with HCV distribution: a marked north–south gradient, a high incidence so that a large proportion of the population would receive parenteral antimalarial drugs at least once, the correct age distribution (more severe in children) and the correct time frame (the frequency of its parenteral treatment presumably increased in parallel with the development of fixed health services, from the 1930s onward).

To determine which interventions had really driven HCV transmission in southern Cameroon, we conducted a survey in the city of Ebolowa, among individuals aged sixty years or more, 56% of whom were HCV-infected, the highest prevalence in the world, while 74% had antitreponemal antibodies, indicating prior yaws or syphilis. We found no evidence that HCV had been transmitted during yaws treatment; many cases occurred during childhood and those treated parenterally received IM rather than IV injections.[62]

However, 80% of the interviewees had experienced at least once in their lifetime an episode of illness for which IV injections were administered, and in about two-thirds of the cases this was for the treatment of malaria. HCV infection was associated with such treatments against malaria and, in the men's case, with having been circumcised traditionally (during collective ceremonies, using knives or broken bottles). Because of its high frequency, the IV treatment of malaria had been the main driver of the transmission of HCV.[62]

We conducted a similar study of elderly individuals in a rural area of south-west Central African Republic (in and around Nola) which used to be, in the 1930s and 1940s, the most virulent focus of African trypanosomiasis. HCV prevalence was much lower than in Cameroun but we found that having been treated for trypanosomiasis in the 1930s and 1940s was associated with HCV, while having received injections of pentamidine for the prevention of trypanosomiasis (between 1946 and 1953) was associated with infection with the HTLV-1 retrovirus. The latter, although much less studied as a blood-borne agent, is an interesting proxy for HIV-1, because it also originated from *Pan trog-lodytes* and infects CD4 lymphocytes (without causing AIDS). We also documented an extraordinary excess mortality amongst individuals who had been treated for sleeping sickness in the 1930s and 1940s. After excluding all other causes, we concluded that this excess mortality was probably caused by the iatrogenic transmission of HIV-1.[63]

Thus several medical interventions were associated with the iatro-genic transmission of blood-borne viruses, and it seems likely that the respective contribution of each varied from place to place, and also over time, depending on the local epidemiology of tropical diseases. And if interventions for the control of tropical diseases contributed to the transmission of HCV and HTLV-1 in Cameroun and AEF in the middle of the twentieth century, the same procedures must have amplified HIV-1 as well, from a single hunter/cook occupationally infected with SIV_{cpz} to several hundred patients treated with arsenicals or other drugs, a threshold beyond which sexual transmission could prosper.

As reviewed in Chapter 4, the number of individuals occupationally infected with SIV_{cpz} around 1921 was probably less than ten, but the probability that these individuals received IV or IM treatment for yaws, syphilis, trypanosomiasis, leprosy or malaria was very high, near 100% for those who lived in the areas hyperendemic for yaws and malaria. Once a second person had been iatrogenically infected with SIV_{cpz}, he/she would develop a high viraemia during primary infection and for a few weeks would be extremely infectious for other patients treated in the same facility with the same hastily sterilised syringes and needles. A vicious circle could result.

In the next chapter, we will examine what happened at the same time in the Belgian Congo. It is unlikely that the original SIV_{cpz}-infected cut hunter lived in this other colony, in which only a tiny fraction of the continent-wide populations of *P.t. troglodytes* were present. Furthermore, there is no evidence that the bonobo, found only in the Belgian Congo, played a role in the emergence of HIV-1. However, the city of Léopoldville was at the heart of the early dissemination of the virus: this is the place where the two oldest HIV-1-containing speci-mens were discovered and the area with the highest genetic diversity of HIV-1 isolates in the world.

9 | The legacies of colonial medicine II: the Belgian Congo

While France was busy running the health systems of more than twenty-five territories in Africa, around the Indian Ocean, in south-east Asia and the Americas, Belgium could concentrate its efforts on its three African colonies, the largest of which by far was the Belgian Congo. Belgium was justifiably proud of its achievements in the Congo, whose health system soon acquired the reputation of being the best in tropical Africa. This led to a substantial improvement in the health of the Congolese people, but also to numerous opportunities for the transmission of blood-borne microbial agents. What happened in and around Léopoldville will be especially relevant, as this is the area where ultimately HIV-1 spread and diversified.

For this part of the story, the best sources of information are in Belgium. Since 1960 the ministry of foreign affairs has kept the archives of the Belgian Congo, which are accessible to researchers. The Royal Library and the university libraries of Brussels, Louvain and Louvain-la-Neuve hold impressive collections of books and journals relating to the country's former colonies. In Antwerp, the tropical medicine institute has made available online the *Annales de la Société Belge de Médecine Tropicale*, in which Belgian medical officers working in the tropics used to publish their findings. More detailed articles were published through the Académie Royale des Sciences Coloniales.

The work of colonial doctors in the Congo was summarised by Jacques Schwetz, a Russian émigré who became a prolific tropical medicine researcher. For somebody to be considered a good doctor, two instruments were essential: a microscope, and a syringe for IV and SC injections. We will see that there were other similarities with the French colonies, but also a few interesting distinctive features.[1]

A patchwork

The first health reports available in the archives start in 1908, the year the colony was bought by Belgium. The health system was rudimentary with small hospitals in Boma, Léopoldville and Stanleyville (Map 6), mostly to provide care to the Europeans. In separate premises, basic care was offered to the soldiers of the Force Publique and some other Africans: mainly the treatment of sleeping sickness with early drugs. The largest facility was the 125-bed Hôpital des Noirs in Boma, the capital, where basic surgery was available. A similar hospital existed in Léo, also with an operating room, while patients with sleeping sickness were treated in the nearby *lazaret*. Patients with syphilis or yaws were given IV arsenicals as early as 1910, by which time there were forty-seven medical doctors in the colony. In the mining areas, private

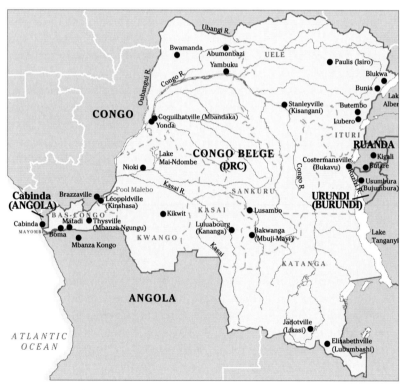

Map 6 Map of the Belgian Congo (current names in brackets).

companies built their own hospitals to care for their workers. Smaller government facilities were developed, with forty clinics or hospitals by 1914.[2]

Mobile teams for the control of sleeping sickness were tested in the Uele and Kwango regions, and then generalised to other endemic areas. These were staffed by expatriate doctors and health agents, as well as Congolese *injecteurs*, people with no formal education who learned over a few months how to do injections and use a microscope to search for trypanosomes. Most trypanosomiasis patients were treated in their own villages by visiting *injecteurs*, who administered eight to twelve weekly injections of arsenicals. In between patients, the syringes and needles were simply rinsed with phenilated water. Later, when sleeping sickness was brought under control, the mobile teams also took care of other endemic diseases such as yaws.[3–5]

Until the mid-1930s, a short course was given in Léopoldville for selected Catholic and Protestant missionaries to enable those working in isolated areas far from any hospital or health post to diagnose and treat a few infectious diseases: trypanosomiasis, yaws and syphilis. They were given a microscope, syringes, needles and arsenical drugs. These missionaries would provide valuable services to underprivileged populations but apparently they were not very good at sending reports. In 1926, there were ninety-three such centres run by volunteer missionaries.

Progressively, the health system was developed as a patchwork of institutions run by the government, Catholic and Protestant missions, philanthropic organisations and private companies. To encourage physicians to go to the Congo, newly qualified Belgian doctors who signed a five-year contract were exempted from their two-year military service. By 1940, there were 302 medical doctors in the Congo: 161 employed by the government, 81 by private companies, 49 by missions or philanthropic institutions and 11 in private practice. In contrast with the French colonies, WWII had little impact on the resources available for health services in the Congo, which functioned like an independent country, exporting large quantities of rubber and minerals needed for the allied war industry. A few doctors and nurses accompanied the 10,000-strong Force Publique units which fought against the Italians in Ethiopia and spent a year in Egypt, but the vast majority of healthcare providers remained in the Congo. Health research continued, and a special journal was published so that new ideas could be disseminated while the colony was cut off from Antwerp.

The development of the health system accelerated after the war, when Belgium felt it had a moral debt towards the Congo, and the annual reports detail an impressive list of capital investments. During the 1950s, ninety-six district hospitals, each with between 120 and 200 beds, were built, and 10% of the colony's regular budget was spent on health care. In 1958, just before the Belgian Congo became independent, there were 2,815 health institutions of all kinds (general hospitals, maternity hospitals, dispensaries, health posts, etc.) with 85,000 hospital beds, more than in the rest of Africa put together, staffed by 703 medical doctors and 1,239 expatriate nurses, but only 128 Congolese medical assistants and 990 Congolese registered nurses. To a large extent, the increases in the number of cases of various diseases which we will review followed this advancement in the availability of health services.[6]

The control of infectious diseases

Starting in the early 1920s, the annual reports of the public health system improved in quality, as did the coverage of the country's population. However, while doctors in the public sector consistently provided data about the number of cases of such and such a disease treated during the previous year, their colleagues in mission hospitals or private companies (the largest of which operated their own healthcare system for their workers and dependants, who in some areas constituted the majority of the population) rarely did so until the early 1930s. Even in the public sector, the cases treated in rural dispensaries without medical supervision were not always tabulated. The incidence data should thus be interpreted as being indicative only of major trends.

As in French territories, sleeping sickness dominated the first few decades of the Belgian Congo. Here again, it is plausible that colonisation and the mixing of populations facilitated the transmission of the parasite. As the public health system increased its reach and implemented case-finding activities following Jamot's model, ever-increasing numbers of cases were diagnosed and treated. In 1920 in the Kikwit territory, a few hundred kilometres east of Léo, 8,922 cases were diagnosed in a single year. As the mobile teams moved eastward into the Kasaï region, other high-prevalence communities were identified, where up to 70% of inhabitants were found to have sleeping sickness, very much like in Cameroun. At some point, overwhelmed by the situation, short of trained microscopists able to spend long periods of time looking for trypanosomes in lymph node aspirates or blood, Schwetz, the head of the mission, decided to do something very unusual: all patients with enlarged cervical lymph nodes were treated without any parasitological assay being performed. In 1924, out of 69,298 cases nationwide, about 20,000 were these 'suspect' cases. Two years later, there were 39,033 suspects among the 64,015 new cases reported. Whether or not these individuals indeed had trypanosomiasis, they received injectable trypanocidal drugs. The practice was discontinued shortly thereafter, and treatment given only to patients with a confirmed diagnosis. In the 1920s, data also took into consideration cases diagnosed during the previous years that needed to receive further treatment, either because they were relapsing or simply to consolidate the initial treatment. Starting in 1930, only new cases with parasitologically confirmed disease were reported. The evolution of the incidence of sleeping sickness in the Congo is shown in Figure 15. As in the French colonies, control measures proved very effective and the number of confirmed cases decreased from 36,030 in 1930 to 1,218 in 1958, the last year for which an annual report was produced. Thus the opportunities for the transmission of blood-borne viruses during the treatment of sleeping sickness were significant mostly during the first three decades of the twentieth century.[1,7,8]

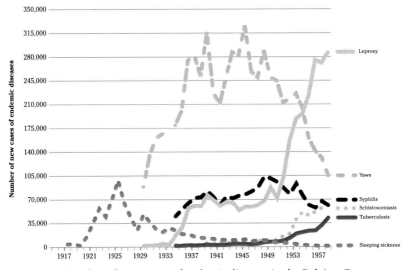

Figure 15 Number of new cases of endemic diseases in the Belgian Congo.

For other endemic diseases, the quality of the health information system improved considerably when, aware that the rational organisation and evaluation of disease control activities required an accurate view of the overall epidemiological situation, medical authorities prompted the colony's governor to issue edicts that forced all healthcare institutions, regardless of their nature, to provide reports on priority diseases. The treatment of some infectious diseases was made compulsory and free. Yaws was the first for which comprehensive information became available in 1930, soon followed by syphilis and tuberculosis.

The Congo's annual reports contained little information about treatments. In general, it seems that therapeutic strategies did not differ much from those adopted in AEF and Cameroun. For leprosy, on top of chaulmoogra another medicinal product was used: hydnocarpus oil, various preparations of which were administered IV, but methylene blue and *Caloncoba* were also popular for a while. For syphilis, in addition to the injections of arsenical or bismuth-containing drugs ('specific treatment'), ointments were applied on the lesions.[9–11]

As shown in Figures 15 and 16, by far the most common endemic disease treated with injectable drugs was yaws, peaking at 325,000 cases in 1945. Its incidence varied dramatically between regions. The highest was in the Costermansville province in the eastern part of the country (later known as Kivu), while yaws was uncommon in Katanga and Kasaï (Figure 17). One of the high-incidence areas was the Mayombe part of Bas-Congo, the only region of the country inhabited by the *Pan troglodytes troglodytes*.[12,13]

Even with the early arsenic- or bismuth-based drugs, the treatment of yaws was so effective, with the skin lesions rapidly regressing, that it was considered a useful public relations measure to attract the natives to the healthcare system, where more important diseases could be diagnosed and treated. The incidence of syphilis was about one third that of yaws, and this STD seemed to have been less common than in the French colonies. This may have reflected an incidence that was truly lower, or perhaps differences in the diagnostic approaches and more rigorous identification of clinically diagnosed cases through more intense medical supervision. There was relatively little regional variation in the incidence of syphilis.

Schistosomiasis was rarely diagnosed initially, exceeding the 10,000 mark only in 1949. Most early patients were treated with IV tartar

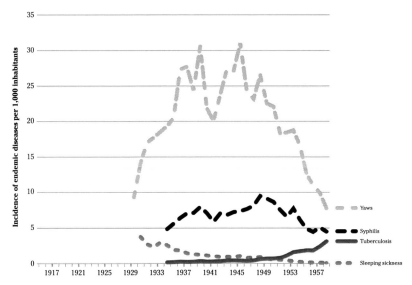

Figure 16 Annual incidence of endemic diseases in the Belgian Congo.

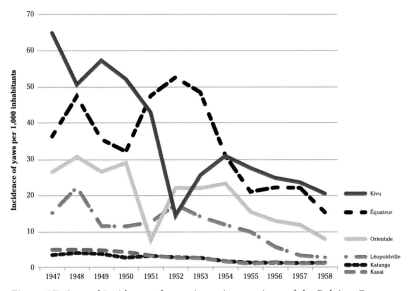

Figure 17 Annual incidence of yaws in various regions of the Belgian Congo.

emetic, as in Egypt. The number of cases reported increased to 40,000–60,000 in the 1950s, but an oral drug artistically called Nilodin (this disease was common in the Nile delta) became popular and may have prompted more dynamic case-finding. Schistosomiasis was prevalent mostly in the eastern end of the country, far from the areas inhabited by the central chimpanzee.[14]

For leprosy, the number of cases reported included a mix of prevalent cases accumulated over the years, and new cases diagnosed within the previous twelve months. The statistics reported those under treatment, loosely defined, and most patients remained in that category for years even if they only had their wounds dressed. There were important geographic variations in the prevalence of leprosy, which was less common in the Mayombe, Bas-Congo and Léopoldville areas. The introduction of sulphone drugs in the early 1950s revolutionised its treatment: oral dapsone was given to patients treated in a leprosarium while fortnightly injections were used for outpatients, who accounted for 86% of cases.[15–16]

Annual reports from the Belgian Congo provided relatively little information about malaria, presumably because the disease was so common that no public health intervention targeting this scourge could be contemplated. Fatalism prevailed. Most deaths occurred among young children, often at home rather than in a health institution. The number of malaria cases reported by government health services increased from 66,038 in 1940 to 938,477 in 1958. This probably did not reflect any genuine change in incidence, but only the degree of penetration and accessibility of health services. The high prevalence of asymptomatic malaria parasitaemia made these statistics somewhat meaningless. In areas where 50% of all healthy looking children have malaria parasites in their blood almost year round, any patient with any febrile illness who gets a blood smear done would have a 50% probability of being smear-positive. Who knows when the febrile episode is really caused by malaria? Based on the prevalence of parasitaemia or splenomegaly (an enlarged spleen) measured during systematic surveys, malaria was most common in the Congo basin and less so in the hilly areas in the east. Antimalarial treatments were used massively and some of these were injectable drugs, mostly IV quinine.[17–21]

The therapeutic virtues of quinine, used by the first physician who worked in Léopoldville (1885–7), were known before the aetiological agent of malaria was identified. Oral quinine was used for the prevention of malaria by Europeans, and proved the most effective intervention in reducing the mortality of colonists in central Africa. The investment in tropical medicine and disease control interventions for the natives eventually paid off: by 1940, the mortality of Europeans in the Congo was marginally higher than that of their kin in Belgium. The plant from which quinine is extracted was grown in the Kivu province so the colony became self-sufficient.[22,23]

The only large-scale immunisation was against smallpox; in the 1950s, between two and five million doses were administered annually. It is thus apparent that, across the entire colony, interventions for the control of sleeping sickness before 1930, and against yaws and to a lesser extent against syphilis after 1930, as well as the parenteral treatment of malaria in hospitals and dispensaries, provided the best opportunities for the iatrogenic transmission of blood-borne agents, including SIV_{cpz}/HIV-1. Focally, the potential role of each disease varied with the local epidemiology and disease control strategies, as we will see shortly for Léopoldville.

A network

As reviewed in Chapter 4, it was suggested that the Stanleyville public health laboratory played a role in the emergence of HIV-1, a hypothesis subsequently disproved. But could other Congolese laboratories have manipulated blood, serum or tissues in a way that would have facilitated the transmission of the virus?

In Léopoldville, a small laboratory set up in 1899 during the EIC period provided diagnostic assays not available elsewhere. The scope of tests gradually expanded: initially only the microscopic examination of stained or unstained specimens, then serology, followed by bacteriological cultures and, in the 1950s, haematological and biochemical assays and even viral cultures. From its early days, the Léopoldville laboratory conducted clinical research on sleeping sickness and experimented with a long list of candidate drugs. With Louise Pearce, a visiting American scientist (always referred to as Miss Pearce rather than Dr Pearce, her unmarried status apparently being more important than her degrees!), starting in 1920 the laboratory carried out the trials that ultimately documented the efficacy of tryparsamide in late-stage sleeping sickness, a major step forward in the treatment of this dreaded disease. The laboratory became a respected world-class research institution with seven Belgian MDs, three biologists, sixteen expatriate laboratory technicians and twenty-five Congolese nurses or medical assistants. In 1937, it moved to a site adjacent to the Hôpital des Noirs and became known as the Princess Astrid Institute of Tropical Medicine (literally, the companion institution of the Prince Leopold Institute of Tropical Medicine in Antwerp). An annex was built to house a sleeping sickness laboratory where trypanosomes could be cultured (very few laboratories could do that at the time, or even today) and tsetse flies bred for experiments on animal models. Some experiments were conducted on monkeys (*Cercopithecus* and *Cercocebus*). A few autopsies were conducted on chimpanzees to look for filariasis, and a single chimpanzee seems to have been inoculated with trypanosomes, but these are the only documented cases of work on apes during more than fifty years of operations. By a strange twist of fate, fifty years later the conference centre of the Léo laboratory would become the site for Projet Sida, the heart of HIV research in Africa in the 1980s.[24-29]

The laboratory prepared vaccines against multiple pathogens: the pneumococcus, gonococcus, meningococcus, staphylococcus, the agents of typhoid, plague, dysentery, tetanus, diphtheria, yellow fever and rabies. A few were imported and conditioned in Léo, while very crude vaccines were produced locally from bacteriological cultures of the targeted pathogens, heat-killed before inoculation, and used as preventive measures among populations with a high incidence of the targeted diseases, or in an attempt to control outbreaks. Some vaccines had therapeutic rather than preventive goals; for example, patients with gonorrhoea were administered the antigonococcal vaccine in the hope that this mix of antigens inoculated in large quantities would result in the production of systemic antibodies that would in turn control the infection in their genital tract. An interesting concept was the *auto-vaccin* (self-vaccine): an isolate of a given pathogen obtained from a given patient would be grown in the laboratory, heat-killed and re-injected in the patient in large quantities, again in the hope of triggering the production of antibodies. Although these bacterial vaccines were probably ineffective, no animal cells were required for their preparation, and the risks of infection were those associated with any other type of injections. The yellow fever and rabies vaccines against viral infections required cells for their production, such as chick embryos.[7,30]

When supplies from Europe were cut off in 1940, the Léopoldville laboratory started preparing therapeutic sera. This continued throughout that decade, to be abandoned only when effective antibiotics such as penicillin became available for patients with pneumonia and meningitis. Therapeutic sera contained, in principle, high levels of antibodies against the pathogen with which the recipient patient was infected. Sera could be produced in animals (which were injected with a large quantity of the bacteria of interest) or obtained from convalescent patients who had just recovered from the disease and were assumed to have developed antibodies. The health services reports indicate that the Léo laboratory produced therapeutic sera against the pneumococcus, meningococcus and the agents of dysentery. Ten years earlier in Katanga, an antimeningococcal serum had been prepared from the inoculation of heat-killed bacteria to mules, due to a dearth of horses. Injected through a lumbar puncture, this was thought to reduce mortality. Horses were available in Léopoldville and were used for the preparation of antisera. The laboratory kept a colony of vipers to extract venom, minute quantities of which were then injected in the same horses to generate an antivenom serum.[7,31,32]

The Léopoldville laboratory also produced a therapeutic serum against poliomyelitis, this time obtained from convalescent patients. The latter disease was relatively rare and the number of recipients must have been small, probably mostly European children. Interestingly, when the first epidemic of highly lethal Ebola fever was recognised in the 1970s, a few patients were treated with convalescent sera obtained from patients who had just survived the infection (whether this measure was effective in reducing mortality is unknown). Necessity is the mother of invention and at the end of WWII the Léo laboratory even produced raw penicillin, presumably from the fungus which was the original source of that revolutionary drug. Across the river, the Brazzaville Institut Pasteur was producing similar bacterial vaccines and therapeutic sera and kept a small colony of monkeys and a few chimpanzees for various experiments, such as verifying the efficacy of its vaccines and antisera.[33]

Smaller provincial laboratories were built in Elisabethville, Stanleyville (the one with the chimpanzee colony), Coquilhatville and Blukwa. The main function of the Stanleyville laboratory, apart from performing diagnostic assays for patients of the Province Orientale and producing crude bacterial vaccines, was yellow fever surveillance and research. There were very few cases of this disease in the Belgian Congo, but it was still considered a potential threat. Hospitals throughout the colony would send to Stanleyville specimens of liver biopsies obtained post-mortem from patients who had died with jaundice or an unexplained febrile illness. An edict made this compulsory if the local doctor decided it was needed; and if the relatives of the deceased thought that part of their loved one was sent abroad for mysterious and possibly magical purposes, it was just too bad. About 2,000 liver specimens were examined each year by a pathologist, and diseases such as schistosomiasis, tuberculosis and liver cancer were far more common than yellow fever. The Stanleyville laboratory performed histopathological examinations on biopsies of other organs and each year diagnosed thirty to sixty cases of Kaposi's sarcoma, a cancer potentially associated with HIV. During the period for which laboratory reports are available, there was no evidence that this cancer was becoming more frequent. In 1953, the laboratory initiated a programme of blood transfusions from volunteer donors, the first in the country. Donors were identified, their blood group determined, and they would be asked by phone to come to the hospital when needed. Until then, relatives or friends of recipients had been donating blood on a case-by-case basis.[34,35]

The Elisabethville laboratory prepared a smallpox vaccine for the whole colony, and more generally worked on viral infections. It had a long-standing interest in poliomyelitis. The Coquilhatville laboratory made chaulmoogra oil from a local plant, to be used in the treatment of leprosy. The small laboratory in Blukwa on Lake Albert focused on plague, and during the 1940s produced large quantities of an antiplague therapeutic serum as well as an antidysenteric serum. During the 1950s, additional laboratories were established in Lubero, Bukavu, Bunia, Butembo, Paulis and Luluabourg.

Despite this wide and creative range of biological activities conducted in ten different sites over several decades, there is no documentary evidence that any of these laboratories manipulated blood or serum in a way or on a scale that could have facilitated the emergence of HIV-1. The Stanleyville laboratory was the only one that used a substantial number of chimpanzees, but we have seen that this is not where HIV-1 originated.

In a class of his own

Between the purchase and transformation of the EIC into the Belgian Congo in 1908 and its accession to independence in 1960, thousands of doctors and nurses left Belgium to work in the Congo. Some only stayed for a few years while others spent most of their career there. None of them left such an indelible mark as Lucien Van Hoof.[36–39]

Born in 1890, a doctor's son, Van Hoof completed his medical degree in Louvain, where he worked for a short time in a bacteriology laboratory. During WWI, he served in military hospitals in Belgium, and volunteered to join the Belgian colonial troops fighting to conquer the then German colony of Tanganyika, arriving in Africa for the first time in 1916. After hostilities ended, the government of the Belgian Congo posted him to Léopoldville, first in the hospital and then in the laboratory. He spent a few years in Boma as director of public health, in Stanleyville as director of the laboratory and in Katanga as the province's chief medical officer. He led a scientific mission in the 'Belgian' Mayombe to investigate an epidemic of dysentery and another in eastern Africa for the League of Nations, concerning the control of trypanosomiasis. He became director of the Léo laboratory in 1930, and was the main architect of its transformation into an institution with an international reputation and spacious, modern premises.

His scientific publications started to appear in 1917. Initially, they covered a wide variety of diseases, as he encountered them in his practice: malaria, onchocerciasis, yaws, dysentery, smallpox, influenza, tuberculosis, meningitis, amoebiasis and relapsing fever. He later focused exclusively on trypanosomiasis, its treatment, epidemiology, transmission, vectors and animal reservoirs. Van Hoof rarely used chimpanzees in his own research, but sent primates to his former mentor, Jérôme Rodhain, in Antwerp for the latter's work on malaria.[40]

In 1934, because of his intellectual ability and knowledge of the colony, Van Hoof was appointed chief medical officer of the Belgian Congo for the usual six-year term. However, WWII intervened and he stayed in this position until 1946. An indefatigable worker without any family obligations (he never married), he led an austere life. His job was to supervise the healthcare system of a huge and complex colony, which employed hundreds of doctors. Under his direction, there was an impressive development, which was barely slowed by the world war. He was also the chief medical officer of the Force Publique and visited the expeditionary forces in Egypt and Nigeria. He never gave up his position in the colonial army and had risen to the rank of general by the end of his career.

A population-based approach was gradually introduced in the Belgian Congo, with ambitious objectives to control certain tropical diseases, like its French neighbours. It was no longer a matter of simply treating cases one by one for the sake of charity, but of reducing the spread of some of the transmissible agents by 'sterilising' their human reservoir. Relatively reliable national statistics were collected for the first time. During his twelve years at the helm, the incidence of trypanosomiasis was reduced by two-thirds. The number of cases of yaws and syphilis doubled because resources were allocated to diagnose, treat and record cases in previously neglected parts of the colony.

Despite a heavy administrative workload, Van Hoof maintained his intense scientific focus and became a leading expert on African trypanosomiasis. To speed up its control, he initiated a series of experiments on the preventive power of pentamidine, a drug that had just been added to the therapeutic arsenal. The idea of preventing trypanosomiasis by chemoprophylaxis (giving a drug systematically and regularly to the entire population of endemic regions) was not new but had never been used on a large scale. Suramin, the only drug utilised for this purpose, had to be given IV every three months, which posed an insurmountable logistical problem.

After a few preliminary tests on guinea pigs, Van Hoof turned to humans. Earlier in 1942, two healthy volunteers had been experimentally infected with a parasite called *Onchocerca volvulus*, the agent of river blindness. The same year, the same two volunteers were given a single IM injection of pentamidine, then trypanosome-carrying tsetse flies were allowed to feed on these men's blood every two or three days. The first developed trypanosomiasis after a year, the second after ten months. They were then treated with suramin, which incidentally allowed Van Hoof to show that this drug was also effective against onchocerciasis. Three more volunteers were subjected to the same tsetse fly feeding three to six months after an injection of pentamidine, and none of them developed the disease. It was concluded that pentamidine had a protective effect that would last at least six months. Without delay, a field experiment was started in the Kwango region, where three-quarters of the whole population were injected with pentamidine while the others served as controls. Over the following year, there were no cases of trypanosomiasis among those who received the pentamidine, while seven cases were documented in the control group. A complete success.[41–45]

These results had a far-reaching effect and sleeping sickness chemoprophylactic campaigns were soon organised in endemic areas not just in the Belgian Congo, but also in the French and Portuguese colonies. In the previous chapter, we saw that, in Oubangui-Chari, these production-line injections facilitated the transmission of HTLV-1, another human retrovirus. The putative role of pentamidinisation in the spread of HIV-1 could only have taken place outside the Belgian Congo, because Van Hoof's beloved colony had very small populations of *P.t. troglodytes*. There were never any chemoprophylactic campaigns in Léo, where sleeping sickness was too rare to justify such an effort. Elsewhere, pentamidinisation campaigns undoubtedly contributed to the decline of trypanosomiasis, even if the theoretical foundations for the intervention (the persistence of the drug in the blood for several months) were incorrect.

In 1946, with the war over and his successor named, a sick Lucien Van Hoof returned to Europe and took his natural place as a professor at the Institute of Tropical Medicine in Antwerp, replacing Rodhain who had recently retired. He developed his vision for the post-war development of the healthcare system in the Belgian Congo, a massive investment that came to be known as the Van Hoof–Duren plan. His reputation had spread far and wide, and he was invited to chair a tropical medicine conference in the US. He also returned to Léopoldville to organise studies on congenital malaria. He died in Antwerp in December 1948.

An epidemic of tuberculosis

In Africa, tuberculosis is by far the most common 'opportunistic' infection among HIV-infected patients. Without HIV, the natural course of infection with *Mycobacterium tuberculosis* is as follows: when the bacillus is inhaled, this generally causes transient and non-specific symptoms, then the pathogen becomes dormant (no replication) somewhere in the lungs, and the patient feels fine until the bacteria are reactivated months or years later. Of 100 persons infected with the pathogen, only 10 will develop tuberculosis in their lifetime while in the other 90 the bacillus will remain dormant in their lungs forever, until they die of something else. The HIV-induced immunosuppression leads to much more frequent reactivation of the dormant infection: from 10% throughout life, the risk becomes 10% each year. In central Africa, where about 5% of the adult population is HIV-infected, 50% of patients with tuberculosis carry the virus.

From the mid-1930s there was a slow but relentless progression in the number of cases of tuberculosis reported, and then a dramatic rise in the 1950s (Figure 15). Is it possible that, in retrospect, this phenomenon reflected the spread of HIV which was already triggering many more cases of reactivation of the tuberculous bacillus? Well, perhaps, but there are several alternative explanations for this increasing incidence. First, medical historians and clinicians of the time agree that the agent of tuberculosis was introduced into central Africa by the Europeans. Very much like HIV, the urbanisation and the development of communication networks facilitated its spread, further enhanced by the promiscuity of urban residents who often had to share a bedroom with several other people. As in many cases where there is a decades-long interval between infection and ultimately developing the disease, more intense transmission in the 1920s would have led to a higher incidence twenty, thirty or forty years down the line. Second, there was a determined drive to develop the health system after WWII, so that ever larger numbers of Congolese had access to a healthcare institution where it was possible to diagnose tuberculosis. Third, the availability of effective drugs starting in the early 1950s made it more attractive for healthcare providers to diagnose tuberculosis: something could be done about it. Fourth, this treatment availability led during the 1950s to the widespread use in urban areas of radiographic surveys aimed at actively detecting cases of tuberculosis. For instance in 1957, the Centre de Dépistage de la Tuberculose in Léopoldville performed 44,234 chest x-rays to look for signs of tuberculosis. X-rays were performed on contacts of cases (all persons living on the same compound), on individuals who looked unwell during the annual medical census and in some parts of town on the whole population. Such aggressive case-finding increased three-fold the number of cases detected.[25,46,47]

Taking good care of free women

We will now examine how a well-intentioned initiative by a non-profit organisation may have contributed to the early spread of HIV-1 in the Congo's capital. An early version of the Croix-Rouge du Congo (CRC) established the first hospitals around 1890 in Boma and Léopoldville, but it was disbanded with the cession of the EIC to Belgium. In 1926, the Belgian Red Cross established a new CRC. Money was raised in Belgium, but also from businesses in the colony. Early on, it was decided that the CRC would focus its efforts on the Province Orientale, and on Léopoldville where two STD clinics were opened with the help of the Belgian National League against the Venereal Threat.[48]

During WWII, the CRC provided support for Belgian families from donations made by colonials still in the Congo. It dispatched correspondence between the Congo and occupied Belgium, sent food and clothes to Belgian war prisoners and funded a home for children of colonial officers who had been caught up in Belgium by the war, away from their parents. However, generosity always has limits, and in this case mulattoes were excluded from the list of children to be supported.

In 1947, the CRC brought to the Congo the country's first paediatrician, Claude Lambotte, along with his wife Jeanne Legrand, also medically qualified. They convinced the CRC to build a 100-bed paediatric hospital, which was inaugurated in 1953. Unfortunately, this facility proved very expensive to operate, which threatened the very survival of the CRC. As the city's endless expansion created a need for more STD clinics, the charity decided rather to withdraw completely from this field and handed over its two clinics to the government. It had also become uncomfortable with the coercive nature of the STD clinics. Reluctant patients being forcibly brought in by the police was inconsistent with the values of the international Red Cross movement.

In 1957, the Croix-Rouge opened a blood transfusion centre in Léo, with a pool of volunteer donors, which was certainly more in line with its traditional responsibilities. Until then, blood had to be given by relatives or friends of the recipient and was transfused within minutes of collection. One of the CRC board members in Belgium, Professor Albert Dubois, warned that strict measures would need to be taken to avoid transmitting diseases such as malaria, trypanosomiasis and viruses during transfusions. 'Don't worry,' he was told, 'our medical officers in Léo will take care of that.' Legrand became the first director of the transfusion centre, but she was caught up in a series of conflicts with doctors at the main hospital (who accused her of stealing their own blood donors), with the volunteer directors of the Léopoldville branch of the CRC, and others. In those days, women working as professionals did not have an easy time. She was fired by the CRC, went into a depression and died in Léo in 1960, with a request to be buried alongside the Africans. It is unlikely that this blood bank contributed to the early dissemination of HIV in Léo because the prevalence among donors must have been rather low and many of the recipients were young children who, had they acquired HIV, would have died before reaching sexual maturity. A year after independence, the Brussels-based CRC disbanded and the blood bank was transferred to other institutions.[49]

However, a specialised institution which warrants greater attention is the Dispensaire Antivénérien (STD clinic). It may have played a crucial role in the iatrogenic transmission of HIV-1 in Léopoldville because it was the main provider of care for free women, all of whom had to show up for the regular examinations necessary for their health card to be stamped. In 1929, the CRC opened a STD clinic in Léo-Est (Barumbu district). Like many such clinics, its official name was later changed to the more innocuous Centre de Médecine Sociale (patients preferred being seen by relatives and neighbours going to a social medicine centre than a venereal disease clinic). Eventually, a smaller satellite clinic was opened in Léo-Ouest. While the annual reports of the CRC provided nice photographs of its leprosarium and hospital in Province Orientale and its paediatric facilities in Léopoldville, the charity was more discreet about its STD clinics.[50,51]

The STD clinics provided free care to women or men who presented spontaneously with a genital complaint (generally a discharge or ulcer) and whose employers did not provide medical care. For men, these would be recent arrivals, the few who were unemployed and all those working for small enterprises or for individuals (domestic staff). As very few women worked in the formal sector, for them the Dispensaire Antivénérien was the only accessible institution. In practice, most free women of Léopoldville, fiscally defined as financially independent adult women not living with a husband, attended at least a few times per year. Contact tracing also generated part of the caseload. Males presenting with an STD had to refer their recent sexual contact(s), otherwise a visiting nurse would come to their compound for this purpose, potentially causing embarrassment. Furthermore, male migrants to Léopoldville had to show up at the same clinics upon arrival in order to comply with health regulations and obtain their *permis de séjour* (they were also required to attend the tuberculosis centre nearby).

The statistics presented in Figure 18 tabulate the totals for the two clinics together, but in practice the Léo-Ouest clinic never got off the ground and 95% of the total number of cases and number of injections correspond to the work done in Léo-Est. The bulk of the caseload

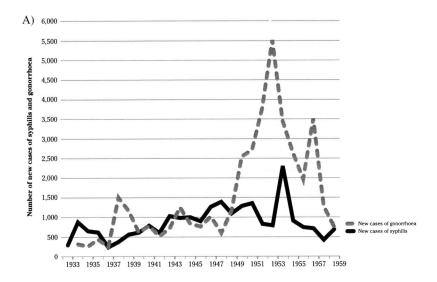

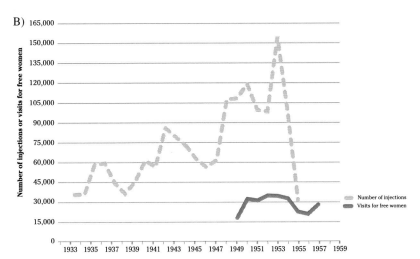

Figure 18 Number of new cases of gonorrhoea and syphilis, injections of various drugs and number of visits for free women at the Dispensaires Antivénériens of Léopoldville.

consisted of thousands of asymptomatic free women who came for screening because they were required to do so by law, in theory every month. At its peak, 32,000 such visits took place each year.

Data on the incidence of new cases of syphilis or gonorrhoea, the number of women and men seen at least once during the year, the number of serological assays for syphilis and the number of injections administered were provided in the annual reports of the Croix-Rouge du Congo, as well as in health service reports. The number of new cases of syphilis or gonorrhoea diagnosed each year varied substantially, reflecting the expansion of the capital's population and changes not just in diagnostic strategies but also in the efforts made to screen free women.[47,51]

Given that those treated for syphilis or gonorrhoea had to attend repeatedly for prolonged courses of injectable drugs but also for a long follow-up, by the early 1950s, as the population of Léo had increased dramatically, up to 1,000 patients attended the Léo-Est Dispensaire Antivénérien each day. The medical officers estimated that they were providing more or less regular check-ups to 3,500 free women. The clinic, which held only four rooms, opened at 4.30 a.m. so men could receive their treatments before going to work. This extremely high turnover of patients made it impossible for syringes and needles to be sterilised properly. In 1952, the Léo-Est facility was enlarged: syphilitics on one side, those with gonorrhoea on the other. STD screening of migrants was abandoned as it was deemed to provide little in the way of results. The blood samples were sent to the Institute of Tropical Medicine for testing. In 1954, 85,654 serological tests for syphilis were performed.

In retrospect, it is extraordinary that the treatment received by most patients of the Dispensaire Antivénérien was useless: wrong diagnoses, ineffective drugs. The reports suggest that, in the late 1940s, the medical officers began to wonder whether these efforts were a waste of time. In the 1949–54 reports, tables show that, of 7,204 new diagnoses of syphilis, only 111, 97 and 29 patients had signs compatible with primary, secondary or tertiary syphilis respectively. All of the others, 97% of patients with so-called syphilis, were given IV or IM drugs merely because they had a positive serology. Even today, the serological assays for syphilis do not discriminate between this latter infection and yaws, the non-venereal disease caused by a closely related bacterium. With both infections, the serological assays remain positive at a low titre for a very long period of time and even for life with some of the best assays. At the time, the medical thinking was that patients needed to be treated repeatedly with rather ineffective drugs until their serology came back completely negative. In 1952, 22% of a random sample of 1,000 adults living in Léo had a positive serology for syphilis/yaws, compared to 34% of free women. Given the high incidence of yaws in the preceding decades in the rural areas where many of these individuals originated, most of these cases with a positive serology probably corresponded to a past episode of yaws, which the patient could not recall because it had occurred in childhood. However, if that person was a free woman or male migrant and happened to be tested at the STD clinic, she/he was always considered to be syphilitic and received long courses of drugs containing arsenic or bismuth until penicillin was introduced around 1954. Even with this wonder drug, half of the patients remained seropositive for 'syphilis'.[51]

The precision of the diagnoses among free women was no better for gonorrhoea. In men, diagnosing gonorrhoea (or chlamydia) is straightforward: pus drips out of the penis. Among women, it is the opposite: most remain asymptomatic and less than 10% of those presenting with a vaginal discharge have gonorrhoea. The STD dispensaries could not cultivate the gonococcus, and did simple stains of the vaginal secretions. Such tests are not very good at identifying those infected as there are non-pathogenic bacteria within the normal vaginal flora that look the same as the gonococcus. Patients thought to have gonorrhoea were treated for up to two months with drugs that aimed to combat the infection by triggering a high fever. They received injections of milk(!), typhoid vaccine(!), a product called Gono-yatren, etc. Starting in 1951, effective antibiotics such as penicillin, sulphonamides or streptomycin were given but only at the end of this 'preparatory' course.

As a result of these debatable diagnostic and therapeutic approaches, during the 1930s and 1940s the STD clinics administered 50,000 injections per year on average (95% of these at the Léo-Est site). About 60% of these injections were given IV. In the 1950s, during the post-war demographic boom, the number of injections fluctuated around 100,000 per year, peaking at the extraordinary level of 154,572 by 1953. This number decreased rapidly thereafter as penicillin was introduced, a course of which required fewer injections than the arsenicals.

It is generally difficult to gather information about the procedures used for the sterilisation of syringes and needles during the colonial era.

In this case, however, it is illuminating to read a paper about hepatitis in Léopoldville written in 1953 by Dr Paul Beheyt, the internal medicine specialist at the Hôpital des Congolais. The author distinguishes epidemic hepatitis from inoculation hepatitis, the latter being defined as a patient developing hepatitis between 45 and 150 days after having received IV injections or transfusions. Inoculation hepatitis must have corresponded mostly to hepatitis B, because acute infection with hepatitis C rarely causes a disease severe enough for the patient to develop jaundice. Of sixty-nine cases of inoculation hepatitis diagnosed during 1951–2, thirty-two had received IV arsenical drugs at the Léo-Est STD clinic, corresponding to 0.9% of the patients treated during the same period by this institution. This measure of risk was greatly underestimated because the reference hospital diagnosed only a fraction of all cases of inoculation hepatitis occurring in Léopoldville, and the iatrogenic infection could only occur among patients who had not been infected with HBV earlier in their lives, at most 5% of adults in central Africa.[52]

It is worth quoting at length from what Beheyt wrote about how his patients were infected:

The Congo contains various health institutions (maternity centres, hospitals, dispensaries, etc.) where every day local nurses give dozens, even hundreds, of injections in conditions such that sterilisation of the needle or the syringe is impossible. At the Dispensaire Antivénérien de la Croix-Rouge in Léopoldville, on average 300 injections are administered each day. The large number of patients and the small quantity of syringes available to the nursing staff preclude sterilisation by autoclave after each use. Used syringes are simply rinsed, first with water, then with alcohol and ether, and are ready for a new patient. The same type of procedure exists in all health institutions where a small number of nurses have to provide care to a large number of patients, with very scarce supplies. The syringe is used from one patient to the next, occasionally retaining small quantities of infectious blood, which are large enough to transmit the disease.[52]

In September 1955, the Croix-Rouge abruptly withdrew from running the STD clinics and the colony took over its clients, nurses and other workers. This must have involved some heated argument because in that year's annual report it appears that the Croix-Rouge transferred responsibility for this activity to the Léopoldville Department of Hygiene following some mutual agreement, while at the receiving end the latter made it clear in its own annual report that the running of the STD clinics had been dumped on it at very short notice.[53]

Nevertheless, the department did its job. By the end of 1957, 3,761 free women were registered, on whom a total of 26,123 screening examinations had been performed. The following year, 4,384 free women were registered, a rather substantial percentage given that the medical officers estimated that there were around 5,000 of them in the city. The number of injections, however, was drastically reduced. Long-acting penicillin completely replaced arsenicals for patients with syphilis, and the indications for such treatment were tightened as physicians acknowledged that it was unnecessary to treat those who probably carried only a 'serological scar' due to a past episode of yaws or a past syphilis which had been adequately treated.[54]

The department of health also ran the annual medical census of the whole population of Léopoldville, for which each and every inhabitant was examined summarily to look for sleeping sickness and leprosy. This represented a substantial effort: between 148,584 (1949) and 322,198 (1958) individuals were examined, all to detect less than 100 cases of sleeping sickness and a few lepers annually. During the last years before independence, in a never-to-be-repeated population measure of the prevalence of symptomatic STDs, the health agents running the medical census required every adult male to drop his pants: of 99,446 men seen in 1958, 163 were found to have gonorrhoea, 335 to have non-gonococcal urethritis (presumably, in retrospect, chlamydia) while only 44 had a chancre suggestive of syphilis.[47,55]

It is remarkable that throughout this period the incidence of other tropical diseases, for which injectable drugs were massively used in the rural areas, including those around Léopoldville, remained minimal in the Belgian Congo's capital. After 1930, there were generally fewer than 100 cases of sleeping sickness diagnosed each year, mostly in migrants from endemic areas, and similar numbers of cases of yaws. To some extent, this was a result of the systematic screening of migrants arriving in Léo so that a large proportion of sleeping sickness cases were identified and treated, which reduced the risk of transmission of the parasite within Léo. This was very good news for its large Belgian population as the risk of being bitten by an infectious tsetse fly was reduced accordingly. Yaws remained uncommon, reflecting an easier access to health care (treatment shortened the duration of infectiousness) and hygienic conditions which, even if far worse than those of the Europeans, were healthier than in rural areas. In the African suburbs, water was readily available, not in each house but at a shared tap for several compounds. Consequently, in Léo the treatment of STDs, especially 'syphilis', provided the best opportunity for the iatrogenic transmission of infectious agents through syringes and needles.

The perfect storm

Less than 0.1% of the total population of the central chimpanzee inhabited the Belgian Congo, so it is unlikely that 'patient zero', the one who started the pandemic, lived there. However, Léo was the most dynamic city in the region, a commercial hub which attracted large numbers of migrants and traders. A SIV_{cpz}-infected cut hunter moving to the city or an HIV-1-infected trader wishing to spend some time in the capital would have to present himself at the STD clinic upon arrival, where he would receive treatment for syphilis if his serological assay was positive, either because of prior syphilis or much more often because of prior yaws. Alternatively, one can imagine that a first HIV-infected free woman sexually infected by one of her patrons would be treated with IV drugs, also because of a positive serology.

Once the virus was introduced within the Léopoldville–Brazzaville conurbation, it would have found an extraordinary opportunity for its amplification through non-sterile syringes and needles at the Dispensaire Antivénérien in the Barumbu district of Léo-Est. There, the caseload of patients was extreme due to the obsession of local physicians with treating anybody with a positive 'syphilis' serology. Iatrogenic transmission of another blood-borne virus, HBV, was well documented in 1951–2 to have occurred as a consequence of the inadequate sterilisation of injection equipment. It does not take much imagination to deduce that if HBV was transmitted iatrogenically, the same must have occurred with SIV_{cpz}/HIV-1 once it was introduced into the cohort of patients treated for presumed STDs at the same Dispensaire Antivénérien. Many of the iatrogenically infected cases would have been free women who had concomitant sexual relationships with several men: it was indeed **the perfect storm**.

Those free women infected parenterally could then transmit the virus sexually to some of their regular clients, who in turn infected other sex workers, or later other women, eventually allowing the virus to move out of the sexual core group. This second part of the amplification process, this time sexual, could proceed at a much faster pace when, during the chaotic years that followed the country's accession to independence in 1960, the face of Léopoldville changed abruptly, with massive migrations, high unemployment rates and the emergence of a different type of prostitution in which some women might entertain up to 1,000 clients per year.

10 | *The other human immunodeficiency viruses*

Although they contribute little to the overall burden of AIDS in the world, the other HIVs (HIV-1 groups O, N and P, and HIV-2) can provide useful insight into the events that led to the emergence of pandemic HIV-1 group M. How was it possible for HIV-2, a different virus that originated from a different simian host, to spread in a different region of Africa at roughly the same time (give or take a few decades) as HIV-1, only to disappear quietly thereafter? And why was HIV-1 group M so successful compared to the others?

HIV-1 groups O, N and P

Highly divergent strains of HIV-1 were described in the 1990s. The first, now known as HIV-1 group O ('O' for outlier), has only 50–65% homology in nucleotide sequences compared to HIV-1 group M, which is why it is considered as a different 'group' rather than a different 'subtype' (subtypes differ by about 20%; in other words, they have 80% homology). The original isolates of HIV-1 group O had been obtained from two Cameroonians living in Belgium, a young woman and her husband. Additional cases were documented among Cameroonians living in France, and in Cameroon itself. Further studies confirmed that Cameroon was the epicentre of HIV-1 group O, where it accounted for 2% of all HIV-1 infections, versus 1% in adjacent Gabon and Nigeria. A few cases were found in other African countries. Within Cameroon, regional variations were noted, with group O representing 6% of all HIV-1 positive sera in Yaoundé but only 1% in northern provinces. When stored sera were tested, group O represented 21% of all HIV-1 positive sera in 1986–8, 9% in 1989–91, 3% in 1994–5 and only 1% in 1997–8. It then remained rather stable at 1–2%.[1–7]

To some extent, this decreasing proportion in the overall burden of HIV-1 infections was mistaken and reflected changes in the quality of diagnostic assays used to sort out group O from group M. But it is also possible that, over the last two decades, HIV-1 group O proved less transmissible than HIV-1 group M, as suggested by its lack of success in spreading outside its central African epicentre. Among more than 10,000 new cases of HIV infection diagnosed in France between 2003 and 2006, only twelve corresponded to HIV-1 group O (nine among Cameroonian migrants, one in a Chadian and two in French nationals). In the laboratory, HIV-1 group O is less 'fit' than group M: it replicates less efficiently in cultures with lymphocytes, which may explain its lower transmissibility.[8-10]

Using the same approaches as for HIV-1 group M, the past dynamics of HIV-1 group O were reconstructed. Remarkably, the most recent common ancestor of all group O isolates was dated around 1920, much the same as for group M but with a wide confidence interval (1890–1940). It is thought that all cases of group O infections resulted from a single cross-species transmission, following which the growth of the infected population was slower than for group M, doubling about every six years. By the late 1990s, of the half million Cameroonians who were HIV-infected, about 7,500 were infected with group O. As could be expected from this limited number of infected individuals, HIV-1 group O displays less genetic diversity than group M, with only three or four subtypes identified so far.[11-13]

HIV-1 group N ('N' for non-M non-O, or new), which was isolated for the first time in 1995 from a Cameroonian with AIDS, had even less success in spreading among humans. Up to now, only thirteen cases have been documented, all in Cameroonians. This may be an under-estimate since it is not easy to sort out group N from group M through serologic tests. Two such cases occurred within a couple, indicating some heterosexual transmission. Nucleotide sequences of group N are similar to those obtained from SIV_{cpz}-infected *P.t. troglodytes* chimps from the same area of southern Cameroon. Group N isolates represent a single lineage with low diversity, perhaps because its introduction in human populations was more recent than groups M and O. The most recent common ancestor of group N HIV-1 isolates has been dated around 1963 (confidence interval: 1948–77).[14-17]

In phylogenetic trees, both groups M and N lie within the radiation of SIV_{cpz} isolates obtained from the *P.t. troglodytes* chimpanzee (Figures 1, 2 and 3) and clearly originated from this same simian host. In contrast, the exact source of group O, the outlier, remained uncertain for some time.

The virus most closely related to group O is the recently described virus of gorillas, SIV_{gor}. It seems likely that gorillas, like their human cousins, were infected from chimpanzees. Given the geographic distribution of groups O and N, there is little doubt that their cross-species transmission event, from ape to man, occurred in Cameroon.[18,19]

Recently, a new group of HIV-1, group P, has been identified following the isolation of a peculiar strain from (again) a Cameroonian living in France. Phylogenetic analyses showed that HIV-1 group P is closest to SIV_{gor}, and actually closer to SIV_{gor} than HIV-1 group O is. The patient herself recalled no exposure to apes and presumably acquired the infection sexually from an infected man. At some point an initial transmission occurred from gorillas to humans, followed by limited inter-human spread. As with group O, the true source of the virus might be the chimpanzee, which could have infected humans and gorillas independently, or infected gorillas which later infected humans. A second case of group P infection has been identified by a diagnostics company in a patient hospitalised in Yaoundé.[20]

These findings about HIV-1 groups O, N and P have at least two implications. First, it shows that other SIV_{cpz} isolates crossed the species barrier in the same geographic region where HIV-1 group M emerged in human populations. In the case of HIV-1 group O this seemed to have happened at roughly the same time as for group M, around 1920, while with group N it was more recent. This supports the idea that cross-species transmissions from chimps to man might have gone on for hundreds of years without triggering a recognisable pandemic and leading only to epidemiological dead ends. One case in point is the HIV-1 group O-infected Norwegian sailor who, in the 1960s, transmitted the virus to his wife who herself infected their child, without any further cases outside this nuclear family. Second, it suggests that one of the reasons behind the dramatic spread of HIV-1 group M might be intrinsic to this specific strain: compared to group O and to HIV-2, HIV-1 group M is better at infecting lymphocytes, which increases its capacity to be transmitted sexually or otherwise from one human to another.

HIV-2 and Guiné Portuguesa

Just a few years after their discovery of HIV-1 as the aetiological agent of AIDS, a different virus, soon to be named HIV-2, was isolated by the

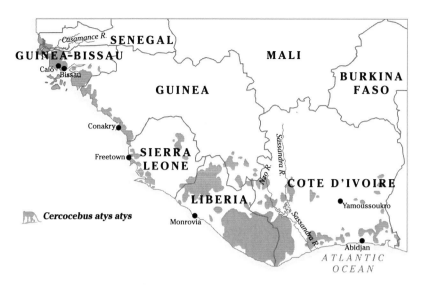

Map 7 Historical range of the sooty mangabey (*Cercocebus atys atys*) in West Africa.

same researchers at the Institut Pasteur from two AIDS patients, one from Guinea-Bissau and the other from Cape Verde. These observations were extended to a larger group of thirty patients recruited in Lisbon with varying degrees of immunosuppression (seventeen with full-blown AIDS), all but two of whom originated from Guinea-Bissau or Cape Verde. This virus had only 30–40% homology with HIV-1 for most of its genes, hence its designation as a different virus rather than just another group of HIV-1. HIV-2 is not just a medical curiosity but illuminates part of the history of HIV-1, because whatever factors were instrumental in the emergence of HIV-1 in central Africa must have existed as well in West Africa, a few thousand kilometres away.[21–22]

The source of HIV-2 was identified as the sooty mangabey (*Cercocebus atys atys*), a small monkey which inhabits parts of coastal West Africa that correspond closely to the geographical distribution of HIV-2 (Map 7). This conclusion was based on the sequencing of simian viruses called SIV_{smm} (smm for sooty mangabey monkey), isolated from this primate, which revealed a high degree of similarity with human HIV-2 isolates. SIV_{smm} does not cause AIDS in its natural sooty mangabey hosts despite replicating at high levels, but causes disease when transferred to other species, especially the macaques, through cage infections. Presumably, when a given SIV has infected a given species

of monkey or ape for a long time, individuals who were more susceptible to the pathogenic effect of the virus, regardless of the underlying
mechanisms, were preferentially removed from the population by death
so that eventually the species became relatively resistant to the ill effects
of this specific virus. One wonders whether the recent decrease in HIV-1
prevalence in some countries of East and southern Africa might to some
extent reflect a similar process of natural selection in human
populations.[23–27]

SIV$_{smm}$ and HIV-2 sequences from animals and humans originating
from the same geographic areas were found to be most related, which
implies local activities as the route of transmission. In Liberia and Sierra
Leone, 22% of free-living sooty mangabeys were infected with SIV$_{smm}$,
compared to only 4% of those kept as household pets, most of which
had been removed from their native troops as infants. Among sooty
mangabeys in the Taï Forest of Ivory Coast, SIV$_{smm}$ prevalence was
even higher at 59%. Because of hunting and destruction of their habitat,
sooty mangabeys are now extinct in Senegal, Guinea-Bissau and parts
of Guinea, while substantial populations remain in Sierra Leone,
Liberia and Ivory Coast.[28–29]

Molecular studies revealed that HIV-2 can be divided into eight
groups, defined according to their degree of genetic diversity. Only
groups A and B managed to spread between humans while groups C
to H represent individual human cases documented in Liberia, Sierra
Leone and Ivory Coast. Each group represents at least one distinct
cross-species transmission event, from the sooty mangabey to man. In
Guinea-Bissau and The Gambia, only HIV-2 group A is found. HIV-2
group B has been detected mostly in and around Ivory Coast. Sierra
Leone, the country with the highest diversity of HIV-2 groups among
humans, also has the lowest HIV-2 prevalence, at 0.02%. The 1,000-
fold higher SIV$_{smm}$ prevalence among sooty mangabeys in the same
country implies that inter-human transmission following an initial
cross-species event was generally ineffective. But cross-species transmission of viruses from sooty mangabeys might have been more common than from chimpanzees, because the former live closer to humans
and can be domesticated as pets.[29]

Epidemiological studies uncovered that the distribution of HIV-2 was
largely limited to West Africa and that its epicentre was Guinea-Bissau,
a tiny country that became independent only in 1974 after a protracted
liberation war against the Portuguese dictatorship, where HIV-2

managed to infect 9% of adults. A lower prevalence (less than 2.5%) was found in other West African countries: Senegal, The Gambia, Cape Verde, Guinea, Liberia, Sierra Leone, Ivory Coast, Burkina Faso, Ghana, Mali and Nigeria. A few cases were documented in distant countries that had had a colonial link with Portugal: Angola, Mozambique and India.

In Guinea-Bissau, an initial survey conducted in Bissau in 1987 revealed a HIV-2 prevalence of 8.9% amongst adults but with a marked age gradient, 20% of those aged forty and over being infected. HIV-1 was absent. Even though HIV-2 does cause AIDS, it is less pathogenic than HIV-1, increasing adult mortality by a factor of two to three while HIV-1 increases mortality ten-fold. In other words, HIV-2 is compatible with prolonged survival in a large portion (perhaps even the majority) of infected individuals, who will ultimately die of something else, in contrast with HIV-1 which kills nearly all untreated subjects within fifteen years. The age distribution of HIV-2, so different from that of HIV-1 elsewhere in Africa, was initially thought to reflect this low mortality and the effect of cumulative exposure over a long period of time.[30–32]

Subsequently, HIV-2 was shown to result in a lower degree of viraemia than HIV-1 and a lesser genital shedding in semen and cervical secretions. As a consequence, HIV-2 is less transmissible than HIV-1, both sexually and from mother to child. This raised the question of how, if the virus is poorly transmissible, prevalence could have reached such a high level in the first place.[33–35]

Serial surveys showed that the infection was so rare among younger people that cumulative exposure could not mathematically explain the high prevalence among the elderly (Table 1). This corresponded rather to what epidemiologists call a 'cohort effect': something peculiar happened to the cohort of individuals born before 1962, which did not apply to those born since. Research then focused on older people. Among women aged fifty and over, HIV-2 was associated with having had sex with a white man, possibly a proxy for prostitution. It was hypothesised that this cohort effect was related to changes in sexual activity (higher promiscuity, more commercial sex) during the 1963–74 liberation war, with the same people becoming less promiscuous after the war came to an end.[30,36–41]

Bissau-Guineans had fought on both sides. Some were *guerilleros* of the liberation movement, which controlled rural areas whose size

Table 1 *HIV-2 prevalence in Guinea-Bissau by age, 1987–2007*[30,36–41]

Age, years	Bissau 1987	Bissau 1989–92	Bissau 1990–2	Caio 1989–91	Bissau 1995–6	Bissau 1998–2000	Bissau 2004–7	Bissau 2005
15–24	0.4%		3.3%	1.8%	1.9%		0.4%	
25–34	11.2%		13.9%	8.6%	6.1%		2.7%	
35–44	13.0%		12.1%	16.0%	14.4%	15.6%	7.4%	
45–54	21.2%	17.1%[a]	11.6%	16.3%	16.3%	13.8%	15.5%	16.0%[a]
≥55	17.4%	11.3%[b]	10.0%	7.8%	16.8%	12.8%	13.8%	10.9%[b]

[a] 50–9 years
[b] ≥60 years

increased as the war progressed, while others had been conscripted into the colonial army, alongside Portuguese soldiers, which controlled the cities. There were problems with this 'promiscuous soldier' theory. First, the initial study showed no associations between HIV-2 infection and either having served in the Portuguese army or the duration of military service. Second, the underlying idea that sexual activity was higher during wartime remained unproven. The conflict in Guinea-Bissau had been a guerrilla war, with fighters from the liberation movement constantly moving to avoid the better armed Portuguese troops and their small aeroplanes. While soldiers stationed in peaceful countries certainly tend to frequent sex workers and acquire STDs, there is little evidence that such prostitution occurs close to combat areas. Recent experiences in Ivory Coast and the DRC revealed, if anything, decreasing HIV-1 prevalence after a period of conflict. When survival becomes the main concern, there is less time and energy for sex, and in disciplined armies rapes are too uncommon to have a measurable effect on HIV transmission. Then Portuguese doctors tested almost 2,000 blood donors who had served in the colonial army in Guinea-Bissau (and who would have been more exposed to prostitutes than their guerrilla opponents): not a single one of them was HIV-2-infected. Either the Portuguese soldiers were extremely virtuous or they were resistant to HIV-2 infection – or the hypothesis was wrong.[36,42–44]

To reconstruct the past dynamics of HIV-2 in Guinea-Bissau, the same approaches were used as for HIV-1. Archival samples obtained in rural areas during a 1980 yellow fever survey were tested. Out of 1,234 specimens, eleven were HIV-2-reactive. Prevalence increased with age and 6% of those more than forty-five years of age were infected. These are the oldest specimens from that country. HIV-2 antibodies were found in a few specimens obtained in the late 1960s or early 1970s in Ivory Coast, Mali, Nigeria, Senegal and Gabon, but not in samples from Liberia, Sierra Leone, Togo, Chad, Niger and Ghana.[45–47]

Cases of HIV-2 AIDS, confirmed by serology, were recognised retrospectively, first in a Portuguese patient who had lived in Guinea-Bissau between 1956 and 1966 and died in 1979. Another case was diagnosed in 1978 in a Portuguese man who had served in the colonial army in Angola between 1968 and 1974 and then travelled between Angola and Mozambique. A Portuguese couple developed AIDS in the early 1980s, and HIV-2 infection could be traced to the man having served in the colonial army in Guinea-Bissau between 1966 and 1969. A Portuguese woman who had received a blood transfusion in Guinea-Bissau in 1967 remained asymptomatic twenty-seven years later, albeit with decreased CD4 lymphocyte counts. These case reports demonstrated that HIV-2 had been present in Guinea-Bissau and other Portuguese colonies at least since the 1960s, and that the incubation period between infection and AIDS was longer than with HIV-1.[48–51]

Molecular clock analyses estimated that the most recent common ancestors for HIV-2 group A existed around 1940, and for HIV-2 group B around 1945, two decades later than for HIV-1 group M. Using mathematical models, it was estimated that in Caio, a high-prevalence village of Guinea-Bissau, a period of exponential growth occurred between 1955 and 1970. A more recent study using slightly different methods dated the most recent common ancestors to 1932 (group A) and 1935 (group B). These findings are in line with the notion that the sooty mangabey became extinct in Guinea Bissau a few decades ago, so that the initial cross-species event must have occurred earlier.[52–53]

The evolution over time in the distribution of HIV-2 infection is also of interest. Surveys in Guinea-Bissau, Ivory Coast and other West African countries over the last two decades reached the same conclusion: HIV-2 is slowly disappearing while HIV-1 becomes prevalent. In countries outside West Africa with past colonial links to Portugal, HIV-2 has already vanished, with the exception of India. In France, out of

164 cases of HIV-2 infection diagnosed in 2003–6, only twenty occurred among French nationals, showing that the virus has had limited epidemiological success despite having been imported into the country by hundreds of migrants from West Africa. In Guinea-Bissau, as the elderly cohorts slowly age and die, HIV-2 prevalence among adults is waning. Among women delivering at the Simao Mendes national hospital, HIV-2 prevalence decreased from 8.3% in 1987 to 2.5% in 2004; over the same period, HIV-1 prevalence rose from 0 to 4.8%. In the Bandim area of Bissau, HIV-2 prevalence among adults dropped from 8.9% in 1987 to 3.9% in 2006 while HIV-1 prevalence increased from 0 to 4.6%. These trends confirmed that HIV-2 is transmitted less effectively than HIV-1 during sexual intercourse. But then, how did it become so prevalent among the generation of elderly Bissau-Guineans?[8,41,54]

To address this question, and exploit the fact that HIV-2 is compatible with prolonged survival (which offers an opportunity to document associations with exposures that took place decades earlier), we conducted a survey of 1,608 individuals aged fifty and over living in Bissau. HIV-2 prevalence was 15% in women and 8% in men. HIV-2 was not associated with previous STDs or with having sold (women) or bought (men) sexual services. Among men, HIV-2 infection was not more common in those who had fought for either side during the independence war. Among women, however, HIV-2 infection was associated with ritual excision of the clitoris. When both genders were combined, HIV-2 was associated with having been treated for sleeping sickness and with having received IM streptomycin for the treatment of tuberculosis. These three independent associations pointed to parenteral rather than sexual modes of transmission, all of which could have played a role only in the distant past.[55]

Sleeping sickness in Guiné Portuguesa peaked in 1952. Most patients were treated with IV melarsoprol (up to fifteen injections, to be repeated if a relapse was diagnosed) while some early cases received IM pentamidine (usually ten injections). The disease eventually disappeared completely so that virtually all participants who reported having previously been treated for trypanosomiasis were in fact treated before the country became independent in 1974. Meanwhile, streptomycin was used to treat tuberculosis until 1992, when a regimen using only oral drugs was adopted. Prior to this change, tuberculosis patients received at least 60 and sometimes more than 100 IM injections of streptomycin. Finally, excision of the clitoris used to be practised in Muslim ethnic groups during the *fanado*, an initiation ritual during which dozens of girls were excised on the same day by elderly women using the same ceremonial knife. These ethnic groups still practise excision, but now during individual procedures rather than collective ceremonies.[56–60]

For a long time, the only purpose of the Guiné Portuguesa health system was to protect the health of the Portuguese colonists and their Guinean employees in the cities. What happened to the sick villagers did not matter to the colonial masters. Ultimately, large-scale medical campaigns for the control of tropical diseases were orchestrated, but only three decades after similar activities started in AEF and Cameroun. For instance, while in 1928 Jamot and his collaborators detected and treated in Cameroun 54,712 cases of sleeping sickness, in Portuguese Guinea (whose population was half a million, one fifth that of Cameroun) fewer than 30 cases were reported. In 1936, the Cameroun health system treated 81,965 cases of yaws, 56,749 cases of syphilis, 4,313 of leprosy and 3,332 of trypanosomiasis. The very same year, in Portuguese Guinea only 232 cases of leprosy and 42 cases of trypanosomiasis were diagnosed, as well as fewer than 100 cases of yaws and syphilis.[56–58,61–65]

The first attempt to organise country-wide public health services came in 1945 with the creation of a vertical programme for the control of sleeping sickness. Predictably, case-finding led to more cases being diagnosed and treated: 404 cases in 1946, 1,272 in 1948, 1,970 in 1950, peaking at 2,169 cases in 1952 and decreasing thereafter as these efforts eventually reduced transmission. Treatment of treponemal infections started on a small scale only after the introduction of penicillin, with 624 cases of yaws and 59 cases of syphilis reported in 1953. Incidence of yaws peaked at 2,644 cases in 1956. Treatment of leprosy also started in the mid-1950s. As cases had been accumulating for decades without treatment, a substantial effort was consented so that 8,389 patients in all were being treated with either IM or oral sulphones by 1958. Leprosy patients treated with IM sulphones received their injections by the side of the road as mobile teams visited their villages every fortnight. As the treatment of leprosy continued over several years, especially for the lepromatous patients with a large quantity of bacteria in their skin and nerves, many lepers received between 50 and 100 such injections.

The most likely scenario is that, until about 1950, occasional cases of HIV-2 infection did occur from occupational exposure to SIV_{smm} but forward transmission was limited, because sexual transmission was relatively ineffective and opportunities for parenteral transmission were scarce. The delay in organising public health services, combined with a lower incidence of yaws and trypanosomiasis in this drier land, resulted in a lower proportion of the population receiving IV injections than in Cameroun. This limited the opportunity for the iatrogenic transmission of blood-borne viruses until the late 1940s. Then, after decades of neglect, health authorities instituted disease control pro-grammes, to demonstrate the benevolent nature of Portuguese coloni-alism in the context of the emergence of African nationalism after WWII, fostered by the anticolonialist stance of the new global super-power, the United States.

This created conditions conducive to the parenteral amplification of HIV-2. From one case of occupationally acquired SIV_{smm} in a cut hunter, a few thousand were created iatrogenically. Although we were able to document only the role of trypanosomiasis and tuberculosis treatments, it is likely that other interventions, including the parenteral treatment of thousands of leprosy patients, contributed to the exponen-tial amplification of the virus between 1950 and 1970. At this stage, some young girls who had been iatrogenically infected with HIV-2 could start their own chains of transmission during the excision rituals. Albeit relatively ineffective, sexual and vertical transmission also con-tributed modestly to the spread of HIV-2 in the overall population.

Subsequent political, social, epidemiological and technological changes resulted in fewer opportunities for the parenteral transmission of HIV-2. When the country became independent in 1974, there was no reason to maintain the disease control programmes of the preceding decades, especially since they had been very effective in reducing the incidence of the targeted diseases. The focus shifted to the provision of primary health care. Apart from the treatment of severe malaria with quinine, few drugs were administered IV since orally administered antibiotics and antiparasitic drugs became available. As the iatrogenic transmission of HIV-2 was much reduced, the relatively ineffective sexual and mother-to-child transmission was not sufficient for the virus to persist: on average, each HIV-2-infected person infected less than one other individual. Very slowly but inevitably HIV-2 will vanish.

The bottom line is that if parenteral transmission played a key role in the emergence of HIV-2 in Guinea-Bissau, the same mechanisms must surely have contributed, in another region of the continent, twenty to thirty years earlier, to the early expansion of HIV-1, a virus associated with a higher degree of viraemia than HIV-2, and thus more transmissible through the sharing of syringes and needles.

11 | *From the Congo to the Caribbean*

We saw in Chapter 1 how geopolitical events, in that case the Cuban intervention in Angola, had a measurable effect on the dissemination of HIV-1 into this Caribbean island. Here, we will see how earlier historical circumstances had even more dramatic impacts on the spread of HIV-1, first in its crucible of central Africa, and then across the Atlantic, by finally creating conditions propitious to the successful dissemination of the virus, after decades of quiescence. Although the next few pages may seem a little bit of a detour, these incidents lie at the heart of our story.

A botched decolonisation

Fifty years later, it is astonishing to read some of the colonial and early post-colonial writings about the Belgian Congo which is described as 'our Congo' or its inhabitants as *Nos Noirs*, our blacks. Belgium exploited this huge country, much to the profit of its banks and large corporations, but the Congolese benefited from the development of the infrastructure. Good roads were built, an impressive health system was put in place and primary school education was offered to many. It was cheaper for the colonial government to subsidise Catholic (and, after WWII, Protestant) missions to take care of the teaching, and its expenditures on education were modest. In contrast with their French and British counterparts, Belgian colonialists elected not to train any Congolese elite, presumably for fear that these educated few would sooner or later challenge the colonial order. Only a tiny proportion would be able to enter secondary schools, and very few apart from Catholic priests would have access to post-secondary education. In 1957–8, out of 494 Congolese students attending post-secondary education, 376 were future priests enrolled in the seminaries. Throughout Africa, the Belgian Congo had the second highest proportion of its population that had attended primary school but the lowest with regard to post-secondary education. Among adults aged twenty and over, 1.7% of men and 0.1% of women had received at least one year of post-primary education, and respectively 0.5% and 0.04% had completed secondary school.[1-2]

The colony's first university, Lovanium, a Catholic institution on the outskirts of Léopoldville, closely associated with Université Catholique de Louvain in the motherland, welcomed its first students in 1954, more than thirty years after universities were established in Dakar and Kampala. By 1960, Lovanium took in only 420 students. It was soon followed by a secular university in Elisabethville, where most students were ... Belgians. In 1958, to provide care for a population of 14 million, the Belgian Congo had 700 medical doctors and not a single one of them was Congolese. Despite six years of post-secondary education, the highest level a Congolese could reach under the Belgian regime was a medical assistant. The Congolese were considered too primitive to become doctors, unable to understand the rules of professional conduct and ethics and the infinite value of human life. Strangely enough, at the same time there were already 600 Congolese priests, who had been through six years of university-level philosophy and theology. When the country became independent, only thirty or so Congolese held university degrees earned at home or abroad.[3-6]

In 1955, Antwerp university professor 'Jef' Van Bilsen proposed a thirty-year programme for leading the country to independence. Unrealistic, overoptimistic, naive, was the response of many in the Belgian establishment. Yet only four years later in February 1960, following a conference in Brussels, the colonial power announced that it would grant independence to the Congo at the end of June. What had happened? The Belgian government belatedly understood that it was fighting a backward and ill-fated opposition to a profound wind of change blowing across most of the world. After India and other Asian countries, African colonies started becoming independent with Ghana in 1957, followed in 1960 by the whole of French Africa, including Congo-Brazzaville across the river. Only the fascist dictatorship of Portugal and the racist regimes of South Africa and Rhodesia did not understand in which direction history was heading.

The prosperity of the early 1950s had brought to the Congo Belgian settlers, mostly Flemish farmers and stockbreeders, whose blatant racism and the large pieces of land they were granted had exacerbated the ever-increasing nationalist fervour of the Congolese. Out of nowhere, dozens of political parties were created, competing for small factions of the future electorate, outdoing each other week after week in their demands for ever-quicker accession to independence. In Léopoldville, the riots of January 1959 had shown that the natives would not tolerate colonial oppression much longer. For the first time a few months earlier, a large number of Congolese had travelled to Belgium during the 1958 Brussels universal exposition. To their amazement, they discovered that there were plenty of poor whites performing menial tasks in the public and private sectors. Oppression is a state of mind in which the oppressed accepts its fate as normal and unavoidable and its inferiority as congenital rather than imposed by past events, and in 1959, the Congolese began to reject this colonial paradigm. A civil disobedience movement emerged, mostly around Léopoldville. Taxes were left unpaid, administrative censuses were boycotted and workers in private and public enterprises went on strike. Other anticolonial riots broke out in Stanleyville and Matadi. After their French neighbours' disastrous colonial wars in Indochina and Algeria, there was no appetite in Belgium for a conflict in which young conscripts might die. Furthermore, the public thought their colonial kin were privileged (better salaries, free housing, cheap domestic staff) and did not want to pay the costs of large-scale interventions aimed at protecting this *status quo*. Opinion polls showed that more than 70% opposed any form of military occupation of the Congo.[7-8]

The Belgian government decided to replace colonialism with neo-colonialism. Let us have a few Congolese as nominal heads of government and ministers and keep them happy with limousines and posh houses while retaining control over what really mattered, the economy, especially the lucrative mining industry in Katanga. Within a few months, a constitution was drafted and adopted by the parliament in Brussels, and legislative elections were held. The first draft of this constitution had proposed that King Baudouin would remain the Congo's head of state but the ungrateful Congolese refused. A power vacuum developed, and at some point Belgium had no fewer than six ministers managing various aspects of the decolonisation process.

The European population, which made up less than 1% of the total, fetched around 50% of all revenues in the Congo; apparently, this was an improvement from ten years earlier. Due to a recession and increasing difficulties in collecting taxes, the Belgian Congo's budget was deeply in the red during the late 1950s, while hundreds of millions of dollars in cash or gold had left the Congo, a process which continued after 1960 and was facilitated by the new country's central bank being conveniently located in Brussels. The Congo was already broke on the day it was born. It would not take long before the nascent government was unable to pay its civil servants and soldiers regularly, a factor which contributed to the impending chaos.[7,9-11]

The rise and fall of Patrice Lumumba

The future Patrice Lumumba was born Elias Okit'Asombo in the Sankuru region in 1925. Educated in missionary institutions, already a rebel and expelled from four successive schools, he managed to complete his middle school education. Aged eighteen, he moved to Stanleyville where he adopted a new name from his mother's side to mark a break with his turbulent past. Lumumba was mainly self-taught, a workaholic and prolific reader of everything he could lay his hands on. He worked as a post office clerk, a part-time journalist and later a salesman for a brewery in Stanleyville and Léo.[12]

Lumumba was first imprisoned for one year in 1955–6 on charges of misappropriating post office funds. It was during this jail term that he became critical of Belgian rule. After his release, he participated in the creation of the Mouvement National des Congolais (MNC), of which he became president. While most other emerging political parties were regional and ethnicity-based, the MNC aimed to be a national non-tribal organisation. Lumumba developed his oratorical skills promoting Polar beer in the many bars of Léopoldville, which enabled him to widen his network of sympathisers. Sent back to jail in October 1959, charged with inciting an anticolonial riot in Stanleyville, his anticolonialism grew more radical. He was released a few days after sentencing to attend the Brussels conference. The MNC rejected Belgium's plans for neo-colonialism and supported a unitary vision for the future country.

Lumumba's party won the most seats in the May 1960 legislative elections, the only free and fair elections to be held in this country during the entire twentieth century. After forming a fragile coalition with smaller parties, Lumumba became prime minister. The members of parliament then voted to elect Joseph Kasavubu as president of the country. The new Congo constitution mirrored that of Belgium, where the prime minister held most of the power. However, unlike Belgium at that time, the Congolese constitution created a federal state divided into six provinces, with substantial powers given to elected provincial governments. The leaders of various secessionist movements soon emerged from these provincial assemblies.

During the ceremony marking the Congo's accession to sovereignty on 30 June, King Baudouin's paternalistic speech started by saying that this day represented the ultimate outcome of the grand undertaking conceived by the genius of Leopold II, not a conqueror but a civiliser. President Kasavubu responded in a polite and appreciative manner. Lumumba, who was not even scheduled to speak, rose and went to the microphone, addressing his words to the 'independence fighters, today victorious'. The tone was set. On his first day as head of government, Lumumba gave a fiercely nationalistic speech, denouncing the colonial oppression of the previous eighty years, the racism, exploitation, humiliations and torture. Even if the second part of his address spoke of reconciliation, human rights and shared prosperity, the Belgian government decided that this man was too dangerous and had to be eliminated as soon as possible.

The day after independence was proclaimed, all territorial district officers, all senior civil servants, all army officers, all private sector management and practically all secondary school teachers remained Belgian. Of the 87,000 Belgian nationals living in the Congo, 10,000 were civil servants of the new government, 17,000 worked in the private sector and 3,000 were missionaries (the rest were their dependants). The high (and naive) expectations of many Congolese towards independence were utterly disappointed. This did not go down well in the army, especially after its commander, general Émile Janssens, famously stated that 'after independence = before independence'. Five days later, a mutiny inside the barracks of Léopoldville and Thysville spread to most of the country. Lumumba sacked Janssens, replaced him with Congolese officers headed by Joseph Mobutu and raised soldiers' wages by giving everybody a promotion, but he could not regain control over the 25,000-strong army, which split along tribal lines.

Rioting crowds killed Belgian nationals here and there, those who happened to be at the wrong place at the wrong time. In some areas, Belgian women were systematically raped. Belgian paratroopers were rushed in to evacuate foreigners. Those living in Léopoldville quickly crossed the river to the safety of Brazzaville. In the strategic port of Matadi, Belgian aeroplanes gunned the city, apparently unaware that almost all expatriates had been safely evacuated, killing scores of

innocent Congolese civilians. This mistake further fuelled the rebellion
of additional units of the army, now joined by civilians as well.

Rarely in history has a country disintegrated so rapidly. The
Lumumba government collapsed as 80% of its expatriate servants
departed within a few weeks, unlike their compatriots in the private
sector who preferred to stay rather than become unemployed in their
homeland. Provinces seceded from the central state, most notably
mineral-rich Katanga on 11 July and southern Kasaï a month later,
encouraged and supported by Belgium, its army and its large corporations. Katanga had been providing half of the central government
income but received only 25% of expenditures. Its secession had been
planned for months: neo-colonialism might be more likely to succeed if
it focused on the resource-rich regions. Lumumba and Kasavubu wrote
to UN secretary-general Dag Hammarskjold asking for immediate help.

The Security Council decided to intervene in the middle of July. UN
troops arrived in Léo the following day and 8,400 were in the country
within ten days. Relations between Lumumba and the UN quickly
deteriorated, the former being convinced that the UN supported
Belgium and the secessionist government of Katanga rather than the
legitimate government of the Congo. By this stage, the impetuous and
uncompromising Lumumba had become paranoid. He travelled to New
York with little success, demanding the UN troops to be under the
control of his government, which the secretary-general could not
accept. President Eisenhower refused to meet him, and State
Department officials thought that Lumumba was mentally unstable.
Although certainly not a communist and only one month after having
made a similar request to the US government, the desperate Lumumba
asked the Soviet Union for help. The Soviets sent planes, along with
their pilots and technical advisers. Most of these were part of the UN
effort, but some were assigned directly to the Lumumba government. In
the midst of the cold war, this was the worst of all of Lumumba's
blunders. The CIA started actively helping the Belgians in their various
plots to get rid of the prime minister. The chief artisan of his own failure,
Lumumba never understood that he did not have the political, military
and economic power needed to sustain his own policies.

In September 1960, Lumumba was dismissed by Kasavubu, and in
turn Lumumba dismissed Kasavubu. The constitution did not allow for
either of these moves. After a few days of confusion, Lumumba was
definitively overthrown in a bloodless military coup led by the very

person he had just appointed head of the army, colonel Mobutu. Lumumba's appeal to Moscow had provided the perfect justification, if one was needed. Mobutu quickly expelled all Soviet advisers. Placed under house arrest, Lumumba tried to escape to Stanleyville where his support remained strong, but he was captured after a few days on the run, imprisoned and then transferred to his arch-enemies in Katanga. One might wonder how the central government in Léo could transfer a prisoner to the Katanga secessionists, against whom they were fighting a low-grade civil war. The explanation is simple: Belgium controlled both ends of the equation, and thought it would be easier to eliminate this dangerous man in Katanga, where he had no political or tribal support. There, in January 1961, five hours after his arrival, he was executed by a firing squad supervised by Belgian policemen. Days later, his body was cut up and dissolved in acid. A state crime had been committed, ordered by the Belgian minister of African affairs, who had cleared this decision with his prime minister. It remains unclear whether the king, a devout Catholic, also approved of this murder. Much to its credit, Belgium formally apologised forty years later for its role in the assassination of Lumumba.[13]

The elimination of Lumumba did not prevent the situation from degenerating into a complex civil war, in which UN troops actively participated in combat in Katanga. The UN secretary-general's plane crashed in northern Rhodesia on its way to a meeting with Katanga's leader, and it remained unclear whether this was the result of foul play or just an accident. Eventually, the Katangese secession was defeated, but other regions tried to fight the central government, especially the Province Orientale where a Lumumbist government was set up, and a large region east of Léopoldville where a left-wing guerrilla attempted to overthrow the regime.

Hundreds of thousands of refugees took shelter in Léopoldville, the economy plummeted, unemployment became the rule rather than the exception, and we have seen in Chapter 6 how this chaos and the ensuing poverty radically changed the face of prostitution in the capital, allowing for the successful sexual amplification of HIV-1, one or two decades after the virus had been given a boost in the same city through parenteral mechanisms. At some point, the number of infected individuals reached a critical stage beyond which the dissemination of HIV-1 into the rest of the Congo, and beyond, became unavoidable.

Nation building, with help from the Caribbean

Mobutu quickly handed power back to the select few civilians with a post-secondary education, but in November 1965, he staged another coup, this time establishing a corrupt dictatorship that would last thirty-two years, later to be described by political scientists as a kleptocracy (a word coined to mean government by thieves). Mobutu's main achievement was to fight successfully the various secessions and rebellions and to end the balkanisation process, eventually reunifying the country and bringing some peace at last. The Congolese government financed its deficits by printing money, which led to a devaluation of the currency and high inflation (often 100% per year). Pay raises were slow to follow. During the first twenty years of nationhood, prices increased 324-fold while salaries rose only 19-fold. In other words, the purchasing power of the average Zairean in 1980 was only 6% of what it had been in 1960. There cannot be a better measure of the pauperisation of this people.[14–16]

During the chaotic post-independence period, most Belgian district administrators, agronomists, doctors and teachers fled the country, fearing for their lives. Promotions were quick in the Congo's administration, and those who had served as low-level officials during Belgian rule, not because of incompetence but because the racial segregation of the colonial system meant that they could not be trained for higher functions, immediately climbed the ladder, far beyond their level of competence. It was more difficult to replace the doctors and teachers. Few Congolese could teach in secondary schools (only one man out of 200 had completed his own secondary school education), and not a single one at the university level. Neither was there a single Congolese medical doctor in 1960. The country asked for and received substantial foreign assistance in these vital sectors.[10,17]

The UN provided the first cohorts of technical assistants in 1960. One year after independence, there were only 240 physicians for the whole country, including 70 sent by the World Health Organization (WHO), compared to 760 before that fateful day. By 1963, the UN had 1,400 civilian technical assistants in the country: 800 teachers and 600 experts in various other fields such as health, communications, agronomy, customs, post office, public works, the judicial system, etc. Some countries also sent technical assistants through bilateral programmes; the Danish surgeon who died of AIDS in 1977 was one of them. In 1964

nearly 2,000 Belgian technical assistants (mostly teachers) were working in the country, but these numbers quickly decreased following
disputes between the Congolese and Belgian governments. Post-
secondary education was provided through scholarships for Congolese
to study overseas and through the creation of specialised national institutions. The WHO funded an accelerated two-year training programme
to turn medical assistants into *bona fide* medical doctors.[17–20]

Many of the UN technicians were hired from the Haitian intellectual
elite, struggling under their own ubuesque dictatorship of François
Duvalier. Haitians presented many advantages: they were black, well
educated, spoke French and were keen to leave Haiti for much better
salaries than those they received at home. Several hundred Haitians
departed for the Congo in the early 1960s as teachers hired by the
United Nations Education, Science and Culture Organization
(UNESCO), the UN agency for education, and as medical doctors
under the umbrella of the WHO. As early as 1960, half of the
UNESCO teachers dispatched to the Congo were Haitians. In 1963–4,
Haitians were the second largest contingent (after the Belgians) among
the UNESCO teachers, with 136 of them working throughout the
national school system. They were also the second largest group (after
the French) in the other fields covered by the UN intervention, with 60
more experts.[17,21]

By some estimates 1,000 Haitians were employed in the Congo in
1963. Progressively, and until the mid-1970s, a larger number of
Haitians came as employees of the Congolese government, which at
the time had the resources (from mining royalties) to hire foreign
teachers that would at last provide young Congolese with the secondary
and higher education denied to their parents. There was a substantial
investment in enhancing educational opportunities, which required
competent teachers willing to work in a rather difficult environment.
Throughout the 1960s, Haitian teachers could be found not only in the
major urban centres but also in smaller district cities that housed a
secondary school. A book on the topic has been written by Camille
Kuyu, a Congolese jurist, who estimated that during that period
approximately 4,500 Haitians worked in the Congo. A census carried
out in Kinshasa in 1967 estimated that about 500 Haitians were living
in the city, so the total number quoted by Kuyu is not far-fetched.[22–25]

Some were single, some were married and brought their families
along, while others, posted into rather unstable regions, preferred to

leave wives and children at home. These efforts eventually paid off, and the most important accomplishment (some would say, the only one) made by the Congo in the two decades after its independence was the dramatic advancement in the education level of the population. In the late 1960s, 20% of the national budget was spent on education. The pedagogical institute of Léopoldville, established in 1961 and initially staffed by UN personnel, produced large enough cohorts of Congolese teachers by the mid-1970s.[17]

Naturally, a number of Haitians entertained liaisons with Congolese women. In his book about the women of Kisangani, Benoit Verhaegen tells the heartbreaking story of a very poor fourteen-year-old girl who, out of necessity, had an affair with a Haitian teacher in 1965. After fathering a child, the teacher claimed that he was going home to show the baby to his mother. They never came back, much as the Europeans had done for a long time. The young woman told the author that her dream was to move to Kinshasa and become a sex worker.[26]

These Haitian technical assistants are the most plausible intermediaries for the next step in the pandemic, the export of HIV-1 out of Africa to the Americas. This process required just one of the 4,500 technical assistants to have acquired HIV-1 sexually or otherwise and for this person to go back to Haiti, either transiently or permanently, to start a chain of sexual transmission in the Caribbean island.

Haitians were not the only foreigners present in substantial numbers in post-independence Congo; there were also thousands of Belgians. Although many went home during the troubles, some stayed or came back, especially those who owned a business or had lucrative jobs in the private sector. Prior to independence, Belgians made up about 80% of the Europeans living in Léo, followed by the Portuguese (7%) and the French (4%). A number of Belgians acquired HIV in the Congo in the 1960s (and probably even earlier), from free women whose sexual services they purchased. This was documented by Jean Sonnet, the former head of internal medicine at the university hospital in Kinshasa, but in these cases forward transmission seems to have been limited to their spouses.[27–28]

Just before and after independence, a few hundred Americans were living in the Léopoldville area. Most were Protestant missionaries, usually married, and thus unlikely to have been sexually exposed to HIV. Fifteen years earlier during WWII, American troops had been stationed in the Congo, including Léopoldville, to beef up the colony's defences, and they were known to have assiduously frequented the bars in the capital, but this occurred too early to fit in well with the rest of the story.[29]

Some of the UN troops who fought against the secessionists in Katanga and other parts of the Congo between 1960 and 1964, 250 of whom were killed in action, could also have been infected as HIV-1 may already have been present outside Léopoldville. At its peak in 1961, the Organisation des Nations-Unies au Congo (ONUC) mission was 20,000 strong. Over the course of the four-year operation, a large part of the Nigerian, Ghanaian, Ethiopian and Malaysian armies cycled through the Congo; 6,200 Irish, 5,600 Indian, 3,250 Moroccan and 3,175 Tunisian soldiers also served, as did smaller numbers of troops from Guinea, Mali, Sudan, Liberia, Sierra Leone, Pakistan, Indonesia, Canada, Norway, Sweden, Denmark, Egypt, etc. The ONUC troops in Katanga have been accused of a number of rapes. Throughout the mission, about 200 Canadian communications officers, mostly franco-phones from Quebec, were stationed in Léo and they frequented assid-uously the city's bars and brothels. No early case of AIDS has been documented retrospectively in the countries that provided the troops, but admittedly some might have remained unrecognised or unreported, resulting in epidemiological dead ends. That being said, the rest of the story that will unfold in the next section strongly suggests that Haiti was indeed the stepping stone for the export of HIV-1 to the Americas.[30–32]

The fourth 'H'

When the first reports describing AIDS appeared in the US in 1981–2, Haitians were quickly identified as a risk group, the fourth 'H' after heroin users, homosexuals and haemophiliacs. Case series of AIDS among Haitians living in Miami, New York, Montreal and Haiti were published. Unlike some of the other risk groups, Haitians were easily identifiable: black persons speaking English with a peculiar accent (or no English at all). Furthermore, many of them were illegal migrants or asylum seekers or, if living legally in the US, not yet American citizens. There had already been some anti-Haitian sentiment building up in Florida, triggered by the recent arrival of thousands of boat people fleeing their dynastic dictatorship.[33–38]

During the first few years of the epidemic, when the modes of trans-mission of the new disease were not understood, mass hysteria became the rule rather than the exception. Before the discovery of HIV as the aetiological agent of AIDS, many different hypotheses were proposed, including the emergence of a Haitian virus perhaps related to bizarre voodoo practices. Haitians living in the US became victims of atrocious discrimination, stigmatisation and prejudice. Some were sacked from their jobs, others were kicked out of their flats, people were even afraid to talk to them, in some clinics they would be asked to queue separately from other patients, Haitian children were taunted at school or even beaten up, Haitian businesses went bankrupt as clients were scared, etc. In Haiti itself, the tourism industry vanished overnight, and thousands lost their source of income. From a high of 144,000 in 1979, the number of visitors decreased to as few as 10,000 in 1982–3. According to medical anthropologist Paul Farmer, it generated an epidemic of discrimination and 'an entire nation of impoverished people had been relegated to the status of a health hazard'.[39–41]

The Haitian community in the US reacted strongly and successfully lobbied the CDC so that Haitians were removed from the list of high-risk groups in 1985, something which was politically sound but epidemiologically debatable. Epidemiologists define a risk group as a subpopulation among whom a disease is more common than in the whole population and at whom specific preventive measures can be targeted. Amongst the first 1,000 cases of AIDS reported to the CDC, fifty-four (5.4%) occurred among Haitians, only three of whom admitted being homosexual; at that time about 0.15% of the US population was born in Haiti. In retrospect, although heterosexual transmission of HIV-1 had already occurred on a similar scale in several African countries, Haitians living in the US represented the first population among whom this was documented and they suffered because other modes of transmission, such as casual contacts, were initially suspected.[42]

As part of their reaction and defence against discrimination, an argument was developed that HIV had actually been exported from the US to Haiti through the sexual tourism of American gay men who bought sex from male prostitutes. This hypothesis was put forward before epidemiological studies were conducted in Haiti but it was plausible. Indeed, thousands of American gay men travelled to Haiti in the 1970s and early 1980s. Homosexual tours were organised out of San Francisco and New York, and some specific hotels (Habitation Leclerc, for example, a walled enclave for those with deep pockets, or Pension Tropicale for the others) catered to this clientele which had a lot of money to spend. The French Canadian airline steward who was linked to many of the early cases of AIDS in the US, and dubbed by some 'patient zero', was one of these visitors. An international gay convention was held in Port-au-Prince in 1979, attended largely by Americans. Herbert Gold, a San Francisco writer, described the gay scene in Port-au-Prince in the late 1970s: the parties were fabulous and apparently some attractive boys were trained for export to the US. This had been going on for quite a while because already in the late 1940s Suzanne Comhaire-Sylvain had described in Kenscoff, near the capital, the existence of homosexuality between some of the café workers and foreign clients, a harbinger of what would later happen on a wider scale.[43–47]

As late as 1982, the Spartacus international travel guide for gay men provided tips such as 'your partners will expect to be paid for their services but charges are nominal'. The going rate seemed to have been $10 to $15. Haitian men were described as 'handsome, very well endowed, highly sexed, uninhibited and affectionate'. In retrospect, however, most people would agree that the statement that 'much of the population is bisexual' may have been somewhat exaggerated. It was noted that the local authorities became less tolerant after 1980 when several youths had been hospitalised following sodomy injuries caused by sadistic Caucasian tourists. At the other end of the island, the Dominican Republic, formerly a 'paradise for gay tourists, particularly paedophiles', had turned into a nightmare due to the bad behaviour of these tourists. Throughout this travel guide, there was certainly a casual attitude towards sex being purchased in Third World countries and a refusal to call it by its true name, prostitution.[48]

In its 1985 edition, a few years into the AIDS epidemic, the Spartacus guide reported that the reaction of the Duvalier government had been to expel from the country foreigners who owned gay bars and hotels, that visitors were now screened at the airport and those who looked gay or whose names were on a list of unwanted aliens were sent back on the same plane. Two years earlier, the Port-au-Prince authorities had announced that all Haitian gay men would be jailed for six months followed by another six months of rehabilitation. A fairly large number were arrested, but they either paid bribes or threatened to name names and most were quickly released.[49–52]

Homosexual prostitution was part of a bigger picture in which, as an unavoidable consequence of an island of deep poverty being located so close to the US, other types of visitors came to Haiti for vacations that included sexual adventures. After the fall of Batista, Cuba was no longer available for such holidays of sun, sand and 'duty-free sex' and another nearby destination was found. Middle-aged American or Canadian women could enjoy a week or two with a Haitian gigolo, and white heterosexual men also had a good time, sometimes with girls in their early teens. Of course, there was a substantial amount of commercial sex for the internal market as well.[41,43,46]

It was postulated for some time that all cases of AIDS among Haitians must have been acquired homosexually, and the fact that many Haitian AIDS patients denied having had sex with another man reflected cultural barriers against acknowledging homosexuality. It is interesting to note that, as a reaction against stigmatisation, the response was to lay the blame on a risk group that had itself been highly stigmatised in the US, long before AIDS.[53–55]

What is the evidence in support of Haiti having been infected from the US or vice versa?

In retrospect, the first probable cases of AIDS in Haiti were recognised in 1978–9. This retrospective chronology is based essentially on diagnoses of Kaposi's sarcoma (KS), a cancer which had rarely been diagnosed in Haiti prior to 1979. This is the form of skin cancer developed in the character played by Tom Hanks in *Philadelphia*, for which he received an Oscar. AIDS-associated Kaposi's sarcoma involves internal organs but patients also display multiple skin lesions which can be easily biopsied, provided the patient has access to a hospital equipped to do histopathological examinations. AIDS-associated KS has to be distinguished from 'endemic Kaposi's sarcoma'. While the former is associated with a profound immunosuppression and a high mortality, the latter is an indolent cancer, compatible with prolonged survival, which has long been recognised as endemic in parts of Africa, including the Belgian Congo, AEF and Uganda. Among eighteen cases of KS diagnosed in Haiti or among Haitians in the US in 1979–81, most died within six months of diagnosis: clearly, this was not the 'endemic' form of the disease. There was a male preponderance.[54–61]

Similarly, cases of probable AIDS with KS among gay men were identified retrospectively in the US in 1978–9. Such temporal coincidence suggests that whichever country got HIV first, the other one got it not long after. The median incubation period from acquiring HIV until developing AIDS is about ten years, but can be shorter in some patients.

These observations suggest that HIV was introduced into both Haiti and the United States at the end of the 1960s or in the early 1970s.[62–65]

However, it does not imply that HIV was introduced into both countries at exactly the same time, for several reasons. KS is not the best marker for retrospectively recognising the emergence of AIDS in a population. Kaposi's sarcoma is a cancer caused by another sexually transmitted virus, human herpesvirus 8. During the early years of the American epidemic, Kaposi's sarcoma as an AIDS-defining illness was much more common in homosexuals than in other risk groups, pre-sumably because human herpesvirus 8 is transmitted better during homosexual than heterosexual intercourse. KS was seen in 21% of homosexuals with AIDS, but in only 6% of male heterosexuals and 1% of haemophiliac men who developed AIDS. Once infected, for some reason males in general are intrinsically more susceptible to the cancer-causing effect of the virus than females (fifty years ago, in central and East Africa, endemic KS was five to thirty-three times more common in men than women). By analogy, changes in the incidence of KS in Haiti probably reflected the introduction of HIV into its homosexual/bisexual community rather than among individuals who acquired HIV through other modes.[59–61,66]

Access to a diagnosis of Kaposi's sarcoma was infinitely better in the US than in Haiti. In the US, it would have been very unlikely for some-body with KS not to have a skin biopsy with histopathological inter-pretation and registration of the case in a cancer registry. In Haiti, it is plausible that some of the early cases of KS were missed. It is interesting to note that a case of AIDS (without KS) was diagnosed in Montreal in 1978, in a Haitian who went to Canada for medical treatment. Since only a tiny proportion of Haitian patients would have had the contacts and resources to travel abroad to seek medical treatment, there must have been earlier cases of AIDS who died quietly in Haiti without a diagnosis. The most frequent HIV-associated opportunistic infection in Haiti would have been tuberculosis, a disease that was already so common in the impoverished island, long before HIV emerged, that any change in its incidence or clinical pattern would have taken years before it was noticed.[67]

As in Africa, scientists tried to locate archival samples of serum. Out of 191 Haitian adults from a rural area tested for dengue fever in 1977–9, none was HIV-positive. Molecular biologists came to the rescue of historians and provided estimates of the respective chronology of the two apparently concomitant epidemics in Haiti and the US. A first study using a molecular clock estimated that the founder of the B subtype in the US originated in 1967 (confidence interval: 1960–71). In the phylogenetic tree, the seven B subtype sequences from Haiti 'branched off' earlier than the other B subtype sequences, which suggested that HIV in Haiti antedated its introduction into the US.[68–69]

More precise measures were generated when researchers recovered HIV-1 sequences from archival specimens collected at a Miami hospital in 1982–3 from Haitian AIDS patients who had recently emigrated to the US and had presumably been infected with HIV-1 while in Haiti. These sequences were compared to isolates from the US and other countries, all of which were HIV-1 group M subtype B. If HIV-1 had arrived in Haiti first, non-Haitian subtype B strains would be expected to be phylogenetically nested within an older and more extensive range of Haitian genetic variations, with Haitian lineages branching off closest to the ancestor. This is exactly what the analysis showed. The probability that subtype B emerged in the US prior to Haiti was estimated at less than one in a thousand.[70]

Analyses supported the hypothesis of a single epidemiologically successful introduction of subtype B from central Africa to Haiti, from where it was re-exported to the US. The time of the most recent common ancestor of subtype B in Haiti was estimated to be 1966 (confidence interval: 1962–70) while the most recent common ancestor for the US epidemic was estimated at 1969 (confidence interval: 1966–72). In other words, HIV was introduced into Haiti around 1966, and from there it moved to the US around 1969, give or take a few years. This was consistent with another study which dated the founder of the US type B epidemic at 1968.[70–71]

These findings represent the best available data concerning the chronology of the introduction of HIV-1 into the Americas. They were contested by Haitian researchers, and one can understand that the wounds of the anti-Haitian stigmatisation of twenty-five years ago have left permanent scars, especially considering that these were superimposed on centuries of domination and exploitation of Haitians by white westerners. However, their arguments were refuted by the authors' reply published in the same journal.[72,73]

There is now little doubt that HIV-1 subtype B was exported from central Africa to Haiti around 1966, from where it was re-exported to the US a few years later. Among the 4,500 Haitians who worked in the

Congo, one of them acquired HIV-1, probably through heterosexual intercourse, and later initiated a chain of transmission upon returning to the Caribbean island, during vacations or at the end of his contract. As in any population of 4,500 adults, there must have been a small minority who were sexually promiscuous and bought sex once in a while. The same behaviours that facilitated acquisition of HIV-1 within the heart of Africa must have contributed to its early spread in Haiti, the returning technical assistant infecting one or more Haitian women, perhaps a sex worker.

Molecular biology and phylogenetics aside, we can be relatively certain of the number of Haitians who introduced HIV-1 into the Americas: a single individual. That is because subtype B, the exclusive subtype present among Haitians and Americans in the early stage of the epidemic, is very uncommon in central Africa where it represents less than 0.5% of all HIV-1 strains that circulate. Thus, it is virtually impossible statistically that more than one Haitian working in the Congo got infected with the same subtype in the early 1960s and brought it back home. This is an extraordinary example of what evolutionary biologists describe as a founder event.

But why was the introduction of HIV-1 into Haiti so epidemiologically successful rather than just another dead end infection, as with the Norwegian sailor and the Belgian expatriates infected in the Congo in the 1960s? How was it possible for a virus imported in 1966, by only one individual, to infect 8% of mothers attending an under-five clinic in the Cité Soleil slum of Port-au-Prince merely a decade and a half later, bearing in mind that such an expansion required more than fifty years in Léopoldville/Kinshasa? There must have been a very effective amplification mechanism early on, but was it sexual or parenteral? This will be the topic of the next chapter.[74]

12 | *The blood trade*

In this chapter, we will examine the possibility that, during the early stage of the Haitian epidemic, a commercial enterprise in Port-au-Prince exponentially and parenterally amplified the number of HIV-1-infected individuals and allowed the virus to thrive. More generally, we will review the role of the blood trade in the globalisation of HIV-1. But first, we need to understand how viruses can be transmitted, not only from donor to recipient, but also from one donor to another during the handling required to prepare certain blood products. The word 'donor' is somewhat misleading here because we are talking mostly about people paid for their 'donations'.

Blood is made of cells (red blood cells, white blood cells and platelets) and plasma, its liquid component. Plasma is made of water and proteins: antibodies, clotting factors and albumin. When a donation is made, the various components are separated to maximise their use. Patients with anaemia or acute blood loss need only receive the red blood cells, those with a low platelet count will be given the platelets and so on. Plasma is highly valuable as it contains many proteins. Therapeutic use of plasma started during WWII as an expander of intravascular volume, to increase quickly blood pressure in patients with serious bleeding. Subsequently, other uses of plasma components were developed, which required the selective processing of specific proteins: albumin (to expand intravascular volume or to patients with low albumin levels), coagulation factors (haemophilia or other coagulation disorders) and immunoglobulins (patients with immune deficiencies or to protect travellers against hepatitis A).

Plasma was also used for the production of the early generation of hepatitis B vaccines, made from the chemical inactivation of the virus present in blood and the purification of its surface antigen. Sources of hepatitis B-positive donors included gay men and prisoners in developed countries, and the general population of Third World nations, where up to 15% of adults chronically carry HBV in their blood. At least 30 million doses of such crude vaccines were administered before being replaced with genetically engineered vaccines.

As the amount of the specific proteins of interest is small in each individual donor's plasma, commercial plasma derivatives must be prepared by pooling plasma from several donors. In particular, the fabrication of coagulation factor concentrates required the pooling of plasma from thousands of donors, such that an infectious agent present in a single donor could make the entire pool infectious and be transmitted to many recipients. Prior to their discovery, transmission of HIV-1 and HCV from coagulation factor concentrates infected thousands of haemophiliacs worldwide, resulting in the tragic death of a large portion of this population. Since then, the infectious risk from coagulation factors has been drastically reduced through the development of sensitive screening assays for donors and better methods for eliminating viruses.

The risk of transmitting HIV was much lower, indeed probably near zero, when the plasma was processed to prepare albumin, because ethanol was used in the fractionation, after which the product was pasteurised by heating. And fortunately, no transmission through immunoglobulins has ever been reported, even if many batches contained antibodies against HIV: again, the ethanol fractionation process inactivated HIV. The early hepatitis B vaccines were not incriminated in the transmission of HIV either; presumably, the methods used to inactivate HBV were effective against HIV as well.[1-2]

In the late 1960s and 1970s, before HIV and HCV were known, the demand for plasma-derived products had escalated rapidly. There was not enough excess plasma from volunteer whole blood donors and paid donors had to be recruited. In order to get more plasma from these paid donors, a technology called 'plasmapheresis' was developed: whole blood was taken from the donor, the plasma quickly separated from the blood cells and the cells re-infused in the donor along with replacement fluids. Thus the donor did not become anaemic and could sell plasma repeatedly, not just twice a year as with donors of whole blood. However, before and even after the infectious risks were understood, viruses could be transmitted not only to the ultimate recipients of the blood products but also between donors participating in plasmapheresis. This required only one breakdown in some component of the process, for instance the re-use of pieces of plastic tubing that had been designed for single use. If a donor with unrecognised HIV infection entered the process and if some precaution was disregarded, this person could infect subsequent plasma donors whose blood was processed by the same machine on the same or following days. In settings where paid donors repeatedly sold their plasma week after week, this would increase the number and proportion of HIV-infected individuals among those selling plasma, further enhancing the risk for the other donors. This vicious circle would result in exponential propagation of HIV between donors, arguably the most effective method for HIV transmission.

The infectious risks for donors in plasmapheresis centres had been known for some time before the HIV epidemic. In 1973, donors at a South Carolina commercial plasmapheresis centre contracted the hepatitis A virus, a microbe which remains present in the bloodstream for only a short period of time. This was caused by the pooling of plasma from multiple donors during its extraction from the cells, allowing the reflux of pooled plasma into the bags of red cells re-infused in the donors. In 1977–8, four outbreaks involved plasma donors who developed 'non-A non-B hepatitis' (later renamed hepatitis C after its aetiological agent was discovered) in plasmapheresis centres in Austria, Germany and Poland, apparently from contamination with plasma of the plastic bags used for re-infusing red blood cells. In the US, paid donors were often recruited in prisons, a substantial percentage of whose populations were previous or current drug addicts at high risk of being infected with HBV or HCV: a chain of transmission could easily be initiated.[3–5]

The first well-documented epidemic of HIV-1 among paid plasma donors occurred in a poor suburb of Mexico City where, in 1986, 281 donors were found to be HIV-infected, especially those that sold plasma ten or more times each month. Re-utilisation of blood collecting material was blamed. At the time there were thirteen plasmapheresis centres in the country, mainly in Mexico City and in states near the Texan border. Most donors were young men living in the peri-urban shanty towns. They could sell their blood as often as every two to three days. By the time that the sale of plasma was prohibited nationwide in 1987, 7% of 9,100 paid donors were HIV-infected. In one of the plasmapheresis centres, HIV prevalence increased from 6% in June to 54% in November 1986. Other outbreaks of HIV transmission among paid plasma donors were reported in Valencia, Spain and Pune, India. In the latter city, among commercial plasma donors, HIV prevalence was 0%

in November 1987 but 78% seven months later, illustrating the exponential transmission of HIV through unhygienic plasma collection practices.[6-11]

These outbreaks, although tragic in their own right, were dwarfed by what happened in China in the early 1990s, several years after the risk of HIV transmission via plasmapheresis was understood, and a decade after the transmission of HCV had been documented in the same Chinese centres. In rural areas, poor farmers were recruited by 'plasma pimps', to sell plasma to increase their meagre income. They received $6 per donation, which could be repeated twice a month in theory, more often if donors attended more than one collection centre. There were several hundred plasma collection stations set up by blood product companies. In the most-heavily affected provinces of Henan, Anhui, Shanxi, Hubei, Hebei, Shandong and Jilin, approximately 250,000 paid donors (a quarter of a million!) acquired HIV.[12-14]

In several plasma collection centres, blood from multiple ABO-matched donors (who were not screened for HIV) was combined for 'more efficient' large volume plasma separation, and then the pooled cell fraction was returned to the donors, along with any infectious agent that had been present in the blood of any of the donors at a given session. The re-use of needles and tubing also facilitated transmission. In some regions, between 9 and 17% of plasma donors became HIV-infected while up to 28% were infected with HCV. It is remarkable that such a high HIV prevalence was reached despite most donors reporting fewer than ten donations per year. Among the small number who sold plasma more than twenty times per year, half became HIV-infected.[12,15]

What do all these stories have in common? Poor people looking for a quick source of income and willing to sell their blood repeatedly. Profit-driven blood collection centres where a small number of entrepreneurs try to make as much money as possible by cutting costs, re-using needles, syringes and tubings, while being unaware of or not caring about the risk of transmitting blood-borne viruses. A lucrative market for these blood products, either locally or internationally. Finally, a 'patient zero' who introduces the pathogen.

The vampire of the Caribbean

Now back to the Caribbean, where the potential for a quick profit in the blood trade had been exploited as well. In Port-au-Prince, a large plasmapheresis centre operated from May 1971 to November 1972 under the name Hemo-Caribbean. This was a joint venture between Joseph Gorinstein, a Miami businessman and stockbroker, a few other American investors and a well-known Haitian politician, Luckner Cambronne.

Luckner Cambronne was born in 1929, the son of a poor Protestant preacher. Starting out as a bank teller, he eventually found a job in the entourage of François Duvalier (Papa Doc), the country doctor elected president in 1957. Initially just a messenger, he then became a bagman. Duvalier liked him and Cambronne quickly rose to become the regime's chief extortionist. He held various ministries (public works, customs, etc.), all of which provided ample opportunity for corruption. His speciality was to intimidate businessmen into making large 'donations', and those who refused had a much shorter life expectancy. Ostensibly, these funds were to be used to rebuild a slum or pave a road but most of it ended up in Duvalier's and Cambronne's bank accounts. This was also the main destination for the funds (deducted from the pay of civil servants) allocated to building a new city, Duvalierville. Only a few bungalows were erected, far from the promised Caribbean Brasilia.[16]

Cambronne was the most feared man in Haiti after his boss for good reason: he was the leader of the infamous Tontons Macoutes, Duvalier's militia, who assassinated thousands of opponents. He became famous for saying that a good Duvalierist is prepared to kill his own children for Duvalier, and also expects his children to kill their parents for him. Cambronne developed many business interests: part-ownership of Air Haiti (which had a monopoly on transportation to Miami), taxi companies, the Ibo Tours travel agency specialising in quick all-inclusive $1,200 divorces for Americans (conveniently, a new divorce law facilitated this enterprise – it was no longer necessary for both parties to be present), fishing facilities, fruit and coffee exports, a supermarket, cannabis plantations and so on. Cambronne also made money by exporting corpses to American medical schools. His plasma commerce would earn him the nickname 'Vampire of the Caribbean'. He became a habitué of the upmarket brothels in Port-au-Prince, a high-stakes poker player in the flashy casinos and a lover of expensive sharkskin suits, hence his other nickname, 'The Shark'.

In January 1972, the *New York Times* reported that Hemo-Caribbean was exporting up to 6,000 litres of plasma to the US each month. Hemo-Caribbean could accommodate 350 donors per day at its two-storey centre on Rue des Remparts, and was building a second facility to increase capacity to 850 donors per day. Run by an Austrian biochemist, Hemo-Caribbean initially had a staff of 110 employees and was open six days a week from 6.30 to 22.00. After the expansion, its payroll doubled to 200 employees including nine full-time medical doctors. Paid donors were among the poorest of a very impoverished nation, described by the *New York Times* as 'many in rags, without shoes'. Most were illiterate. They would show up once a week and receive between $3 and $5 per donation, a process described by some as 'plasma farming'. A local doctor commented: 'The plasma cows are rather tired, but they don't have a job anyway.' When sold in the US, the same quantity of plasma would fetch around $35. An author estimated that ultimately around 6,000 Haitians sold their plasma to Hemo-Caribbean. That seems reasonably accurate because Gorinstein claimed that in late 1972 Hemo-Caribbean was paying donors an average of $70,000 each month: at $4 per donation, this corresponds to 700 different donors each day and about 4,200 through an average week.[17–26]

Of course, only plasma was utilised and the red cells were re-infused in the donor to enable him/her to come back quickly for a further donation. The frozen plasma was exported on Air Haiti, Cambronne's company, and sold to four American enterprises (according to the *New York Times*: Armour Pharmaceutical, Cutter Laboratories, Dade Reagents and Dow Chemical) as well as to clients in Germany and Sweden.[17]

After the death of Papa Doc in 1971, when nineteen-year-old Jean-Claude (Bébé Doc) succeeded his father, Cambronne was the most powerful man on the island as minister of interior and national defence. The following year, he fell into disgrace and had to flee from Haiti. Whether this was related to the fact that he had allegedly been the lover of Simone Duvalier (Manman Simone) after the death of Papa Doc remains unclear. He also had a conflict with Marie-Denise, Jean-Claude's powerful eldest sister, who helped to oust Cambronne while Manman Simone happened to be in Miami. Jean-Claude Duvalier was afraid that Cambronne wanted the top job, and unhappy with the bad publicity generated by the *New York Times* report, not just outside but also within Haiti (the Haitian Catholic Church had issued a pastoral letter condemning the trade as unjustified exploitation of a poor people). In November 1972, he ordered Hemo-Caribbean to be closed and the divorce law was modified so that both parties had to be represented in Port-au-Prince. Gorinstein tried to relocate his plasma business into Puerto Rico. Cambronne ended up in Miami where he died peacefully in 2006.

Although it has been stated that no case of HIV infection in Haiti was ever found among the thousands of people who had sold their plasma, it is far from clear that the first cohorts of Haitian AIDS patients, diagnosed in Port-au-Prince or in the US, were ever asked this question. Since Hemo-Caribbean was closed in 1972, and since the interval between HIV infection and death is generally around ten years, perhaps slightly less in impoverished countries, the opportunity to document such an association did not last long.[27]

The earliest reports of AIDS among Haitians merely described the new disease, the variety of opportunistic infections and the immunological findings. When the HIV aetiological agent was identified, investigators started looking for risk factors, but many of the early Haitian AIDS studies lacked a comparison group. Factors investigated were those already identified in the US: homosexuality, bisexuality, intravenous drug use, transfusions, haemophilia and contaminated injections, heterosexual promiscuity, sex with prostitutes or past STDs. To these were added potential factors of local interest: the use of medicinal roots or herbs, history of malaria, travel to the US or sex with Americans. Men accounted for three-quarters of these early patients, and many lived in Carrefour, a poor suburb of Port-au-Prince known to be a hotbed of prostitution. The 1982 Spartacus Gay Guide recommended that travellers to Haiti should, 'above all, avoid any establishment' in the crowded slum area of Carrefour, where theft was rampant, sometimes accompanied by violence. The preponderance of males among early cases of AIDS could reflect either homosexual transmission, heterosexual transmission in which a small number of female prostitutes infected a large number of male clients, or perhaps a preponderance of men among the paid donors of Hemo-Caribbean. Elsewhere in the world, the sex distribution of paid plasma donors varied: in Mexico, three-quarters were men while in China it seemed more evenly distributed between genders.[28-36]

In the first study in which AIDS cases diagnosed between 1979 and 1984 were compared to controls (same-sex siblings or friends), researchers asked questions about homosexuality, bisexuality, transfusions, intravenous drug use, number of IM injections in the last five years, source of injections (medical personnel versus non-qualified *piquristes*), level of education, place of residence, income, occupation and foreign travel. But apparently they did not ask any questions about the sale of plasma. One third of the men with AIDS acknowledged having had homosexual intercourse, which indicated that this mode of transmission was significant. Heterosexual promiscuity and receiving injections, especially from a non-medical source, were also more common in cases of AIDS than in controls.[37]

A similar study was conducted in 1984 among Haitians diagnosed with AIDS in Miami and New York, and healthy seronegative Haitians of the same age and sex as controls. Among forty-three men with AIDS, having bought sex from prostitutes, a history of gonorrhoea, a positive serological test for syphilis, low socioeconomic status and a recent arrival in the US were more common than in controls, but only one admitted to having had sex with another man. Whether, as was alleged later, this reflected a cultural barrier between patients and interviewers is doubtful as the questionnaire was administered in Creole by Haitian interviewers. It is certainly possible, however, that some men were reluctant to acknowledge their homosexuality. The small group of women with AIDS was more likely than controls to have been offered money for sex and to have a friend who was a voodoo priest! Cases and controls did not differ for a long list of factors: transfusions, drug use, prostitution with tourists, education, occupation, area of residence in Haiti before coming to the US, travel to central Africa, receiving injections in Haiti, going to an injectionist, self-injections, sharing a razor, tattoos, voodoo practices, history of malaria, animal bites, use of folk healers, etc. No data were collected about the sale of plasma. Nor was such information collected in a survey of pregnant women in the Cité Soleil slum area of Port-au-Prince.[38,39]

In follow-up studies, the proportion of AIDS patients diagnosed in Haiti who admitted to homosexuality decreased from 50% in 1983 and 27% in 1984, to as little as 8% in 1985, 4% in 1986 and 1% in 1987. That was a very quick drop indeed, one very hard to explain and never seen elsewhere in the world. Again, no mention was made of the sale of plasma as a risk factor. During the same interval, the proportion of cases seemingly acquired during a transfusion decreased from 23 to 7%. In a 1991 review article about AIDS in Haiti, the risk of transmission via the Red Cross and public blood banks was discussed, without any mention of the past activities of Hemo-Caribbean.[40–42]

To summarise, the Hemo-Caribbean plasmapheresis centre in Port-au-Prince could have been the perfect venue for the rapid parenteral amplification of a strain of HIV-1 subtype B recently imported from the Congo, and potentially for its re-export to other countries through the international trade in blood products. Hemo-Caribbean operated in 1971 and 1972, at exactly the right time, a few years after the virus had been imported into Haiti. The examples of India, Mexico and China suggest that if HIV-1 was introduced into the cohort of the Port-au-Prince paid donors, transmission could have been swift. Most of these individuals would have died before or shortly after AIDS was recognised in Haiti, and unfortunately the early epidemiological studies did not look for this specific risk factor.

Would it be possible to verify this hypothesis epidemiologically, assuming that some of the paid donors who did not get HIV were infected with HCV instead? Unfortunately, the chaotic situation of the last twenty-five years made it very difficult to conduct medical research in this small country, and those dedicated and courageous enough to do so have focused, quite rightly so, on the treatment of HIV-1 infection. The catastrophic earthquake may have buried definitively any possibility of sorting this out.

The red gold

Meanwhile, at the receiving end of the plasma equation, technological advances contributed to the dissemination of the virus. Haemophiliacs have a genetic deficiency in a coagulation factor (usually, factor VIII) which, in the absence of treatment, leads to their early death, generally from bleeding inside the brain. Blood transfusions and, in the 1950s, administration of plasma were not very effective because they contained little of the missing coagulation factor. Starting in the mid-1960s, 'cryoprecipitates' were used: the freezing and thawing of plasma led to some concentration of factor VIII, which was recuperated after such cycles. One treatment required cryoprecipitates obtained from three to six donors. Unfortunately, the titre of factor VIII in cryoprecipitates varied substantially from lot to lot. Furthermore, they had to be stored at –40°C and thawed slowly before being administered.

These shortcomings were solved around 1972 with the marketing of factor VIII concentrates, in which the quantity of the coagulation factor was high and fixed, and the product conserved as a dry powder, a revolution in the treatment of haemophilia. From the mid-1970s, concentrates were even used preventively and administered regularly (forty to sixty times per year) to some high-risk haemophiliacs. However, the production of factor VIII concentrates required the pooling of plasma obtained from between 2,000 and 25,000 donors, implying that the recipients would be potentially exposed during each treatment to any infectious agent present in the plasma of thousands of individuals. A given lot would be administered to dozens of recipients. Even if much diluted through this pooling process, HIV which had been present in a single donor would be found in many of the vials prepared: in Scotland, eighteen of thirty-two haemophiliacs who had been exposed to a single HIV-infected batch developed HIV infection.[43–46]

It is likely that some of the plasma sent to the US by Hemo-Caribbean was used to produce albumin and immunoglobulins (products whose manufacturing processes inactivated HIV, in contrast with coagulation factors), and the Port-au-Prince company was shut down before factor VIII concentrates became widely used. It could have been worse.[17]

When Hemo-Caribbean was forced out of business, plasma traders used other sources, one of which was Managua, Nicaragua, where one centre was owned by the dictator Anastasio Somoza and a Cuban entrepreneur. For a few years, the Compania Centroamericana de Plasmaferesis was the largest plasma collection centre in the world. With two dozen doctors and a few hundred employees, it could process plasma from up to 1,000 donors per day. Somoza ordered the 1978 killing of the editor of a local newspaper, Pedro Joaquin Chamorro, also a prominent opponent of Somoza's rule, who had dared to criticise this blood trade. At the latter's funeral, a riotous crowd burned down the plasma centre and that was the beginning of the end for Somoza. Chamorro's widow later became president of the country.[22,23]

In the 1970s, about 20% of the plasma produced in the US came from the Third World. A considerable proportion of commercial plasma used in North America and Western Europe was bought and sold by brokers. The largest plasma brokers were a Montreal company called Continental Pharma Cryosan, and Brandenberger AG in Zurich. During the heyday of the plasma trade in the early 1970s, plasma was bought in at least twenty-five developing countries to be exported to pharmaceutical companies in the industrialised world. Apart from those already mentioned, the list included Belize, Brazil, Colombia, Costa Rica, the Dominican Republic, El Salvador, Guatemala, Puerto Rico, Taiwan, Thailand and even

African countries such as Lesotho. In Latin America, blood became known as *el oro rojo*, the red gold.[47]

A large and respected French company had another interesting idea: extracting plasma from placentas, which came from France but were also imported from other countries. All of this slowed down after 1975 when the WHO's annual assembly of health ministers unanimously adopted a resolution condemning such practices and urging member states to enact legislation to protect blood donors and blood recipients. Plasma trafficking became illegal in some countries, and the traders who continued risked fines and/or jail terms. These did not deter everybody, given the anticipated hefty profits. For instance, plasma was exported from South Africa to Belgium, Austria, China and India well into the 1980s and 1990s.[47–49]

Such wheeling and dealing necessarily meant that the ethical standards of non-profit corporations were not respected. Following investigations by the Royal Canadian Mounted Police, Continental Pharma Cryosan pleaded guilty in 1980 to charges that it had mislabelled the source of some plasma that it traded. An internal draft memo written in 1977 by a Health Canada official had commented, concerning the same company: 'It is evident we are dealing with more than technical violations, but rather a calculated and deliberate business designed to take advantage of legal loopholes providing possibly hazardous products on the world market.' This was referring to the fact that Canadian regulations did not apply to blood products that were to be re-exported from the country. The Krever Commission inquiry into Canada's blood supply established that Continental Pharma Cryosan had bought plasma from American prisoners in 1983 and resold it to a number of clients, including Connaught Laboratories in Toronto, the sole Canada-based plasma fractionator. Such practices were discouraged by the US Food and Drug Administration (FDA) because prisoners were already thought to be at greater risk of being infected with the putative aetiological agent of AIDS. In June 1983, Health Management Associates, a company buying plasma from prisoners in Arkansas, informed Continental Pharma Cryosan that thirty-eight units of plasma had been obtained from four prisoners who had previously tested positive for HBV antigen and should have been excluded, even if their more recent test was negative.[50,51]

As a measure of the ongoing international circulation of plasma two years into the AIDS crisis, four of these thirty-eight units had been sold by Continental Pharma Cryosan to Connaught, while the other thirty-four had been vended to companies in Switzerland, Spain, Japan and Italy. Continental Pharma Cryosan did not inform Connaught of the problem. Eventually Health Management Associates recalled the thirty-eight units and informed the FDA, which then informed Health Canada, which in turn informed Connaught. Up to that time, Connaught apparently did not know that it was processing plasma obtained from prisoners. Because the process required the pooling of a large number of donations, small quantities of plasma from the four HBV-infected donors was now present in 2,409 vials of coagulation factor concentrates, only 417 of which could be retrieved. The others had already been administered.

Then, a fifth Arkansas donor was found to have been HBV-positive in the past. This prisoner had sold plasma thirty-four times over ten months. Only twenty-seven out of 1,968 vials that included plasma from this man could be recalled. That was too much for the Canadian Red Cross, the national distributor of blood products, which cancelled its contract with Connaught. The Krever Commission also revealed that Connaught had earlier processed plasma from inmates in four Louisiana prisons. There, prison plasma collection centres were exploited by Community Plasma Center Inc., which sold the plasma to Health Management Associates, which resold it to Continental Pharma Cryosan, which then resold it to Connaught between November 1982 and January 1983.[51]

A class action lawsuit initiated by HCV-infected haemophiliacs against the Canadian Red Cross, Connaught Laboratories and Continental Pharma Cryosan was eventually settled as part of a larger arrangement that included several other parties, after the defendants collectively agreed to pay a multi-million dollar compensation to the plaintiffs, most of which had been raised by the Canadian Red Cross selling some of its assets.

We will never know for sure how often and from what sources HIV entered this transcontinental network. However, the point is that, throughout the 1970s and the early 1980s, any virus present in plasma samples could have travelled thousands of miles in all directions within days or weeks of being collected, and ended up in the veins of many recipients.

13 | *The globalisation*

The early spread

Here we will review how, from its central African crucible, HIV managed to disseminate throughout Africa, at the same time as it did so across the Atlantic. But first we need to review two epidemiological terms. As explained in Chapter 1, 'incidence' is a measure of new cases of HIV that occur among previously uninfected subjects over a period of time. The same individuals have to be tested repeatedly: this is time-consuming, expensive and rarely used. 'Prevalence' is the proportion of individuals who have HIV at some point in time, a snapshot that indicates the current distribution. As the median interval between HIV infection and death in Africa is about ten years, measures of HIV prevalence reflect an accumulation of individuals infected from as little as a few weeks ago to more than ten years earlier. Over time, prevalence in a population increases if the number of new infections since the previous survey was greater than the number of individuals who died from HIV or other causes. Prevalence decreases when the reverse occurs, i.e. the number of deaths is higher than the number of new infections.

Information about the dynamics of HIV-1 in the 1960s–1970s can be inferred by analyses of archival samples, as well as by surveys carried out in the first few years after the identification of HIV-1. Among samples from the adult population, not a single case of HIV-1 was found in Gabon or among the Congo-Brazzaville pygmies. It is surprising, however, that two cases of HIV-2 infection were found in 1967 in samples from Gabon, a country not endemic for this retrovirus, and one wonders what the results would be if these sera were tested with modern methods. No HIV-infected person was identified among 250 individuals at the Yonda leprosarium of the DRC, whose blood had been stored since 1969. The HIV-1 positive samples from that early period came from Kinshasa where 0.25% of women attending a well-baby clinic in 1970 were HIV-1-infected, and from the village of Yambuku where prevalence was 0.8% in 1976.

By 1980, among a similar group of Kinshasa mothers, 3.0% were HIV-1-infected.[1-4]

Thus in countries inhabited by the *P.t. troglodytes* source of HIV-1, prevalence probably remained minimal for most of the fifty years that followed cross-species transmission around 1921, too low to be detected in more than a handful of retrospectively diagnosed cases but high enough for the virus to persist. This is not contradictory. In Western Europe and North America, HIV-1 prevalence in the general adult population has remained around 0.1–0.2% for the last twenty-five years, and it is the much more effective transmission within small subgroups (gay men, injection drug users) which allows HIV-1 not to disappear. In central Africa between 1921 and 1970, HIV-1 prevalence was probably of the same order of magnitude for the overall adult populations but higher among the core groups of urban free women and their clients and among patients attending specific health institutions where iatrogenic transmission occurred. These sanctuaries allowed HIV-1 to persist, and eventually to disseminate when conditions were ripe.

In 1980–4, not a single case was found among adults from the Sangha region of Congo-Brazzaville or the Campo area of Cameroon. At the same time, in Lambaréné (the region of Gabon of Albert Schweitzer fame), three cases of HIV-1 infection were documented among 1,407 patients attending the hospital and one more among 1,313 adults living there. In 1984–5, in Franceville and other rural regions of Gabon, only three out of 1,648 villagers were HIV-1 infected. We can be pretty sure that Gabon, despite its large population of *P.t. troglodytes*, is not the site where HIV-1 emerged: prevalence thirty years ago was too low, especially considering that sampling patients attending health institutions overestimated the true prevalence.[3-5]

In 1985–6, among samples of 300–500 individuals representative of the adult (fifteen to forty-four years) male and female population, HIV-1 prevalence remained minimal in rural Gabon, Equatorial Guinea, Yaoundé, Douala and smaller cities of Cameroon (all around 0.3%) as well as in Port-Gentil (0.5%). However, prevalence was 1.4% in Franceville, 1.8% in Libreville, 4.4% in Bangui and 4.6% in Brazzaville. In the same cities, HIV-1 prevalence among pregnant women was either identical to the former measures (Brazzaville, Bangui, rural Gabon), a bit higher (Yaoundé: 1.3%) or a bit lower (Libreville: 0.5%). This modest prevalence in Douala and Yaoundé suggests that these urban centres were not involved in the early dissemination of the virus. In Kinshasa, among pregnant women, hospital employees and blood donors tested in 1984–5, prevalence varied between 5 and 8%, figures which were similar to those documented in Brazzaville, reflecting the strong links between the twin cities.[4,6]

At the time, Kigali, the capital of Rwanda, had the highest HIV-1 prevalence in the world: between 15 and 20% among blood donors, factory employees and hospital workers, 50% among STD patients and 80% or more among prostitutes. Bujumbura, the capital of Burundi, was not far behind, with 16% of pregnant women infected. The gender imbalance that we described in Léopoldville as the main driver of prostitution also existed in Kigali. In 1972, out of the 60,000 inhabitants of this small town, 2,000 were free women selling sexual services: the city was basically a large brothel. By the early 1980s, the male/female ratio among adults aged twenty to thirty-nine years was 1.57 in Kigali, 1.50 in Nairobi and 1.39 in Bujumbura compared to 0.98 in Kinshasa. In Kigali, the excess of males was driven largely by local customs rather than by the former coloniser's policies (which is why it persisted long after freedom from colonial rule). Traditionally in Rwanda, men marry at a much older age than women, and the age group corresponding to the unmarried cohort was also the one that moved to the capital in search of a better life. Since marriage or other types of romantic consortship were impossible, sex was purchased and the supply followed the demand. Of the 10,000 inhabitants of Butare, the second largest city of Rwanda and the site of its national university, 293 were prostitutes, 80% of whom were already HIV-1-infected in 1983–4, as were 28% of men presenting with an STD. The lack of male circumcision further fuelled transmission.[4,7–11]

Nobody kept ancient collections of sera which could have been tested to document when the virus arrived. However, in Rwanda, 85% of isolates belong to subtype A while, in Burundi, 81% belong to subtype C. This marginal diversity implies that the virus was certainly introduced in Kigali and Bujumbura a long time after Léopoldville. The explosive epidemics in these two small adjacent countries resulted from the introduction from the Congo basin of two different founder HIV-1 subtypes, with very successful subsequent dissemination locally. The dramatic prevalences reflected a high incidence in the previous years rather than a slow spread.[12–14]

In the DRC, by 1986 the virus was widespread. For instance, among sex workers in small towns of the Equateur province, prevalence varied between 9% and 13%. In the remote Nioki hospital where I had worked, 2% of blood donors and 3% of trypanosomiasis patients were HIV-1-infected, and having travelled to Kinshasa was the strongest risk factor. In Kimpese, a Protestant mission 225 kilometres west of Kinshasa, 4% of pregnant women were HIV-1-infected, with considerable diversity and a predominance of subtype A, much like in the capital. Such diversity with a predominance of subtype A was also noted in Mbuji-Mayi, Kisangani and Bwamanda while at the extreme southeast of the country, in Lubumbashi near the Zambian border, 1,400 kilometres from Kinshasa, subtype C accounted for 51% of isolates, suggesting a more recent introduction of the virus. Because of the decay of the roads, travel between Lubumbashi and Kinshasa had to be by plane, much more expensive than the river boat to Kisangani.[15–19]

Surveys of sex workers during the late 1980s revealed high prevalences in Kinshasa (27–40%), Brazzaville (34%) and Pointe-Noire (46%), an intermediate prevalence in Bangui (12–21%), but much lower figures in Douala (6.5%) and Yaoundé (7.5%). As prostitutes represent a sentinel population in which HIV (along with other sexually transmitted pathogens) is amplified at the outset of an epidemic, these data suggest that the virus was introduced into this core group earlier in Kinshasa, Brazzaville and Pointe-Noire than in the major cities of Cameroon. Once more, Cameroon can be ruled out as the site of the early spread of the virus, even if 'patient zero' might very well have been Cameroonian.[4]

From its DRC bridgehead, the virus slowly managed to propagate into other regions of the continent. Using molecular methods, it was estimated that HIV-1 reached parts of East Africa in the 1970s, where subtype A was probably introduced from the Zairean city of Kisangani. By the mid-1980s, the virus had infected 1–2% of pregnant women in Nairobi and Dar es Salaam, 8% in Lusaka and 11% in Kampala.[4,20]

Meanwhile, HIV-1 subtype C spread to southern Africa via Lubumbashi in the Katanga province of the DRC, through adjacent Zambia. In Zimbabwe, HIV-1 group C was introduced in the early 1970s; after a short period of slow growth, the number of infected individuals expanded rapidly during 1979–81, coinciding with the return of tens of thousands of refugees and freedom fighters at the end of the liberation struggle. The best documentation of the emergence of HIV-1 comes from the Karonga district of northern Malawi, where a large collection of blood samples had been collected for long-term studies of leprosy. Of about 1,000 adults bled in

1981, none was HIV-infected. The following year, 4 of 4,354 specimens (0.1%) were HIV-reactive. By 1988, 1.1% of adults were HIV-infected. Testing of these archived samples showed that initially (1982–4) HIV-1 subtypes A, C and D were introduced, with subsequent explosive growth of subtype C but only limited spread of the others, reinforcing the idea that subtype C might be more transmissible. Later, history would repeat itself: the gender imbalance in the mining towns of South Africa led to rapid HIV transmission between prostitutes and miners, who brought it back, during their annual leaves, to their home areas in South Africa, Mozambique, Lesotho and Swaziland. This epidemic would eventually dwarf all others.[20–23]

At the other end of the continent, the economic metropolis of Abidjan was the hub around which HIV-1 disseminated in West Africa. Testing of stored samples did not show evidence of HIV-1 before 1980, while two persons were infected with HIV-2 in 1966. The viruses then spread exponentially among sex workers, half of whom were infected by the mid-1980s. Quickly, HIV-2 was superseded by HIV-1, whose sexual transmission is more effective, and the dominant HIV-1 strain came to be CRF02_AG, which was rare in the DRC but relatively common in Gabon and Cameroon, implying a northward progression towards West Africa. Abidjan, a booming city that attracted migrants, especially male agricultural workers from Burkina and Ghanaian female sex workers, was the only major city in West Africa with a gender imbalance. Its male/female ratio among adults aged twenty to thirty-nine was 1.23 in 1983 (1.38 in 1955), compared to ratios close to 1.0 in urban Ghana, Senegal, Mali and Benin. Prostitution flourished, the best possible breeding ground for HIV-1.[4,11,24]

To summarise, during the 1970s and into the early 1980s, the virus disseminated silently but relentlessly throughout the African continent, at about the same time that it crossed the Atlantic to establish a foothold first in Haiti, and then in the US. At this stage, its subsequent transformation into a global epidemic became unavoidable.

The subsequent spread

As the number of infected persons had expanded considerably, there could now be multiple introductions of the virus into various other parts of the world, rather than single founder effects. The same methods that allowed a reconstruction of the epidemic history in Africa, Haiti and the US were deployed to track down retrospectively what had occurred elsewhere. The history of the global and mainly post-1981 dissemination of HIV-1 could fill a whole book. I will present here just a brief overview of selected foci, as an illustration of the epidemiological genius of this retrovirus and of the power of currently available tools in evolutionary biology.

Starting in the early 1980s, HIV-1 group B was successfully re-exported from the US to Western Europe, through several channels. First, there were multiple introductions by European homosexuals who vacationed in San Francisco or New York (and a few in Port-au-Prince), or the other way around by American gay men who had a good time in Europe. As an example, in the United Kingdom, between 1981 and 1987 there were at least six independent successful introductions of HIV-1 group B followed by exponential transmission within the gay community until the early 1990s, while several other introductions became epidemiological dead ends. Second, the exportation of unheated contaminated plasma: HIV prevalence among haemophiliacs of various European countries in the late 1980s paralleled the proportion of their coagulation factors that had been imported from the US. And third, through drug addicts, a small fraction of whom were rich enough to inject their heroin or cocaine on both sides of the Atlantic. Within these three Western European subpopulations, nearly all HIV-1 infections were initially caused by subtype B, which could only have originated from the US. The same country also re-exported HIV-1 to Canada, most of Latin America, Australia and even to the white gay community of South Africa.[25–29]

Although some other subtypes were introduced at roughly the same time, it is only in the 1990s that non-B subtypes spread within Western Europe. These infections were initially documented among travellers and migrants from endemic countries, especially sub-Saharan Africa. Eventually, in some European countries, non-B subtypes managed to get transmitted within the local population and became predominant. For instance in Greece, subtype A is now the most common subtype, having been imported from East Africa and re-exported to Albania.[30–31]

Meanwhile in India, the country with currently the third highest number of HIV-infected individuals in the world (after South Africa and Nigeria), HIV was first recognised in 1986, but certainly had been present for a few years. It spread swiftly, especially among the core group of sex workers and their clients, but also among intravenous drug users. Subtype C represents around 95% of all Indian HIV-1 infections, and seems to have been introduced from South Africa, which is not surprising given the latter country's large Indian population that must travel intermittently to its homeland.[32–36]

Throughout south and south-east Asia, intravenous drug use played a major role in the dissemination of several subtypes of HIV-1 along heroin trafficking routes. In Thailand, a variant of subtype B (Thai B or B') and the recombinant CRF01_AE were introduced simultaneously and recognised around 1985–7. The former, imported from North America or Europe, spread among IDUs while the latter, originating from Africa, disseminated via heterosexual transmission. Exponential spread among IDUs and female prostitutes followed almost immediately, in 1988–9. Eventually CRF01_AE had much more success and became the predominant strain, even among IDUs, which allowed it to be re-exported quickly to Vietnam, while B' reached Myanmar.[37–40]

In China, phylogenetic analyses showed that HIV-1 subtype B' was introduced around 1985 or shortly thereafter through intravenous drug users, from the Golden Triangle region, the opium-producing area that covers the boundaries of Burma, Laos, Thailand and China. A few years later, around 1991, the same subtype reached the cohorts of paid plasma donors, among which it propagated exponentially, as described in Chapter 12.[41–42]

Beyond these main events, a large number of country-specific or risk group-specific importations of each and every subtype and recombinant have been documented across the six continents, from the remote regions of Brazil to the former republics of the Soviet Union. Never in human history has the global dissemination of a pathogen been studied so thoroughly. This bewildering diversification of the virus will make it even harder to develop an effective vaccine, or at least one that could be distributed globally.

The response

We will now examine the early response to this emerging pandemic through a short biography of one of its most prominent and colourful characters. Jonathan Mann was born in Boston in 1947. He studied history at Harvard and did a year of political science (1967–8) in Paris.

We do not know if he was affected by the French student rebellion in May 1968 ('No forbidding allowed'), but his proficiency in French would serve him well in the future. He obtained his MD in 1974. Having received a scholarship from the Public Health Service, he had to work for the government for two years and he entered the Epidemic Intelligence Service training programme of the Centers for Disease Control. He was sent to Santa Fe and soon gave up his plans to become an ophthalmologist.[43,44]

As a public health doctor in New Mexico, he developed an interest in viral hepatitis, rabies, botulism, measles and especially bubonic plague, which had fascinated him since he was a teenager, when he had read Albert Camus' masterpiece *The plague*. According to his sister, Jonathan identified with the hero Dr Rieux, as he struggles against the devastating epidemic, which symbolises fascism, the corruption of minds and evil. The plague was mildly endemic in the American south-west, and Mann devoted a dozen scientific articles to it.[43,45]

In 1984, the CDC needed an epidemiologist who spoke French to head up an AIDS research project, 'Projet Sida', in Kinshasa, Zaire. Looking for a new challenge, Mann got the job, which would change his life. He only stayed two years but it was a very productive period. Projet Sida was a collaboration between American, Belgian and Congolese institutions, the first long-term, Africa-based research project devoted exclusively to this new disease. Prior to that, embryonic AIDS research in Africa was of the 'safari' type: expeditions of a few weeks to gather specimens, which were then processed in the West. Projet Sida set up a laboratory in Kinshasa and other resources to analyse locally its findings. Mann and his team, many of whom were young Congolese doctors without any research experience, published about twenty articles on the epidemiology of HIV-1 in Kinshasa. Their work may seem rudimentary today but at the time it systematically broke new ground.[46,47]

Projet Sida showed that the main mode of transmission of the virus in Africa was heterosexual sex, which debunked the theories inherited from the early years of the epidemic in industrialised countries, where this mode of infection was thought to be ineffective. The impact was devastating: it meant that every sexually active person was at risk. The prevalence of HIV-1 in Kinshasa was 5–8% in the general adult population, already a generalised epidemic, and the first to be characterised. The Projet Sida team also began to document that Congolese children acquired the infection from their mothers and sometimes from blood transfusions, but not from mosquitoes. The populations studied included not just the patients and staff at Hôpital Mama Yemo but also prostitutes, 27% of which were HIV-1-infected. Project SIDA also investigated the role of medical injections in HIV transmission. Several of their studies documented that HIV-infected individuals had received more injections than seronegatives, but they could not tell which came first, HIV or the injections.

Jonathan Mann showed an innate sense of diplomacy, which was remarkable given his lack of previous African experience. He maintained cordial relations with numerous health ministers, who were constantly replaced at the whim of the 'enlightened leader' and 'founding president' of the Mouvement Populaire de la Révolution. Every one of Projet Sida's scientific presentations to any group, every one of its publications, had to be pre-approved by the minister. Mann scrupulously followed the rules, which allowed his team to continue doing their research in Kinshasa at a time when it was virtually taboo to mention AIDS in many African capitals. He navigated easily through the muddy waters and vicissitudes of daily life in Zaire, where corruption was rampant and galloping inflation could in a matter of weeks make the salaries of the Projet Sida staff virtually worthless.[47]

Charismatic, eloquent, energetic and a visionary, Mann soon came to the attention of the director of the WHO, Halfdan Mahler, who, in late 1986, offered him to lead the new WHO Global Programme on AIDS (GPA). Previously WHO had thought AIDS was not its concern since it was limited to particular groups in a few industrialised countries. Realising that this was a huge mistake, it worked hard to make up for lost time. Financially and organisationally, GPA grew like lightning, due in large part to Mann's skills as a communicator and diplomat and his intense lobbying of donor organisations. GPA expanded from a few employees in 1986 to hundreds in 1990, with an annual budget of over $100 million.[44,47]

Mann travelled constantly and was active on all fronts. Having no confidence in the WHO's African bureaucracy in Brazzaville, GPA brought in country-level staff who reported directly to Geneva. The first medium-term plans to fight AIDS were developed by GPA consultants, for implementation by ministries of health, at least in theory. At a first special meeting of dozens of health ministers in London, these politicians understood that AIDS was truly a 'pandemic', literally 'affecting all peoples'. This sounded the death knell for the denial phase – with the tragic exception of South Africa.

Mann's flamboyant personality and high profile, disregard for the UN's complex bureaucracy and rules and independence from senior officials would sooner or later cause him grief. When Mahler retired in 1988 and was replaced by Hiroshi Nakajima, it did not take the latter long to put spokes in Mann's wheels and pressure him to leave. Nakajima was appointed and reappointed largely due to lobbying by Japan, which promised substantial aid to southern hemisphere countries that supported its nominee (and threatened to cancel its aid if they did not). Nakajima would ultimately leave behind him a demoralised organisation that had run out of steam. Tired of all the harassment, Mann resigned amid much ado in 1990.

He was offered a chair at the Harvard School of Public Health, a demotion if a very honourable one. His team published two editions of *AIDS in the world*, a review of the state of the pandemic. But the main mission he set himself was to champion the fight against AIDS from the perspective of human rights, which he had started to advocate while still at the WHO. Since AIDS is linked to poverty, injustice, exploitation, vulnerability and all kinds of inequities, all these determinants of the epidemic needed to be addressed simultaneously. This was dreaming in technicolour. However, Mann seemed to enjoy the character he had created for himself as a university humanist in a bowtie. In early 1998, he accepted the position of founding dean of the School of Public Health at Drexel University in Philadelphia.[48–50]

Jonathan Mann was a leading figure in the first decade of the struggle against AIDS in Africa. His epidemiological work in Kinshasa increased our understanding of the magnitude of the problem and of the mechanisms of transmission. His time at the WHO helped to make the international community aware of the extent to which AIDS had already become a global problem. It was not restricted to a few marginal groups in the West, and would continue to spread inexorably through heterosexual sex. His unflagging denunciation of the stigmatisation of and discrimination against those infected with HIV certainly helped the victims to be ultimately accepted by their societies, governments and families.[44]

He also had a real impact on many developing countries that were initially tempted to bury their heads in the sand and were gradually persuaded to adopt a more intelligent approach. 'Close down the city!'

the authorities in Oran were ordered when the city was hit by bubonic plague, and many governments (starting with the US) were tempted to react to AIDS the same way, not knowing that it was already much too late: the virus was everywhere. It is impossible to fight a disease if one refuses to admit it exists. Mann managed to get across this simple truth to politicians on all continents.

In retrospect, however, Jonathan Mann's efforts, first at the WHO and then in academia, probably had little impact on the dynamics of the virus. He often talked about three epidemics: first the spread of HIV infections, then AIDS a decade later, swiftly followed by an epidemic of discrimination and rejection. He seems to have become obsessed with the third aspect to the detriment of the first, as if he thought it was impossible to limit the transmission of the pathogen. Public health measures that had a significant impact in the second half of the twentieth century in sub-Saharan Africa were all simple, effective and inexpensive, so that they could be replicated continent-wide: vaccination against measles, oral rehydration, management of respiratory infections and insecticide-treated mosquito bednets. Obviously there was no magic bullet against AIDS, but Mann does not seem to have realised that, especially at the end of the 1980s, millions of infections could have been prevented by the systematic implementation, across the continent, and in southern Africa in particular, of preventive measures targeting prostitutes and their clients. In all infectious disease control programmes, the first step is to identify high-risk groups and focus efforts on these, at least initially. In the case of HIV, this principle was ignored. Pilot projects demonstrated the feasibility and efficacy of interventions for sex workers, but this was never promoted as a programme to be implemented in all cities, big and small, across Africa. Such an intervention, involving the vigorous and often authoritarian imposition of the use of condoms throughout the sex trade, reversed the course of the epidemic in Thailand in the 1990s.

In Algeria, Rieux did not have antibiotics to treat plague sufferers, and it remained unclear whether the experimental serum developed by one of his colleagues was effective. Mann did not have inexpensive antiretrovirals, and the treatments for opportunistic infections that complicated AIDS in Africa were pathetic. The Oran hospital was simply a place to die, like the African hospitals overflowing with AIDS patients at the end of the twentieth century. Many Oran doctors died of the plague contracted on the job, as did physicians, surgeons and nurses in Africa, who got HIV from their patients. And just like Rieux, coura-geous and compassionate but not knowing how to control the epidemic, Mann seems to have considered the spread of HIV as unstoppable. The genius who created Rieux, Albert Camus, died prematurely in a car accident in 1960. Jonathan Mann died in 1998, in the crash of Swissair Flight 111, on his way to Geneva to attend a conference. Camus' novel ends with the phrase 'perhaps the day will come when to the misfortune or enlightenment of humanity, the plague will again bestir its rats and send them forth to die in a happy city'.[45]

14 | *Assembling the puzzle*

After reviewing the many elements of the puzzle piece by piece throughout this book, it is now time to assemble them into a coherent summary of the events that led to the transformation of SIV$_{cpz}$ into HIV-1, triggering the worst pandemic of modern times. Several pieces of this puzzle are irrefutable, while others remain the most plausible hypotheses explaining parts of the story, given the currently available circumstantial evidence. However, as the years go by, it becomes less and less likely that researchers will uncover novel information that could substantially alter this narrative.

We have seen in Chapter 2 that, for at least several hundred years, the *Pan troglodytes troglodytes* chimpanzee of central Africa has been infected with a simian immunodeficiency virus, SIV$_{cpz}$, which is genetically identical to HIV-1. The distribution of SIV$_{cpz}$ among chimpanzees in the pre-colonial era was probably not much different from what it is today. Apart from the higher level of threat from humans, the social and sexual behaviour of chimps has not changed over time. SIV$_{cpz}$ is mainly transmitted within well-defined troops of chimpanzees, presumably through sexual intercourse, but only sporadically to other communities, with which contacts are infrequent. This resulted in a heterogeneous distribution of SIV$_{cpz}$, absent from some communities while infecting a third of the members of other troops. Overall, around 6% of *P.t. troglodytes* chimps are infected with SIV$_{cpz}$. Some naturally infected chimps develop a disease reminiscent of AIDS, but only after several years during which their intense sexual promiscuity allowed them to spread the virus. It is clear that the other three subspecies of *Pan troglodytes* are not the source of HIV-1. The other chimpanzee species, the *Pan paniscus* bonobo, has been less investigated but there is so far no evidence that it is infected with SIV.[1]

Human populations of central Africa have been in contact with *P.t. troglodytes* for as long as they have lived there, around 2,000 years for the Bantus and longer for the pygmies, and in contact with SIV$_{cpz}$-infected chimps for as long as the virus has been present among apes. Why did not SIV_{cpz} emerge into HIV-1 sooner? First, human contacts with chimpanzee blood may have been less common during the pre-colonial era as the lack of firearms made it more difficult to hunt for apes, and the dearth of even rudimentary roads in densely forested areas reduced the interactions between humans and chimps (Chapter 4). Secondly, the conditions that would later facilitate the large-scale sexual and/or parenteral amplification of SIV_{cpz}/HIV-1 did not yet exist. At the time there was little opportunity for the parenteral transmission of blood-borne viruses, apart from traditional scarifications and ritual circumcisions. And there were no cities where high-risk prostitutes would have sex with more than 1,000 men each year. Thus, when pre-colonial hunters or cooks acquired SIV_{cpz}, such infections remained epidemiological dead ends: the hunter infected his wife or wives, the cook infected her husband, both would die of AIDS ten years later, and that would be the end of it. The number of cases would be too low for the virus to be transported during the slave trade on a scale that would have made it recognisable 300 years later, epidemiologically or phylogenetically, or for the disease to be identified among many others by the pioneers of tropical medicine in the early twentieth century. Then, around 1921, the date of the most recent common ancestor of pandemic HIV-1 strains, the situation changed. Not so much that many more people had contacts with chimpanzee blood, although small firearms were by then readily available, but the mechanisms that would allow the exponential amplification of the infection appeared.

In the following pages, I will try to estimate the probability that a number of events did or did not occur. There are many sources of error and many assumptions had to be made. Therefore, these figures should be seen as generally indicative of what may have happened rather than as precise mathematical measures. Even if one doubles or halves this or that number, it does not materially alter the conclusions.

We have seen in Chapter 4 that, around 1921, 1.35 million adults lived in areas inhabited by *P.t. troglodytes*: Cameroun Français, Gabon, Moyen-Congo, Oubangui-Chari, Guinea Espanola, the Cabinda enclave of Angola and the small part of the Belgian Congo that lies north of the Congo River. Presuming that the frequency of exposure to chimpanzee blood was the same as in recent times, 0.1% of these adults had been exposed to blood potentially containing SIV_{cpz} at least once in their lives. If we multiply the total number of adults by 0.1% and multiply this by the 5.9% SIV_{cpz} prevalence among *P.t. troglodytes* chimps, we can calculate that eighty adults were exposed to the virus while hunting or handling chimpanzee carcasses. With a 1% risk of transmission during occupational exposure through the skin, we end up with one human infected from chimps, or three if transmission per exposure was closer to 3% (these estimates of risk of transmission are based on extrapolations from healthcare workers exposed to HIV-infected blood). To facilitate the subsequent calculations, let us use the median number and say that in 1921 there were two SIV_{cpz}-infected humans, probably both men, living in one of the countries inhabited by *P.t. troglodytes*.[1–2]

Then, if we were to assume that urbanisation and urban prostitution were the only amplifying mechanisms (the current standard theory on the emergence of HIV-1), we need one of these SIV_{cpz}-infected hunters to infect a first prostitute in a colonial city, perhaps Yaoundé, Bangui, Libreville, Brazzaville or Léopoldville, for a chain of sexual transmission to be initiated. A number of factors made such a process a bit unlikely. First, the proportion of the population of central Africa that lived in urban areas around 1921 was at most 5%. Second, those who were more likely to be SIV_{cpz}-infected, the illiterate villagers who had occupational contacts with chimpanzees, must have been less prone to move into urban areas than individuals with at least a few years of primary school education, who spoke some French and could be hired by the colonial administration, private companies or expatriates. Third, not all men living in the cities had sex with prostitutes. So if we start with two SIV_{cpz}-infected men, assume a 2.5% probability of moving to a colonial city, and also assume that half of the city dwellers bought sex from free women, the probability that at least one of the two might have had sex with a free woman would be something like one in forty. However, the probability of male-to-female transmission of HIV-1 is not 100%. There are many serodiscordant couples in Africa (and elsewhere), in which one remains seronegative despite hundreds of unprotected intercourses with the seropositive spouse. In general, the risk of HIV-1 transmission is estimated at about one per 1,000 intercourses. Transmission is more effective, however, in the presence of an STD, especially those causing genital ulcers, and if the man is not circumcised. If we assume that the SIV_{cpz}-infected man had repeated intercourses over many years with free women, the cumulative probability of at least one forward transmission of HIV-1 would be around 50%. So the 1:40 probability becomes 1:80. It is entirely possible that this did occur and that the pandemic was in essence caused by an unpredictable factor: bad luck.

Would the odds have been different if the first chains of sexual transmission had not occurred in the cities but in the camps housing the unfortunate men conscripted into forced labour for building the Congo–Océan railway, as described in Chapter 3? If we exclude those from Tchad (no *P.t. troglodytes*), about 110,000 men from Moyen-Congo and Oubangui-Chari were forced to work on the railway between 1921 and 1932, which was roughly 16% of all adult men living within the *P.t. troglodytes* habitat. If we do the same maths as above, we end up with a 1:7 probability that one of them was infected with SIV_{cpz}. Let us say that half had sex with local free women, but for a shorter period (unlike the urban migrants, most CFCO workers would not spend much more than a year or two *in situ*), thus with a lower risk of forward transmission. So we would probably end up with the same type of odds, something like 1:40 or 1:80.[3]

However, this chain of events would have been infinitely more likely, even unavoidable, if there had been, somewhere in one of these countries, an initial phase of parenteral amplification of SIV_{cpz}/HIV-1 through re-usable syringes and needles for the treatment of tropical diseases. For this to happen, we would need one of the two SIV_{cpz}-infected men to be diagnosed with a tropical disease and to receive an IV drug. For villagers, this was much more probable than migrating to a city and infecting a prostitute. They did not have to move at all: the mobile disease control teams came to their villages with their microscopes, syringes, needles and drugs. For the Congo–Océan workers, rudimentary hospitals provided care along the railway, and many workers would need their services, however primitive these were.

Opportunities for the parenteral transmission of blood-borne viruses first arose with the campaigns against sleeping sickness, then with the early treatments of leprosy, at exactly the right place and time (Chapter 8). A few years later, massive iatrogenic transmission of HCV occurred in south Cameroon through the parenteral treatment of malaria when fixed health centres and hospitals, which could administer intravenous quinine, were established in the 1930s. In some regions, transmission of HCV may have been enhanced by large-scale campaigns for the control of yaws and syphilis, which used mostly parenteral drugs. The areas highly endemic for malaria and yaws happened to correspond to the forested areas inhabited by *P.t. troglodytes*.

For instance in the Ntem, Kribi and Sanaga-Maritime regions of Cameroun, as well as in most of Gabon and Moyen-Congo, population incidence of yaws was often greater than 200 per 1,000 per year between 1930 and 1950, and most humans would be bitten by a mosquito carrying the malaria parasite every other day. Over a period of a few years, almost the entire population, including our two SIV_{cpz}-infected individuals, would be treated with injectable drugs.

The efficacy of transmission of SIV_{cpz} from one patient to another would have been comparable to what has been described in many parts of the world, mostly after 1981, among drug addicts. As reviewed in Chapter 7, once the virus is introduced into such groups who share syringes and needles, it spreads quickly, and up to 50% of addicts can acquire HIV-1 within a few years.[4] Transmission of HIV-1 is ten times more effective through the sharing of needles and syringes than via sexual intercourse because the minute quantity of blood from the first user which remained in the syringe or needle is then injected IV, directly into the next user's blood, where HIV-1 can easily spread to the latter's lymphocytes. When a second person, an addict or, in our case, another individual treated for the same tropical diseases, developed primary HIV-1 infection, a very high degree of viraemia ensued, reaching 10^5 to 10^7 viral copies per ml. After two or three weeks at this level, viraemia slowly decreased over four to six months until it reached a steady state, generally around 10^4 viral copies per ml. During this brief peak, the second person's blood was highly infectious so that the risk of transmission to a third person must have been higher than 1% per episode of needle/syringe sharing. Further injections of antitreponemal, antitrypa-nosomiasis or antimalarial drugs with the syringe or needle used for this second patient would expose to HIV-1 other patients who were treated on the same or following day. Inevitably, a third person would become infected, further increasing the risk for the other patients treated at the same health facility or disease control mobile clinic. The tragic iatro-genic epidemics of HIV-1 in Romania and Libya, which, long after HBV, HCV and HIV were identified, occurred in countries with far more resources than those available in central Africa during the early twentieth century, demonstrated the potentially devastating efficacy of health care in spreading HIV-1 parenterally.

The fact that in parts of Cameroun and Gabon up to 50% of some birth cohorts were infected iatrogenically with HCV suggests that if SIV_{cpz}/HIV-1 was ever introduced into the group of patients receiving injections in a given healthcare facility, the amplification must have been substantial. So from one SIV_{cpz}/HIV-1-infected patient, there could have been hundreds after a few years. Such amplification was probably limited geographically to the patients receiving medical care in the same hospital, dispensary or disease control mobile clinic as the first SIV_{cpz}-infected patient. However, once the number of HIV-1-infected individuals had increased to a few hundred, the probability of at least one of them moving to a city, infecting a free woman and initiating a chain of sexual transmission increased proportionally. From a long shot this became an unavoidable certainty.

Such an initial phase of parenteral amplification was necessary for the emergence of HIV-2 in West Africa, a virus whose sexual transmission is rather ineffective but which still managed to infect tens of thousands of individuals, as summarised in Chapter 10. HIV-2 slowly faded away when the opportunities for its parenteral transmission decreased: the number of newly infected subjects ultimately became less than the number of long-infected individuals who died of AIDS or some other disease. This contrasts with HIV-1 group M which, after benefiting from the parenteral amplification, also proved its superior ability to infect lymphocytes and other cells, a characteristic that would facilitate its sexual transmission. Part of the epidemiological success story of HIV-1 group M was thus probably biological and intrinsic to this virus. HIV-1 group N did not benefit from such parenteral amplification, because it crossed species in a more recent era when IV drugs had been replaced by oral meds for the treatment of many tropical diseases, with the result that it remained limited to a very small number of infected individuals.

While the initial phase of parenteral amplification of HIV-1 group M must have occurred in an area inhabited by *P.t. troglodytes*, the next phase of sexual dissemination followed migration and trading routes. From a rural area, HIV-1 moved into the nascent cities of central Africa. On a purely geographic basis, the most likely candidates for such urban spread were Yaoundé, Douala, Libreville, Bangui, Brazzaville and Léopoldville. However, given the very low HIV-1 prevalence measured in Cameroonian and Gabonese cities in the mid-1980s, among the general adult population but also sex workers (Chapter 13), the early sexual propagation probably did not occur there. The clear preponderance in Cameroon and Gabon of CRF02A_G, a recombinant which could not have emerged in the early years of the epidemic, further rules out these locations as the site of the initial spread. We cannot rule out Bangui, where prevalence was already a significant 4.4% in 1986. It is unfortunate that no archival serum samples from Bangui or southern Central African Republic were ever found in the local Institut Pasteur or that if such work was done it was not published. The lower genetic diversity of HIV-1 subtypes in Bangui compared to Kinshasa and Brazzaville (Chapter 1) suggests that the virus has been circulating in the latter area for a longer period of time than on the banks of the Oubangui. Furthermore, only a small part of the Central African Republic is inhabited by *P.t. troglodytes* and the genetic diversity of HIV-1 is similar to that in Chad, a country without any *P.t. troglodytes*. These two countries' intermediate genetic diversity of HIV-1 isolates probably represents an ancient import of subtypes which had already been differentiating somewhere else.[5–6]

Several arguments suggest that the Léopoldville/Brazzaville urban area was central in the dissemination of HIV-1 (Chapters 1 and 13). First, the extraordinary diversity of HIV-1 in samples obtained from Kinshasa and Brazzaville, where all known subtypes and many recombinants are present. Second, the two oldest samples containing HIV-1 obtained in 1959–60 both came from Léopoldville. Third, the retrospective description of five clear-cut cases of AIDS that corresponded to infections probably acquired in the DRC in the late 1960s or early 1970s. Fourth, the presence of HIV-1 antibodies in samples obtained in 1970 from women representing the general adult population of Kinshasa (mothers bringing their children to an under-five clinic), even if at a low prevalence of 0.25%. Fifth is the finding that in 1980, among a similar sample of women, prevalence was already at 3.0%. Sixth, the surveys conducted in representative samples of the adult population of various central African cities in the mid-1980s showed low prevalences in Gabon and Cameroon but rather high prevalences (4–8%) in Kinshasa and Brazzaville. Finally, the status of the Léopoldville/Brazzaville conurbation, for a long time the commercial and administrative heart of central Africa attracting thousands of migrants each year into an ever larger melting pot of all ethnic groups.[7–15]

What was the geographical origin of the first cases of HIV-1 imported into Léopoldville/Brazzaville? There is a remote possibility that the source was from within the Belgian Congo. The part of the Bas-Congo region north of the river was inhabited by *P.t. troglodytes*, and there were

excellent road and rail communications between Boma, Matadi and
Léopoldville. However, this area is small, with limited *P.t. troglodytes*
populations, and we do not know whether local communities of chimps
are infected with SIV$_{cpz}$. Far more likely, the virus managed to reach
Brazzaville first, with its subsequent implantation in Léopoldville just
across the river. As reviewed in Chapter 5, Brazzaville became the administrative centre of the AEF federation, the terminus for navigation on the
Congo and the departure point of the train to Pointe-Noire and the
Atlantic coast. These factors implied constant movements of Africans
and Europeans between the capital city and the territories of Oubangui-
Chari, Moyen-Congo and Gabon. Initially concentrated within Moyen-
Congo, these population movements reached further inland and on a
massive scale when forced labour was brought in for the construction of
the Congo–Océan railway in the 1920s. Furthermore, the part of south-
east Cameroun with the highest prevalence of SIV$_{cpz}$ among its chimps,
and whose strains of SIV$_{cpz}$ are closest to HIV-1 group M, has rivers, the
Dja and the Ngoko, that drain into the Congo system through the
Sangha, which also drains part of southern Oubangui-Chari inhabited
by *P.t. troglodytes*. For these populations, trading was easier towards the
Congo than to Yaoundé and Douala, and ever since the German colonisation, steamboats would regularly make the journey between south-
east Cameroon and Brazzaville/Léopoldville.

   Once HIV-1 reached Brazzaville, it would not take long for it to move
into Léopoldville. Some traders from the AEF hinterland visited both
cities on the same or successive journeys, depending on where they
thought they could fetch the highest prices for their goods.
Alternatively, there might have been a little local transmission within
Brazzaville before the virus was introduced into Léopoldville. There
was a ferry as well as smaller boats departing every half hour for the
twenty-minute journey. Before independence, commerce was brisk
between the two cities, as traders, many of them women, managed to
find a price differential for some goods that would make the short trip
profitable. And after independence in 1960, when the economic situation deteriorated in the DRC, trading if anything increased as agricultural products from the Bas-Congo could be sold at higher prices in
Brazzaville, where smart traders could then use their CFA francs to buy
goods that Léopoldville was short of, guaranteeing a hefty profit. Free
women also moved back and forth between the two capitals while other

migrants settled on the other side of the river for longer periods in search of a better life (Chapters 5 and 6).[16]

Once HIV-1 was present in both cities, the conditions in Léopoldville were more favourable to its successful sexual propagation than in Brazzaville. Early in colonial history, a gross gender imbalance was created in Léopoldville by the Belgian colonists, on a scale far worse than across the river, as we have examined in Chapter 5. For a few decades, Léopoldville was an urban work camp where women and children were unwelcome. This was fertile ground for prostitution to develop on a large scale, and develop it did. Even when colonial policies were softened after WWII, Léopoldville was such a booming town that it constantly attracted a flux of migrants from the adjacent rural areas and young men would come first, perpetuating the imbalance. On both sides of the trade, prostitution involved mainly the unmarried and within this subgroup as late as the 1950s there were more than five men for each woman in Léopoldville.

For the first few decades of its presence in Léopoldville, the dissemination of HIV-1 was slow and limited. According to mathematical models, for a long time there was something like 100 infected individuals in the city (Chapter 3). The type of sex trade that existed during the colonial era corresponded to what is currently referred to as concomitant partnerships or semi-prostitution rather than hard-core prostitution (Chapter 6). A free woman would have a few regular clients, perhaps three on average, to whom she provided a variety of services, not just sex. If that woman got infected with HIV-1, she could only transmit the virus to one of her other steady clients, who might eventually infect another free woman. This setting was good enough for the persistence of the infection, possibly a very slow growth of the infected population up to a few hundred, but nothing like the exponential transmission of HIV-1 that was to be documented in Kenya in the early 1980s.

It is likely that some of the initial transmission of HIV-1 to free women in Léopoldville occurred iatrogenically and not just sexually. For a long time, starting in the early 1930s, free women were forced to attend the Dispensaire Antivénérien in Léo-Est for regular STD screening (Chapter 9). Those with a positive syphilis serology (many of whom carried such antibodies not because of syphilis but because they had had yaws in their childhood) were treated with injectable drugs, most often administered IV. In 1953, more than 150,000 injections were administered just in this one institution, which treated up to 1,000 patients each day. Documentary evidence reveals that syringes and needles were not sterilised but only rinsed between patients, with the result that many cases of iatrogenic hepatitis B acquired in this STD clinic were recognised by a clinician at the main hospital of Léopoldville, even in a setting where only a small minority of adults was susceptible to infection with HBV. This situation created an extraordinary opportunity for the spread of HIV-1: the women infected iatrogenically were semi-prostitutes, who could in turn transmit the infection, now sexually, to some of their regular clients. And thus a perfect storm developed.[17]

More widespread sexual transmission became possible when the face of prostitution in Léopoldville was dramatically altered around 1960–1. The political chaos and civil war in parts of the Congo brought hundreds of thousands of internal refugees into the capital, resulting in massive unemployment and poverty (Chapter 11). As documented by several observers, high-risk prostitution appeared, with sex workers providing sexual services to a few men every day, potentially more than 1,000 per year, in downmarket brothels which were little more than glorified shacks. For a number of years, it remained a concentrated epidemic, with a higher prevalence among prostitutes than among their clients. As long as the gender imbalance persisted, that is until the early 1970s, there were relatively few opportunities for dissemination outside this initial core group, because for many men it was not easy to find a female partner to marry or with whom they could at least sustain a romantic relationship. The transition from a concentrated to a generalised epidemic occurred between 1970 and 1980, a period during which HIV prevalence among mothers at a well-baby clinic in Kinshasa increased from 0.25 to 3.0%. If these prevalences were representative of the whole adult population of Kinshasa, the number of HIV-1-infected individuals in the city rose from about 1,400 in 1970 to some 36,000 ten years later. That is why in the mid- to late 1970s physicians at the Mama Yemo and at the university hospitals started seeing cases of what would be later recognised retrospectively as AIDS.[13,14,18–21]

Once the number of HIV-infected persons in Léopoldville expanded, it was unavoidable that it would spread outside the capital, which was the political and economic centre of a large country with endless movement of traders, bureaucrats and all kinds of economic migrants between the various regions of the Belgian Congo, the DRC and later Zaire. HIV-1 eventually reached Kigali, Rwanda, where it found extremely favourable conditions for its sexual transmission in this small city with a gross surplus of uncircumcised men and a thriving sex industry (Chapter 13). A similar process, albeit with a different founder strain, happened in Bujumbura, Burundi. In other countries of central Africa, HIV-1 arrived at the same time or even earlier, but as conditions were less propitious its spread was slower. From central Africa, HIV then progressively moved into other regions of the continent. Southern Africa was infected by the extension of subtype C infection from the Katanga province of the DRC to Zambia, and then further south to Zimbabwe, Malawi and eventually South Africa. East Africa was infected via Kisangani while West Africa was infected by the extension of the CRF02A_G recombinant northwards along the coast, from Gabon and Cameroon to Nigeria, Ivory Coast and so on.

At some point between 1960 and 1966, among the 4,500 teachers dispatched to Congo-Léopoldville, a single Haitian technical assistant was infected with HIV-1 group M subtype B (Chapter 11). Around 1966, this person went back to Haiti and stayed long enough to start a local chain of sexual transmission. There, this rare subtype of HIV-1 had to be amplified exponentially early on, otherwise it would have been impossible for a virus introduced in 1966 to infect 8% of women in Port-au-Prince sixteen years later, reaching a level seen in Léopoldville–Kinshasa only several decades after its introduction.[22–23]

Did this amplification occur sexually, within the small homosexual/bisexual community of male Haitians selling sex to American tourists, as suggested by some? I doubt it very much, for a simple reason: American gay tourists did not stay in Port-au-Prince or elsewhere in Haiti for long enough. For exponential amplification to occur through the homosexual route, as documented later in San Francisco, New York and many other locations, a first HIV-infected person needs to transmit the virus to one or two individuals, then each of these second-generation cases needs to infect a few more, and each of these third-generation cases to infect a few more, and so on, with a short interval (three or four months) between each cycle of transmission. Most American tourists who acquired HIV-1 subtype B from a Haitian male prostitute probably went back to the US within a couple of weeks, before they developed the high viraemia and high infectiousness which is characteristic of primary HIV infection and which drives the sexual amplification of HIV. Thus, these tourists had little opportunity to infect a second Haitian male prostitute for such a vicious circle to be initiated but a much greater chance of infecting other American gay men back home. Some

American gay tourists undoubtedly infected Haitian male sex workers, or acquired HIV-1 from these same prostitutes, and some homosexual prostitutes infected each other, but it does not seem plausible that this caused a massive spread of the virus within the small Haitian bisexual community severe enough for the infection to spill over quickly into the heterosexual population.[24–26]

Admittedly, this part of the story remains unproven, but there are good reasons to believe that the Hemo-Caribbean plasmapheresis centre (Chapter 12) could have been the perfect breeding ground for a quick increase in the number of HIV-infected Haitians, to a level where sexual transmission would then inevitably but more slowly allow for its further dissemination. Extremely rapid transmission of HIV-1 was documented among individuals selling their blood in commercial plasmapheresis centres in China, Mexico and India. Once the virus is introduced among paid plasma donors, up to three-fourths can get infected within a year. It seems unlikely that the procedures that should have prevented the transmission of blood-borne viruses were more stringent in Port-au-Prince than in all these other places, quite the contrary. Haitian plasma sellers were even poorer than their counterparts in other countries and they had to put up with whatever was done at the Hemo-Caribbean clinic. For this disaster to have happened, we need just one HIV-1-infected person to have entered the cohort of plasma sellers; within the next year, from a handful of HIV-1-infected persons on the island, there could have been several hundred. At this stage, the number of infected persons in Haiti had reached the critical mass which enabled it to disseminate successfully among sex workers, male and female, and then into the general adult population.

If indeed this happened, then the export of the plasma to the US, where it was bought and processed by large pharmaceutical companies, could have allowed for some spread of HIV-1 subtype B into the Americas and Western Europe. Once a shipment of plasma entered the stock of a plasma broker, it could be sold and resold in several countries on both sides of the Atlantic within a short period of time (Chapter 12). We do not know whether all of the plasma sent to the US or Europe by Hemo-Caribbean was processed into albumin and immunoglobulins (with no risk of HIV transmission), or if some lots were used to prepare factor VIII cryoprecipitates, in which case this business could have contributed to the spread of the virus. Either through this route or via American gay tourists, HIV-1 was introduced into the US. It was already present, albeit at a low prevalence, among drug addicts in the mid-1970s, a population within which HIV spread quickly: by 1979, one third of addicts in New York were infected.[27–28]

Following the 1969 Stonewall riots, a gay rights movement emerged in the US, and San Francisco became its focal point where 5,000 homosexuals migrated each year, in search of freedom and tolerance. By 1978, 6% of gay men in San Francisco were HIV-infected. The same year, through some of them who donated blood, HIV entered the local blood supply. The extraordinary level of sexual promiscuity within this population, recently liberated from centuries of repression and stigmatisation, led to an exponential homosexual amplification of HIV-1. Many of the initial cohorts of HIV-1-infected gay men had 100–200 sexual partners per year, most often during anonymous encounters in bathhouses. HIV prevalence among San Francisco gay men increased to 19% in 1979, 33% in 1980 and 44% in 1981. The incidence peaked around July 1981, when 1.4% of gay men acquired HIV infection each month.[25,29–31]

HIV infections were identified retrospectively among American haemophiliacs starting in 1978, but the virus may have been present at a low prevalence for some years. It was already infecting some British haemophiliacs by 1979. In a cohort of American haemophiliacs, just a few with stored serum going back to 1976, the first case of HIV infection appeared in 1978, with rapid spread in 1981–2. More than half of haemophiliacs in Georgia were HIV-infected by 1981, as were 85% of their Californian counterparts by 1984. The first cases of AIDS among haemophiliacs were recognised in early 1982.[32–35]

Thus by the late 1970s in the US several modes of HIV transmission acted concomitantly, to a large extent independently of each other but with occasional interconnections. Haemophiliacs who happened to be gay might have sexually infected other gay men and homosexually infected men might have been volunteer blood donors or paid plasma donors. This latter step diversified the sources of HIV-1 which from multiple sites now entered the complex process that led to the production of coagulation factor concentrates made from pools of plasma collected from thousands of donors, by then hugely popular among haemophiliacs and their physicians. The all-male haemophiliacs were otherwise healthy and, if old enough, sexually active. Some infected their female spouses (who in turn could infect their infants) but, because the average number of concomitant sexual partners was low, these became epidemiological dead ends. Although a tragedy with almost half of the 20,000 American haemophiliacs infected, this had only a modest impact on the overall picture. Whole blood transfusions did not contribute much to the overall dissemination of the virus either, because most recipients were sick or elderly individuals undergoing heart surgery or being treated for leukaemia or some other nasty disease, who were not active sexually in the ensuing months. Furthermore, because of the massive infective dose, transfusion recipients developed AIDS and died within just a few years. HIV-1 transmission among drug addicts was more consequential: to generate the income needed for their dope, some addicts sold sexual services or became paid plasma donors, others happened to be gay and infected their sexual partners, and female addicts could infect their offspring.

During the 1970s, there was much dissemination of HIV by gay men visiting other cities where they had unprotected sex. The case of the Air Canada flight attendant, the so-called 'patient zero', who was linked to many early cases of AIDS in various American cities, has been described in detail elsewhere. Mobility and promiscuity proved excellent breeding grounds for a sexually transmitted virus, allowing exponential transmission by men who continued having sex with other gay men shortly after they developed a high viraemia during their primary HIV period. Transmission was further facilitated by the high prevalence of other sexually transmitted pathogens within the homosexual community. In this early phase of the epidemic in the US, in all risk groups combined, each HIV-infected person infected another person every year or so. From the United States, the virus was re-exported to many parts of the industrialised world.[36,37]

Eventually, after an incubation period of roughly ten years during which their CD4 lymphocytes were progressively destroyed, these early American patients developed a variety of opportunistic infections and a new disease was recognised by the physicians who published the landmark *MMWR* short article in 1981. And thus AIDS was born.

15 | *Epilogue: lessons learned*

Twenty-nine million deaths later, are there any useful lessons that can be drawn from this tragedy? Or was it just an extraordinary confluence of chance events, unlikely ever to be repeated? In retrospect, two factors probably drove the emergence of SIV_{cpz} into HIV-1. Even if their respective contributions will never be fully sorted out, there is little doubt that without them the pandemic would not have developed.

The first was the profound social changes that accompanied the European colonisation of central Africa, eventually leading to sexual behaviours far different from those of traditional societies which had lived there for 2,000 years. A relatively small number of women had sex against remuneration, initially with a few regular clients, and then, after 1960, with a large number of men, a process which amplified the transmission of sexually transmitted pathogens, both the traditional ones (gonorrhoea, syphilis, etc.) and the emerging one, HIV-1. This is just another example of the complex relationships between social changes and diseases. Tuberculosis emerged as an important cause of adult mortality in nineteenth-century Europe, when the industrial revolution brought many poor peasants to the cities where they lived in crowded, unhealthy conditions conducive to the transmission of this respiratory pathogen. More recently, in the last decades of the twentieth century, an unprecedented epidemic of obesity has developed in industrialised countries as a consequence of our sedentarisation, itself driven by the ever-increasing availability of motor vehicles, televisions, video games, the Internet, and so on. Upcoming changes in the lifestyle of future generations will impact on the incidence of various diseases, in a way which is hard to predict and which cannot be avoided. Some of these changes could be detrimental to the human race, while others will represent progress. For instance, the progressive reduction in the use of fossil fuels and their replacement by greener sources of energy should eventually lower the incidence of the respiratory diseases associated with air pollution.

The second factor in the emergence of SIV_{cpz} into HIV-1 was its parenteral amplification through poorly sterilised syringes and needles, re-used on many patients. In central Africa, this may have jump-started the epidemic by increasing the number of infected humans to a level where sexual transmission could thrive. In retrospect, this iatrogenic amplification resulted from a lag of only about fifty years between the development of therapeutic agents that required their IV administration and the realisation that infectious agents, especially viruses, could be transmitted by this route. When humans manipulate nature in a way that they do not fully understand, there is always a possibility that something unpredictable will occur.

This is a reminder that the most dangerous threat to the long-term survival of the human species is the human race itself. Of course, this has been obvious for some time. My generation and the one before us grew up with the fear of a nuclear holocaust. Even though the number of nuclear missiles has been reduced, the list of countries possessing this technology has grown, and with it the probability that one day somebody will push the button. My children's generation has grown up with the threat of global warming, a process whose consequences could be as destructive, albeit much slower. The human race is not very quick to understand novel threats. Just a few years ago, the president of the United States refused to ratify the Kyoto protocol on the basis that the 'American way of life is not negotiable', as if the core of American civilisation and values were the four-wheel drive vehicles produced by three large corporations that barely survived the end of this president's term in office.

In this context, the one new message that the HIV epidemic, as chronicled in this book, should bring home is that well-intentioned human interventions can have unpredictable and disastrous microbiologic consequences. Mankind has emerged through a process of natural selection over billions of years. Apart from ourselves, there is probably no other living organism on earth that could destroy us completely, because if such organisms had existed, we would not have managed to reach our current status in the first place. But as I write these lines, there is renewed interest in sending humans on a wonderful voyage to Mars and back. The kids who watched Neil Armstrong's small steps on the moon are now engineers, pilots, administrators and politicians. They think that their own generation also needs to push back a new frontier, that this is part of the human experience, and perhaps something that will provide an answer to perennial questions about the meaning of life. For a long time I have thought that space adventures were very unwise. What is the point of setting up a small human colony somewhere in orbit around the earth or even further away, when we are systematically destroying, day in and day out, the only planet which can sustain human life? Would it not be smarter to spend our resources and ingenuity on scientific adventures whose purpose would be to protect our earth rather than taking the risk of importing into our cherished planet a completely different form of microscopic life, perhaps not even based on DNA, and whose innocuous nature has not been proven by billions of years of natural selection and co-evolution with us?

References

Introduction

1. Gottlieb M et al. *Pneumocystis carinii* pneumonia – Los Angeles. *MMWR* (1981), **30**: 250–2.
2. Shilts R. *And the band played on. Politics, people and the AIDS epidemic.* New York: Penguin Books, 1987.
3. UNAIDS. *Global Report. UNAIDS report on the global AIDS epidemic – 2010.* Geneva, 2010.
4. UNAIDS. *AIDS epidemic update 2009.* Geneva, 2009.
5. Garrett L. *The coming plague. Newly emerging diseases in a world out of balance.* New York: Penguin Books, 1994.
6. Illiffe J. *The African AIDS epidemic. A history.* Athens: Ohio University Press, 2006.
7. Fassin D. *When bodies remember. Experiences and politics of AIDS in South Africa.* Berkeley: University of California Press, 2007.
8. Mukudi E et al. *HIV/AIDS in Africa. Challenges and impact.* Trenton: Africa World Press, 2008.
9. Nolen S. *28 stories of AIDS in Africa.* Toronto: Vintage Canada, 2008.
10. Denis P et al. *L'épidémie du sida en Afrique subsaharienne.* Paris: Karthala, 2006.
11. Hooper E. *The river. A journey back to the source of HIV and AIDS.* London: Little Brown and Company, 1999.
12. Pepin J et al. Parenteral transmission during excision and treatment of tuberculosis and trypanosomiasis may be responsible for the HIV-2 epidemic in Guinea-Bissau. *AIDS* (2006), **20**: 1303–11.
13. Schmid GP et al. Transmission of HIV-1 infection in sub-Saharan Africa and effect of elimination of unsafe injections. *Lancet* (2004), **363**: 482–8.

1 Out of Africa

1. Piot P et al. AIDS in a heterosexual population in Zaire. *Lancet* (1984), **2**: 65–9.
2. Van de Perre P et al. Female prostitutes: a risk group for infection with HTLV-III. *Lancet* (1985), **2**: 524–7.

3. Quinn T et al. AIDS in Africa: an epidemiologic paradigm. *Science* (1986), **234**: 955–63.
4. Desmyter J et al. Anti LAV-HTLV-III in Kinshasa mothers in 1970 and 1980. Paris: International Conference on AIDS, June 1985.
5. Nzila N et al. The prevalence of infection with HIV over a 10-year period in rural Zaire. *N Eng J Med* (1988), **318**: 276–9.
6. Byers R et al. Estimating AIDS infection rates in the San Francisco cohort. *AIDS* (1988), **2**: 207–10.
7. Foley B et al. Apparent founder effect during the early years of the San Francisco HIV-1 epidemic (1978–79). *AIDS Res Hum Retrovir* (2000), **15**: 1463–9.
8. Moore JD et al. HTLV-III seropositivity in 1971–72 parenteral drug abusers – a case of false positives or evidence of viral exposure. *N Eng J Med* (1986), **314**: 1387–8.
9. Garrett L. *The coming plague. Newly emerging diseases in a world out of balance.* New York: Penguin Books, 1994.
10. Anonymous. Ebola haemorrhagic fever in Zaire, 1976. Report of an international commission. *Bull World Health Organ* (1978), **56**: 271–93.
11. Wendler I et al. Seroepidemiology of HIV in Africa. *Br Med J* (1986), **293**: 782–5.
12. Kawamura M. HIV-2 in West Africa in 1966. *Lancet* (1989), **1**: 385.
13. Chiodi F et al. Screening of African sera stored for more than 17 years for HIV antibodies by site-directed serology. *Europ J Epidemiol* (1989), **5**: 42–6.
14. US Census Bureau. *HIV/AIDS surveillance data base*. Washington, 2006.
15. Otu A et al. Antibody to the AIDS virus in Kaposi's sarcoma in Nigeria. *J Surg Oncol* (1988), **37**: 152–5.
16. Levy J et al. Absence of antibodies to HIV in sera from Africa prior to 1975. *Proc Natl Acad Sci U S A* (1986), **83**: 7935–7.
17. Tabor E et al. Did HIV and HTLV originate in Africa? *JAMA* (1990), **264**: 691–2.
18. Sher R et al. Seroepidemiology of HIV in Africa from 1970 to 1974. *N Eng J Med* (1987), **317**: 50–1.
19. Piot P et al. Retrospective seroepidemiology of AIDS virus infection in Nairobi populations. *J Infect Dis* (1987), **155**: 1108–12.
20. Vangroenweghe D. The earliest cases of HIV-1 group M in Congo-Kinshasa, Rwanda and Burundi and the origin of AIDS. *Phil Trans R Soc Lond B* (2001), **356**: 923–5.
21. Lyons H et al. *Pneumocystis carinii* pneumonia unassociated with other disease. *Arch Intern Med* (1961), **108**: 929–36.
22. Hooper E. *The river. A journey back to the source of HIV and AIDS.* London: Little Brown and Company, 1999.

23. Shilts R. *And the band played on. Politics, people and the AIDS epidemic.* New York: Penguin Books, 1987.

24. Froland S. HIV-1 infection in a Norwegian family before 1970. *Lancet* (1988), **1**: 1344–5.

25. Jonassen T et al. Sequence analysis of HIV-1 group O from Norwegian patients infected in the 1960s. *Virol* (1997), **231**: 43–7.

26. Bygbjerg I. AIDS in a Danish surgeon (Zaire 1976). *Lancet* (1983), **1**: 925.

27. Nemeth A et al. Early case of AIDS in a child from Zaire. *Sex Transm Dis* (1986), **13**: 111–13.

28. Rogan E et al. A case of AIDS before 1980. *Can Med Assoc J* (1987), **137**: 637–8.

29. Sonnet J et al. Early AIDS cases originating from Zaire and Burundi (1962–1976). *Scand J Infect Dis* (1987), **19**: 511–17.

30. Clumeck N et al. AIDS in African patients. *N Eng J Med* (1984), **310**: 492–7.

31. Motulsky A et al. Population genetics study in the Congo. I. Glucose-6-phosphate deficiency, hemoglobin S, and malaria. *Am J Hum Genet* (1966), **18**: 514–37.

32. Nahmias A et al. Evidence for human infection with HTLV-III/LAV-like virus in Central Africa, 1959. *Lancet* (1986), **1**: 1279–80.

33. Zhu T et al. An African HIV-1 sequence from 1959 and implications for the origin of the epidemic. *Nature* (1998), **391**: 594–7.

34. Worobey M et al. Direct evidence of extensive diversity of HIV-1 in Kinshasa by 1960. *Nature* (2008), **55**: 661–4.

35. Geretti A. HIV-1 subtypes: epidemiology and significance for HIV management. *Curr Opin Infect Dis* (2006), **19**: 1–7.

36. Butler I et al. HIV genetic diversity: biological and public health consequences. *Curr HIV Res* (2007), **5**: 23–45.

37. Los Alamos National Laboratory. The circulating recombinant forms. www.hiv.lanl.gov/content/sequence/HIV/CRFs/CRFs.html.

38. Paleebu P et al. Effect of HIV-1 envelope subtypes A and D on disease progression in a large cohort of HIV-1 positive persons in Uganda. *J Infect Dis* (2002), **185**: 1244–50.

39. John-Stewart G et al. Subtype C is associated with increased vaginal shedding of HIV-1. *J Infect Dis* (2005), **192**: 492–6.

40. Novitsky V et al. Viral load and CD4+ T-cell dynamics in primary HIV-1 subtype C infection. *JAIDS* (2009), **50**: 65–76.

41. Vidal N et al. Distribution of HIV-1 variants in the Democratic Republic of Congo suggests increase of subtype C in Kinshasa between 1997 and 2002. *JAIDS* (2005), **40**: 456–62.

42. Salemi M et al. Different epidemic potentials of the HIV-1 B and C subtypes. *J Mol Evol* (2005), **60**: 598–605.

43. van Harmelen J et al. An association between HIV-1 subtypes and mode of transmission in Cape Town, South Africa. *AIDS* (1997), **11**: 81–7.

44. Taylor B et al. The challenge of HIV-1 subtype diversity. *N Eng J Med* (2008), **358**: 1590–602.

45. Peeters M et al. Genetic diversity of HIV in Africa: impact on diagnosis, treatment, vaccine development and trials. *AIDS* (2003), **17**: 2547–60.

46. Hemelaar J et al. Global and regional distribution of HIV-1 genetic subtypes and recombinants in 2004. *AIDS* (2006), **20**: W13–W23.

47. Nadal Y et al. HIV-1 epidemic in the Caribbean is dominated by subtype B. *PLoS ONE* (2009), **4**: e4814.

48. Cuevas M et al. High HIV-1 genetic diversity in Cuba. *AIDS* (2002), **16**: 1643–53.

49. Falk P. Cuba in Africa. *Foreign Affairs* (1987), **65**: 1077–96.

50. Kahn O. Cuba's impact in southern Africa. *J Interam Stud World Aff* (1987), **29**: 33–54.

51. Abecasis A et al. HIV-1 genetic variants circulation in the north of Angola. *Infect Genet Evol* (2005), **5**: 231–7.

52. Bartolo I et al. Highly divergent subtypes and new recombinant forms prevail in the HIV/AIDS epidemic in Angola: new insights into the origins of the AIDS pandemic. *Infect Genet Evol* (2009), **9**: 672–82.

53. Nkengasong J et al. Genotypic subtypes of HIV-1 in Cameroon. *AIDS* (1994), **8**: 1405–12.

54. Delaporte E et al. Epidemiological and molecular characteristics of HIV infection in Gabon, 1986–94. *AIDS* (1996), **10**: 903–10.

55. Mboudjeka I et al. Genetic diversity of HIV-1 group M from Cameroon and Republic of Congo. *Arch Virol* (1999), **144**: 2291–311.

56. Ortiz M et al. Molecular epidemiology of HIV-1 subtypes in Equatorial Guinea. *AIDS Res Hum Retrovir* (2001), **17**: 851–5.

57. Muller-Trutwin M et al. Increase of HIV-1 subtype A in Central African Republic. *JAIDS* (1999), **21**: 164–71.

58. Vidal N et al. High genetic diversity of HIV-1 strains in Chad, West Central Africa. *JAIDS* (2003), **33**: 239–46.

59. Vidal N et al. Unprecedented degree of HIV-1 group M genetic diversity in the Democratic Republic of Congo suggests that the HIV-1 pandemic originated in Central Africa. *J Virol* (2000), **74**: 10498–507.

60. Kalish M et al. Recombinant viruses and early global HIV-1 epidemic. *Emerg Infect Dis* (2004), **10**: 1227–34.

61. Niama F et al. HIV-1 subtypes and recombinants in the Republic of Congo. *Infect Genet Evol* (2006), **6**: 337–43.

2 The source

1. Peterson D. *Jane Goodall. The woman who redefined man*. Boston: Houghton Mifflin, 2006.
2. Greene M. *Jane Goodall. A biography*. Westport: Greenwood Press, 2005.
3. Goodall J. *Through a window. My thirty years with the chimpanzees of Gombe*. Boston: Houghton Mifflin, 1990.
4. Wildman DE et al. Implications of natural selection in shaping 99.5% nonsynonymous DNA identity between humans and chimpanzees: enlarging genus *Homo. Proc Natl Acad Sci U S A* (2003), **100**: 7181–8.
5. International Union for Conservation of Nature. *West African chimpanzees. Status survey and conservation action plan*. Gland, 2004.
6. Teleki G. Population status of wild chimpanzees (*Pan troglodytes*) and threats to survival. In Hetne P and Marquardt L (eds.), *Understanding chimpanzees*. Harvard University Press, 1989.
7. Mathis M. *Vie et moeurs des anthropoides*. Paris: Payot, 1954.
8. Mathis C. *L'œuvre des Pastoriens en Afrique Noire, Afrique Occidentale Française*. Paris: Presses Universitaires de France, 1946.
9. Wilbert R et al. 'Pastoria', centre de recherches biologiques et d'élevage de singes. *Bull Soc Pathol Exot* (1931), **24**: 131–48.
10. Leroy E et al. Multiple Ebola virus transmission events and rapid decline of central African wildlife. *Science* (2004), **303**: 387–90.
11. Tutin C et al. Nationwide census of gorilla (*Gorilla g. gorilla*) and chimpanzee (*Pan t. troglodytes*) populations in Gabon. *Am J Primatol* (1984), **6**: 313–36.
12. Tutin C et al. *Regional action plan for the conservation of chimpanzees and gorillas in Western Equatorial Africa*. www.primate-sg.org//PDF/ApesRAP.French2.pdf.
13. Manson J et al. Intergroup aggression in chimpanzees and humans. *Curr Anthropol* (1991), **32**: 369–90.
14. Vigilant L et al. Paternity and relatedness in wild chimpanzee communities. *Proc Natl Acad Sci U S A* (2001), **98**: 12890–5.
15. Tutin C. Saving the gorillas (*Gorilla g. gorilla*) and chimpanzees (*Pan t. troglodytes*) of the Congo basin. *Reprod Fertil Dev* (2001), **13**: 469–76.
16. Peeters M et al. Isolation and partial characterization of an HIV-related virus occurring naturally in chimpanzees in Gabon. *AIDS* (1989), **3**: 625–30.
17. Huet T et al. Genetic organization of a chimpanzee lentivirus related to HIV-1. *Nature* (1990), **345**: 356–9.
18. Janssens W et al. Phylogenetic analysis of a new chimpanzee lentivirus $SIV_{cpz-gab2}$ from a wild-captured chimpanzee from Gabon. *AIDS Res Hum Retrovir* (1994), **10**: 1191–2.

19. Peeters M et al. Isolation and characterization of a new chimpanzee lentivirus (simian immunodeficiency virus isolate cpz-ant) from a wild-captured chimpanzee. *AIDS* (1992), **6**: 447–51.

20. Vanden Haesevelde M et al. Sequence analysis of a highly divergent HIV-1 related lentivirus isolated from a wild captured chimpanzee. *Virology* (1996), **221**: 346–50.

21. Gao F et al. Origin of HIV-1 in the chimpanzee *Pan troglodytes troglodytes*. *Nature* (1999), **397**: 436–41.

22. Gilden R et al. HTLV-III antibody in a breeding chimpanzee not experimentally exposed to the virus. *Lancet* (1986), **1**: 678–9.

23. Corbet S et al. *env* sequences of simian immunodeficiency viruses from chimpanzees in Cameroon are strongly related to those of HIV group N from the same geographic area. *J Virol* (2000), **74**: 529–34.

24. Santiago M et al. SIV$_{cpz}$ in wild chimpanzees. *Science* (2002), **295**: 465.

25. Keele B et al. Chimpanzee reservoirs of pandemic and nonpandemic HIV-1. *Science* (2006), **313**: 523–6.

26. Santiago M et al. Foci of endemic SIV infection in wild-living eastern chimpanzees (*Pan troglodytes schweinfurthii*). *J Virol* (2003), **77**: 7545–62.

27. Sharp P et al. SIV infection in chimpanzees. *J Virol* (2005), **79**: 3891–902.

28. Li Y et al. Molecular epidemiology of SIV in eastern chimpanzees and gorillas. Abstract presented at the 17th Conference on Retroviruses and Opportunistic Infections, San Francisco, February 2010.

29. Prince A et al. Lack of evidence for HIV type 1-related SIV$_{cpz}$ infection in captive and wild chimpanzees (*Pan troglodytes verus*) in West Africa. *AIDS Res Hum Retrovir* (2002), **9**: 657–60.

30. Van Heuverswyn F et al. Genetic diversity and phylogeographic clustering of SIV$_{cpz}$ in wild chimpanzees in Cameroon. *Virology* (2007), **368**: 155–71.

31. Neel C et al. Molecular epidemiology of simian immunodeficiency virus infection in wild-living gorillas. *J Virol* (2010), **84**: 1464–76.

32. Van Heuverswyn F et al. SIV infection in wild gorillas. *Nature* (2006), **444**: 164.

33. Takehisa J et al. Origin and biology of SIV in wild-living western gorillas. *J Virol* (2009), **83**: 1635–48.

34. de Waal F et al. *Bonobo. The forgotten ape.* Berkeley: University of California Press, 1997.

35. de Waal F. Behavioral contrast between bonobo and chimpanzee. In Heltne P and Marquardt L (eds.), *Understanding chimpanzees.* Harvard University Press, 1989.

36. Kaon T. The sexual behaviour of pygmy chimpanzees. In Heltne P and Marquardt L (eds.), *Understanding chimpanzees.* Harvard University Press, 1989.

37. Van Dooren S et al. Lack of evidence for SIV infection among bonobos. *AIDS Res Hum Retrovir* (2002), **18**: 213–16.

38. Lowenstine LJ et al. Seroepidemiologic survey of captive old-world primates for antibodies to human and simian retroviruses, and isolation of a lentivirus from sooty mangabeys (*Cercocebus atys*). *Int J Cancer* (1986), **38**: 563–74.

39. Sharp P et al. The evolution of HIV-1 and the origin of AIDS. *Phil Trans R Soc B* (2010), **365**: 2487–94.

3 The timing

1. Illiffe J. *The African AIDS epidemic. A history.* Athens: Ohio University Press, 2006.

2. Kapita B. *Sida en Afrique.* Kinshasa: Éditions Centre de Vulgarisation Agricole, 1988.

3. Pales L. État actuel de la paléopathologie. Contribution à l'étude de la pathologie comparative. Thèse pour le doctorat en médecine. Université de Bordeaux, 1929.

4. Gabai M. *L'ambulance chirurgicale légère 222 du Corps d'Armée coloniale dans la guerre 1939–1940.* Paris: Jouve et Cie, 1941.

5. Trezenem E. *L'Afrique Équatoriale Française.* Paris: Éditions Maritimes et Coloniales, 1955.

6. Archives Nationales d'Outre-Mer, Aix-en-Provence. Files 3H7, 3H9, 3H12, 3H13, 3H14, 3H34, 3H36, 3H37, 3H52, 3H53.

7. Sautter G. Notes sur la construction du chemin de fer Congo–Océan (1921–1934). *Cah Etud Afr* (1967), 7: 219–99.

8. Coquery-Vidrovitch C. *Le Congo au temps des grandes compagnies concessionnaires 1898–1930.* Paris: Éditions de l'École des hautes études en sciences sociales, 2002.

9. Headrick R. *Colonialism, health and illness in French Equatorial Africa, 1885–1935.* Atlanta: African Studies Association Press, 1994.

10. Lefrou G. Contribution à l'étude de l'utilisation de la main d'œuvre indigène. Considérations médicales sur le personnel des chantiers de construction du chemin de fer Congo–Océan. *Ann Med Pharm Col* (1927), **25**: 5–51.

11. Pales L. Les lésions anatomopathologiques de la pneumococcie en AEF d'après 85 autopsies. *Bull Soc Pathol Exot* (1933), **26**: 1182–91.

12. Pales L. Les lésions anatomopathologiques de la pneumococcie en AEF d'après 85 autopsies. *Bull Soc Pathol Exot* (1934), **27**: 45–55.

13. Pales L. La tuberculose des Noirs vue d'Afrique Équatoriale Française. *Revue de la Tuberculose* (1938), **4**: 190–8.
14. Auclert J. Contribution à l'étude de la tuberculose des Noirs et de ses lésions anatomiques en Afrique Équatoriale Française. Thèse pour le doctorat en médecine, Université de Marseille, 1937.
15. Korber B et al. Limitations of a molecular clock applied to considerations of the origin of HIV-1. *Science* (1998), **280**: 1868–71.
16. Korber B et al. Timing the ancestor of the HIV-1 pandemic strains. *Science* (2000), **288**: 1789–96.
17. Yusim K et al. Using HIV-1 sequences to infer historical features of the AIDS epidemic and HIV evolution. *Phil Trans R Soc London B* (2001), **356**: 855–66.
18. Sharp P et al. The origins of acquired immune deficiency syndrome viruses: where and when? *Phil Trans R Soc London B* (2001), **356**: 867–76.
19. Mokili J et al. The spread of HIV in Africa. *J Neurovirol* (2005), **111** (suppl 1): 66–75.
20. Weiss RA. Natural and iatrogenic factors in HIV transmission. *Phil Trans R Soc London B* (2001), **356**: 947–53.
21. Worobey M et al. Direct evidence of extensive diversity of HIV-1 in Kinshasa by 1960. *Nature* (2008), **55**: 661–4.
22. Wertheim JO et al. Dating the age of the SIV lineages that gave rise to HIV-1 and HIV-2. *PLoS Comput Biol* (2009), **5**: e1000377.

4 The cut hunter

1. Calattini S et al. Simian foamy virus transmission from apes to humans, rural Cameroon. *Emerg Infect Dis* (2007), **13**: 1314–20.
2. Wolfe N et al. Naturally acquired simian retrovirus infection in central African hunters. *Lancet* (2004), **363**: 932–7.
3. Switzer W et al. Frequent simian foamy virus infection in persons occupationally exposed to non-human primates. *J Virol* (2004), **78**: 2780–9.
4. Briat RL. *Cameroun, Togo*. Paris: Encyclopédie coloniale et maritime, 1951.
5. Anonymous. Le chimpanzé. *Congo Illustré* (1894): 23–4.
6. Tutin C. Écologie et organisation sociale des primates de la forêt tropicale africaine: aide à la compréhension de la transmission des rétrovirus. *Bull Soc Pathol Exot* (2000), **93**: 157–61.
7. Ndembi N et al. HIV-1 infection in Pygmy hunter gatherers is from contact with Bantu rather than from nonhuman primates. *AIDS Res Hum Retrovir* (2003), **19**: 435–9.
8. Leplae E. *La chasse et la pêche au Congo Belge*. Louvain: Ceuterick, 1939.

9. Tutin C. Saving the gorillas (*Gorilla g. gorilla*) and chimpanzees (*Pan t. troglodytes*) of the Congo basin. *Reprod Fertil Dev* (2001), **13**: 469–76.

10. Gouvernement français. *Rapport annuel du gouvernement français sur l'administration sous mandat des territoires du Cameroun pour l'année 1922.* Paris, 1923.

11. Ministère des colonies. *Rapport annuel sur l'administration de la colonie du Congo belge pendant l'année, présenté aux Chambres législatives.* Brussels, 1927, 1945.

12. Leplae E. *Les grands animaux de chasse du Congo Belge.* Brussels, Ministère des Colonies, 1925.

13. De Limbourg J. La faune congolaise en péril. *Bulletin du Centre d'Études des Problèmes Sociaux Indigènes* (1957), **39**: 27–45.

14. Frechkop S. *Mammifères et oiseaux protégés au Congo Belge.* Brussels: Institut des Parcs Nationaux du Congo Belge, 1936.

15. Guernier E. *Afrique Équatoriale Française.* Paris: Encyclopédie coloniale et maritime, 1950.

16. Perrois L. *Peuples et civilisations de la grande forêt.* Paris: ORSTOM, 1967.

17. Ngoma B. Herméneutique de quelques interdits et structures de défoulement en société yombe. *Zaire-Afrique* (1976), **16**: 489–500.

18. Staner P. *Chasse et pêche au Congo belge.* Brussels: Larcier, 1948.

19. Wolfe N et al. Exposure to non-human primates in rural Cameroon. *Emerg Infect Dis* (2004), **10**: 2094–9.

20. Neel C et al. Molecular epidemiology of simian immunodeficiency virus infection in wild-living gorillas. *J Virol* (2010), **84**: 1464–76.

21. Ondoa P et al. In vitro susceptibility to infection with SIV_{cpz} and HIV-1 is lower in chimpanzees than in human peripheral blood mononuclear cells. *J Med Virol* (2002), **67**: 301–11.

22. Sharp P et al. SIV infection in chimpanzees. *J Virol* (2005), **79**: 3891–902.

23. Kestens L et al. Phenotypic and functional parameters of cellular immunity in a chimpanzee with a naturally acquired SIV infection. *J Infect Dis* (1995), **172**: 957–63.

24. Novembre F et al. Development of AIDS in a chimpanzee infected with HIV-1. *J Virol* (1997), **71**: 4086–91.

25. Novembre F et al. Rapid CD4 T-cell loss induced by HIV-1 in uninfected and previously infected chimpanzees. *J Virol* (2001), **75**: 1533–9.

26. O'Neill S et al. Progressive infection in a subset of HIV-1-positive chimpanzees. *J Infect Dis* (2000), **182**: 1051–62.

27. Santiago M et al. Foci of endemic SIV infection in wild-living eastern chimpanzees (*Pan troglodytes schweinfurthii*). *J Virol* (2003), **77**: 7545–62.

28. Keele BF et al. Increased mortality and AIDS-like immunopathology in wild chimpanzees infected with SIV$_{cpz}$. *Nature* (2009), **460**: 515–19.

29. Heeney J et al. Transmission of simian immunodeficiency virus SIV$_{cpz}$ and the evolution of infection in the presence and absence of concurrent HIV-1 infection in chimpanzees. *J Virol* (2006), **80**: 7208–18.

30. Ondoa P et al. Longitudinal comparison of virus load parameters and CD8 T-cell suppressive capacity in two SIVcpz-infected chimpanzees. *J Med Primatol* (2001), **30**: 243–53.

31. Brenner BG et al. High rates of forward transmission events after acute/early HIV-1 infection. *J Infect Dis* (2007), **195**: 951–9.

32. Ippolito G et al. Occupational HIV infection in health care workers: worldwide cases through September 1997. *Clin Infect Dis* (1999), **28**: 365–83.

33. Cardo D et al. A case-control study of HIV seroconversion in health care workers after percutaneous exposure. *N Eng J Med* (1997), **337**: 1485–90.

34. Hooper E. *The river. A journey back to the source of HIV and AIDS.* London: Little Brown and Company, 1999.

35. Plotkin S. Chimpanzees and journalists. *Vaccine* (2004), **22**: 1829–30.

36. Plotkin S. CHAT oral polio vaccine was not the source of HIV-1 group M for humans. *Clin Infect Dis* (2001), **32**: 1068–84.

37. Osterrieth P. Oral polio vaccine: fact versus fiction. *Vaccine* (2004), **22**: 1831–5.

38. Blancou P et al. Polio vaccine samples not linked to AIDS. *Nature* (2001), **410**: 1045–6.

39. Poinar H et al. Molecular analyses of oral polio vaccine samples. *Science* (2001), **292**: 743–4.

40. Berry N et al. Vaccine safety: analysis of oral polio vaccine CHAT stocks. *Nature* (2001), **410**: 1047.

41. Worobey M et al. Contamination polio vaccine theory refuted. *Nature* (2004), **428**: 820.

42. Gilks C. AIDS, monkeys and malaria. *Nature* (1991), **354**: 262.

43. Blacklock D et al. A parasite resembling *Plasmodium falciparum* in a chimpanzee. *Ann Trop Med Parasitol* (1922), **16**: 99–106.

44. Blacklock D et al. The pathological effects produced by *Strongyloides* in a chimpanzee. *Ann Trop Med Parasitol* (1922), **16**: 283–91.

45. Troisier A. Le groupe sanguin II de l'homme chez les chimpanzés. *Ann Inst Pasteur (Paris)* (1928), **42**: 363.

46. Contacos P et al. Experimental adaptation of simian malarias to abnormal hosts. *J Parasitol* (1963), **49**: 912–18.

47. Rodhain J et al. Sur la spécificité des plasmodiums des anthropoides de l'Afrique centrale. *Compt Rend Soc Biol* (1938), **127**: 1467–8.

48. Rodhain J. Les plasmodiums des anthropoides de l'Afrique centrale et leurs relations avec les plasmodiums humains. *Ann Soc Bel Med Trop* (1940), **20**: 489–505.

49. Rodhain J. Les plasmodiums des anthropoides de l'Afrique centrale et leurs relations avec les plasmodiums humains. Réceptivité de l'homme au *Plasmodium malariae* (*Plasmodium rodhaini* Brumpt) du chimpanzé. *Compt Rend Soc Biol* (1940), **133**: 276–7.

50. Rodhain J. Les plasmodiums des anthropoides de l'Afrique centrale et leurs relations avec les plasmodiums humains. *Bull Acad R Med Belgique* (1941), **6**: 21–60.

51. Rodhain J et al. L'infection à *Plasmodium malariae* du chimpanzé chez l'homme. Étude d'une première souche isolée de l'anthropoide Pan satyrus verus. *Ann Soc Bel Med Trop* (1943), **23**: 19–46.

52. Rodhain J et al. Contribution à l'étude du *Pl. schwetzi* E. Brumpt (3ème note). L'infection à *Plasmodium schwetzi* chez l'homme. *Ann Soc Bel Med Trop* (1955), **35**: 757–75.

53. Pettit A. *Sérothérapie antipoliomyélitique d'origine animale.* Paris: Masson, 1936.

54. Réal J. *Voronoff.* Paris: Stock, 2001.

55. Anonymous. *Le prix du singe.* Paris: Le Figaro, 27 October 1922.

56. Anonymous. *On avait même songé à ça.* Brazzaville: L'Étoile de l'AEF, 18 January 1934.

57. Voronoff S et al. *Testicular grafting from ape to man.* London: Brentano's, 1929.

5 Societies in transition

1. Ndaywel è Nziem I. *Histoire générale du Congo. De l'héritage ancien à la République Démocratique.* Paris: Duculot, 1996.

2. Curtin P. *The Atlantic slave trade. A census.* Madison: University of Wisconsin Press, 1969.

3. Klein H. *The Atlantic slave trade.* Cambridge University Press, 1999.

4. Eltis D et al. *The trans-Atlantic slave trade. A database on CD-ROM.* Cambridge University Press, 1999.

5. Hotez PJ et al. The neglected tropical diseases of Latin America and the Caribbean: a review of disease burden and distribution and a roadmap for control and elimination. *PLoS Negl Trop Dis* (2008), **2**: e300. doi:10.1371/journal.pntd.0000300.

6. Lammie P et al. Eliminating lymphatic filariasis, onchocerciasis, and schistosomiasis from the Americas: breaking a historical legacy of

slavery. *PLoS Negl Trop Dis* (2007), **1**: e71. doi:10.1371/journal. pntd.0000071.

7. Morgan J et al. *Schistosoma mansoni* and *Biomphalaria*: past history and future trends. *Parasitology* (2001), **123**: S211–S228.

8. Marr J. Merchants of death: the role of slave trade in the transmission of disease from Africa to America. *Pharos of Alpha Omega Honor Medical Society* (1982): 31–5.

9. Martial J. Hepatitis C virus (HCV) genotypes in the Caribbean island of Martinique: evidence for a large radiation of HCV-2 and for a recent introduction from Europe of HCV-4. *J Clin Microbiol* (2004), **42**: 784–91.

10. Andernach IE et al. Slave trade and Hepatitis B virus genotypes and subgenotypes in Haiti and Africa. *Emerg Infect Dis* (2009), **15**: 1222–8.

11. Verdonck K et al. HTLV-1: recent knowledge about an ancient infection. *Lancet Infect Dis* (2007), **7**: 266–81.

12. Rego F et al. HTLV-1 molecular study in Brazilian villages with African characteristics giving support to the post-Columbian introduction hypothesis. *AIDS Res Hum Retrovir* (2008), **24**: 673–7.

13. Casseb J et al. Lack of *tax* diversity for tropical spastic paraparesis/ HTLV-1 associated myelopathy development in HTLV-1 infected subjects in Sao Paulo, Brazil. *Mem Inst Oswaldo Cruz* (2006), **101**: 273–6.

14. Van Dooren S et al. Evidence for a post-Columbian introduction of HTLV-1 in Latin America. *J Gen Virol* (1998), **79**: 2695–708.

15. Gessain A et al. Low degree of HTLV-1 genetic drift in vivo as a means of monitoring viral transmission and movement of ancient human populations. *J Virol* (1992), **66**: 2288–95.

16. Pakenham T. *The scramble for Africa. White man's conquest of the dark continent from 1876 to 1912.* New York: HarperCollins, 2003.

17. De St-Moulin L. Contribution à l'histoire de Kinshasa. *Zaire-Afrique* (1976), **108**: 461–73.

18. Hochschild A. *King Leopold's ghost. A story of greed, terror and heroism in colonial Africa.* Boston: Mariner Books, 1999.

19. Ngalla DN. *Les missions catholiques et l'évolution sociale au Congo Brazzaville de 1880 à 1930 (l'œuvre d'éducation).* Brazzaville: Éditions Presse et Culture, 1993.

20. Goyau G. *Monseigneur Augouard.* Paris: Librairie Plon, 1926.

21. Beslier G. *L'apôtre du Congo. Mgr Augouard.* Paris: Éditions de la Vraie France, 1946.

22. Mathieu M. *Monseigneur Augouard. Un poitevin roi du Congo.* La Crèche: Geste Éditions, 2006.

23. Frey R. *Brazzaville. Capitale de l'Afrique Équatoriale Française.* Paris: Encyclopédie mensuelle d'outre-mer, 1954.

24. Coquery-Vidrovitch C. *Le Congo au temps des grandes compagnies concessionaires 1898–1930*. Paris: Éditions de l'École des hautes études en sciences sociales, 2002.

25. Martin J. *Savorgnan de Brazza, 1852–1905*. Paris: Les Indes Savantes, 2005.

26. Villien F et al. *Bangui, capitale d'un pays enclavé d'Afrique centrale. Étude historique et géographique*. Bordeaux: CRET, 1990.

27. Ngando BA. *La France au Cameroun 1916–1939. Colonialisme ou mission civilisatrice*. Paris: L'Harmattan, 2002.

28. Maurel A. *Le Congo. De la colonisation belge à l'indépendance*. Paris: L'Harmattan, 1992.

29. Naval Intelligence Division. Geographical Handbook Series. *The Belgian Congo*. Oxford, 1944.

30. Headrick R. *Colonialism, health and illness in French Equatorial Africa, 1885–1935*. Atlanta: African Studies Association Press, 1994.

31. Gouvernement français. *Rapport annuel adressé par le gouvernement français au conseil de la Société des Nations conformément à l'article 22 du pacte sur l'administration sous mandat du territoire du Cameroun pour l'année 1931*. Paris, 1932.

32. Gondola C. *The history of Congo*. Westport: Greenwood Press, 2002.

33. Franqueville A. *Yaoundé. Construire une capitale*. Paris: ORSTOM, 1984.

34. Lotte A. Aperçu sur la situation démographique de l'AEF. *Med Trop* (1953), **13**: 304–19.

35. Pouquet J. *L'Afrique Équatoriale Française et le Cameroun*. Paris: Presses Universitaires de France, 1954.

36. Capelle E. *La cité indigène de Léopoldville*. Léopoldville: Centre d'Étude des Problèmes Sociaux Indigènes, 1947.

37. Baumer G. *Les centres indigènes extracoutumiers au Congo belge*. Paris: Éditions Domat-Monchrestien, 1939.

38. Leleux A. *La cité indigène de Kinshasa*. Léopoldville: Courrier d'Afrique, 1934.

39. Romaniuk A. *La fécondité des populations congolaises*. Paris: Mouton, 1967.

40. Gondola C. Oh, rio-ma! Musique et guerre des sexes à Kinshasa, 1930–1990. *Rev Fr Hist O-M* (1997), **84**: 51–81.

41. Comité Franco-Belge d'Études Coloniales. *La crise économique au Congo Belge et en Afrique Équatoriale Française*. Paris, 1931.

42. Jewsiewicki B. The great depression and the making of the colonial economic system in the Belgian Congo. *Afr Econ Hist* (1977): 153–76.

43. Comhaire-Sylvain S. *Food and leisure among the African youth of Leopoldville (Belgian Congo)*. University of Cape Town, 1950.

44. Gondola C. *Villes miroirs. Migrations et identité urbaines à Kinshasa et Brazzaville 1930–70.* Paris: L'Harmattan, 1997.
45. La Fontaine JS. *City politics. A study of Léopoldville, 1962–63.* Cambridge University Press, 1970.
46. Shapiro D. *Kinshasa in transition. Women's education, employment, and fertility.* University of Chicago Press, 2003.
47. Devauges R. *Le chômage à Brazzaville en 1957.* Paris: ORSTOM, 1959.
48. McDonald G et al. *Area handbook for the People's Republic of the Congo (Congo Brazzaville).* Washington: The American University, 1971.
49. Vanderlinden J. *Pierre Ryckmans 1891–1959. Coloniser dans l'honneur.* Brussels: De Boeck Université, 1994.
50. De St-Moulin L. L'effort de guerre 1940–1945 au Zaire. *Zaire-Afrique* (1985), **142**: 91–104.
51. Van Wing J. Quelques aspects de l'état social des populations congolaises. *Bulletin des séances de l'Institut Royal Colonial Belge* (1947), **18**: 185–201.
52. Van Wing J. Le Congo déraille. *Bulletin des séances de l'Institut Royal Colonial Belge* (1951), **22**: 1–8.
53. Trezenem E. *L'Afrique Équatoriale Française.* Paris: Éditions Maritimes et Coloniales, 1955.
54. MacGaffey G et al. *US Army area handbook for the Republic of Congo (Leopoldville).* Washington: The American University, 1962.
55. Biaya TK. La culture urbaine dans les arts populaires d'Afrique: analyse de l'ambiance Zairoise. *Can J Afr Stud* (1996), **30**: 345–70.
56. Gondola C. O, Kisasa makambo! Métamorphose et représentations urbaines de Kinshasa à travers le discours musical des années 1950–60. *Le Mouvement Social* (2003): 109–29.
57. Colin P. *Un recensement des activités indépendantes à la cité indigène de Léopoldville.* Léopoldville: Éditions de la Direction de l'Information, 1956.
58. Comhaire-Sylvain S. *Femmes de Kinshasa, hier et aujourd'hui.* Paris: Mouton, 1968.
59. Centre d'études des questions économiques africaines. *Le revenu des populations indigènes du Congo-Léopoldville.* Université Libre de Bruxelles, 1963.
60. Romaniuk A. *Démographie congolaise au milieu du XXe siècle.* Presses Universitaires de Louvain, 2006.
61. Baeck L. Léopoldville, phénomène urbain africain. *Zaire* (1956), **10**: 613–36.
62. Denis J. *Le phénomène urbain en Afrique centrale.* Brussels: Académie Royale des Sciences Coloniales, 1958.

63. Lamal F. L'exode massif des hommes adultes vers Léopoldville. *Zaire* (1959), **13**: 365–77.

64. Congo Belge. *Enquêtes démographiques. Cité Léopoldville.* Léopoldville, 1957.

65. Raymaekers P. *L'organisation des zones de squatting. Élément de résorption du chômage structurel dans les milieux urbains des pays en voie de développement. Application au milieu urbain de Léopoldville.* Paris: Éditions Universitaires, 1964.

66. Akoto Mandjale E et al. Démographie zairoise. In Janssens PG (ed.), *Médecine et Hygiène en Afrique centrale de 1885 à nos jours.* Brussels: Fondation Roi Beaudoin, 1992.

67. McDonald G et al. *Area handbook for the Democratic Republic of the Congo (Congo-Kinshasa).* Washington: The American University, 1971.

68. Bernard G. L'Africain et la ville. *Cah Etud Afr* (1973), **13**: 575–86.

69. Mbumba N. *Kinshasa 1881–1981. 100 ans après Stanley. Problèmes et avenir d'une ville.* Kinshasa: Centre de Recherches Pédagogiques, 1982.

70. Pain M. *Kinshasa. La ville et la cité.* Paris: ORSTOM, 1984.

71. République démocratique du Congo. *Étude socio-démographique de Kinshasa 1967.* Kinshasa, 1969.

72. Ziavoula RE. *Brazzaville, une ville à reconstruire.* Paris: Karthala, 2006.

73. Gondola C. Kinshasa et Brazzaville: brève histoire d'un mariage séculaire. *Zaire-Afrique* (1990), **249**: 493–501.

74. Anonymous. Entre Kin et Brazza: le 'pont Fima'. *Zaire*: 18–23.

75. Gouvernement français. *Rapport annuel du gouvernement français à l'assemblée générale des Nations-Unies sur l'administration du Cameroun placé sous la tutelle de la France. Année 1957.* Paris, 1958.

76. Franqueville A. *Une Afrique entre le village et la ville.* Paris: ORSTOM, 1987.

6 The oldest trade

1. Côté AM et al. Transactional sex is the driving force in the dynamics of HIV in Accra, Ghana. *AIDS* (2004), **18**: 917–25.

2. Alary M et al. The central role of clients of female sex workers in the dynamics of heterosexual HIV transmission in sub-Saharan Africa. *AIDS* (2004), **18**: 945–7.

3. Piot P et al. Retrospective seroepidemiology of AIDS virus infection in Nairobi populations. *J Infect Dis* (1987), **155**: 1108–12.

4. Lauro A. *Coloniaux, ménagères et prostituées au Congo belge (1885–1930).* Loverval: Éditions Labor, 2005.

5. Gouvernement français. *Rapport au Ministre des Colonies sur l'administration des territoires occupés du Cameroun pendant l'année 1921.* Paris, 1922.

6. Songué P. *Prostitution en Afrique. L'exemple de Yaoundé.* Paris: L'Harmattan, 1986.
7. Rich J. Une Babylone noire: interracial unions in colonial Libreville, c.1860–1914. *Fr Colon Hist* (2003), **4**: 145–70.
8. Colle P. *Les Baluba (Congo Belge).* Brussels: Dewit, 1913.
9. Torday E et al. *Notes ethnographiques sur des populations habitant les bassins du Kasai et du Kwango oriental.* Brussels: Musée du Congo Belge, 1922.
10. West R. *Brazza of the Congo. Exploration and exploitation in French Equatorial Africa.* London: Jonathan Cape, 1972.
11. Romaniuk A. *La fécondité des populations congolaises.* Paris: Mouton, 1967.
12. Martin P. *Loisirs et société à Brazzaville pendant l'ère coloniale.* Paris: Karthala, 2005.
13. Castellani C. *Les femmes au Congo.* Paris: Flammarion, 1898.
14. Vermeersch A. *La femme congolaise. Ménagère de blanc, femme de polygame, chrétienne.* Brussels: Dewit, 1914.
15. Eynikel H. *Congo belge. Portrait d'une société coloniale.* Gembloux: Duculot, 1984.
16. Jeurissen L. Quand le métis s'appelait mulâtre. *Cah Migr* (2003), **29**: 14–44.
17. Coppens P. Le problème des mulâtres. *Zaire* (1947), **1**: 733–53.
18. Bolamba AR. A propos de la prostitution. *Voix du Congolais* (1952): 330–2.
19. Biaya T. La culture urbaine dans les arts populaires d'Afrique: analyse de l'ambiance Zairoise. *Can J Afr Stud* (1996), **30**: 345–70.
20. Hunt NR. STDs, suffering, and their derivatives in Congo-Zaire: notes towards an historical ethnography of disease. In Becker C et al. (eds.), *Vivre et penser le sida en Afrique/Experiencing and Understanding AIDS in Africa.* Paris: Codesria, Karthala, IRD, 1999.
21. Congo Belge. Hôpital des Noirs de Boma. *Rapport annuel.* Boma, 1909.
22. Congo Belge. *Rapport sur l'Hygiène Publique.* Boma, 1912.
23. Congo Belge. Hôpital des Blancs de Léopoldville. *Rapport annuel.* Léopoldville, 1912.
24. Gouvernement français. *Rapport annuel du gouvernement français sur l'administration sous mandat des territoires du Cameroun pour l'année 1922.* Paris, 1923.
25. Gouvernement français. *Rapport annuel du gouvernement français sur l'administration sous mandat des territoires du Cameroun pour l'année 1923.* Paris, 1924.

26. De Baudre. *Le danger vénérien*. Yaoundé: Imprimerie du Gouvernement, 1928.

27. Gouvernement français. *Rapport annuel du gouvernement français aux Nations-Unies sur l'administration du Cameroun placé sous la tutelle de la France. Année 1947*. Paris, 1948.

28. Rousseau. Les maladies transmissibles observées dans les colonies françaises et territoires sous mandat pendant l'année 1927. *Ann Med Pharm Col* (1929), **27**: 237–41.

29. Ledentu. Les maladies transmissibles observées dans les colonies françaises et territoires sous mandat pendant l'année 1929. *Ann Med Pharm Col* (1931), **29**: 661–851.

30. Marque. Les maladies transmissibles observées dans les colonies françaises et territoires sous mandat pendant l'année 1931. *Ann Med Pharm Col* (1933), **31**: 123–322.

31. Ledentu. Les maladies transmissibles observées dans les colonies françaises et territoires sous mandat pendant l'année 1933. *Ann Med Pharm Col* (1935), **33**: 552–815.

32. Territoire du Moyen-Congo. *Rapport annuel*. Brazzaville, 1945.

33. Territoire du Moyen-Congo. Rapport médical annuel. Deuxième partie (partie médicale). *Commentaires*. Brazzaville, 1954.

34. Afrique Équatoriale Française.Colonie du Gabon. Service de Santé. *Rapport médical annuel*. Libreville, 1932.

35. Afrique Équatoriale Française.Colonie du Gabon. Service de Santé. *Rapport médical annuel*. Libreville, 1933.

36. Afrique Équatoriale Française.Oubangui-Chari. Service de Santé. *Rapport annuel*. Bangui, 1929.

37. Afrique Équatoriale Française. Territoire de l'Oubangui-Chari. Service de Santé. *Rapport médical*. Bangui, 1945.

38. Afrique Équatoriale Française.Oubangui-Chari. *Rapport médical annuel*. Bangui, 1932.

39. Sautter G. Notes sur la construction du chemin de fer Congo–Océan (1921–1934). *Cah Etud Afr* (1967), **7**: 219–99.

40. Coquery-Vidrovitch C. *Le Congo au temps des grandes compagnies concessionnaires 1898–1930*. Paris: Éditions de l'École des hautes études en sciences sociales, 2002.

41. Headrick R. *Colonialism, health and illness in French Equatorial Africa, 1885–1935*. Atlanta: African Studies Association Press, 1994.

42. Gondola C. *Villes miroirs. Migrations et identité urbaines à Kinshasa et Brazzaville 1930–70*. Paris: L'Harmattan, 1997.

43. Congo Belge. *Rapport sur l'Hygiène*. Brussels, 1932.

44. Capelle E. *La cité indigène de Léopoldville*. Léopoldville: Centre d'Étude des Problèmes Sociaux Indigènes, 1947.

45. Pons V. *Stanleyville. An African urban community under Belgian administration.* Oxford University Press, 1969.

46. Verhaegen B. *Enquête démographique par sondage 1955–57 – Province Orientale – District de Stanleyville – District du Haut-Uele.* Brussels: Les cahiers du CEDAF, 1978.

47. Verhaegen B. *Le centre extra-coutumier de Stanleyville (1940–45).* Brussels: Les cahiers du CEDAF, 1981.

48. Comhaire-Sylvain S. *Food and leisure among the African youth of Leopoldville (Belgian Congo).* University of Cape Town, 1950.

49. Mwepu B. La vie des femmes légères, dites 'libres', au centre extra-coutumier d'Elisabethville. *Bulletin du Centre d'Études des Problèmes Sociaux Indigènes* (1951), **17**: 175–83.

50. Bongolo H. A propos des 'coutume indigènes' qui se pratiquent à la cité indigène de Léopoldville. *Bulletin du Centre d'Études des Problèmes Sociaux Indigènes* (1948), **5**: 36–46.

51. Van Wing J. La polygamie au Congo Belge. *J Int Afr Inst* (1947), **17**: 93–102.

52. La Fontaine JS. The free women of Kinshasa: prostitution in a city of Zaire. In David J (ed.), *Essays in honour of Lucy Mair.* London: Athlone Press, 1974.

53. Denis J. *Le phénomène urbain en Afrique centrale.* Brussels: Académie Royale des Sciences Coloniales, 1958.

54. Bruaux P et al. La lutte contre les infections vénériennes à Léopoldville. *Ann Soc Bel Med Trop* (1957), **37**: 801–13.

55. Tshingi K. *Kinshasa à l'épreuve de la désagrégation nationale.* Paris: L'Harmattan, 2007.

56. Romaniuk A. *L'aspect démographique de la stérilité des femmes congolaises.* Léopoldville: Éditions de l'Université, 1963.

57. Morison L et al. Commercial sex and the spread of HIV in four cities in sub-Saharan Africa. *AIDS* (2001), **15**: S61–S69.

58. Ngandu E. La prostitution ronge le Congo. *Voix du Congolais* (1945): 209–21.

59. Mupenda JE. Prostitution et polygamie. *Voix du Congolais* (1947): 821–2.

60. Wassa F. Liberté de la femme noire et prostitution. *Voix du Congolais* (1947): 71–2.

61. Omari AJ. Remèdes contre la prostitution. *Voix du Congolais* (1951): 59–63.

62. Omari AJ. Les conséquences de la prostitution sur les mariages. *Voix du Congolais* (1952): 134–5.

63. Mathieu M. *Monseigneur Augouard. Un poitevin roi du Congo.* La Crèche: Geste Éditions, 2006.

64. Ngalla DN. *Les missions catholiques et l'évolution sociale au Congo Brazzaville de 1880 à 1930 (l'œuvre d'éducation)*. Brazzaville: Éditions Presse et Culture, 1993.

65. Balandier G. *Sociologie des Brazzaville noires*. Paris: Presses de la Fondation Nationale des Sciences Politiques, 1985.

66. Soret M. *Démographie et problèmes urbains en AEF. Poto-Poto – Bacongo – Dolisie*. Brazzaville: Mémoires de l'Institut d'Études Centrafricaines, 1954.

67. Balandier G. *Ambiguous Africa. Cultures in collision*. New York: Pantheon Books, 1966.

68. Mokondzi O et al. Halte à la prostitution. *La Semaine de l'AEF*, 23 July to 24 September 1955.

69. Schwarz A. Illusion d'une émancipation et aliénation réelle de l'ouvrière zairoise. *Can J Afr Stud* (1972), **6**: 183–212.

70. Raymaekers P. *L'organisation des zones de squatting. Élément de résorption du chômage structurel dans les milieux urbains des pays en voie de développement. Application au milieu urbain de Léopoldville*. Paris: Éditions Universitaires, 1964.

71. Gondola C. Bisengo ya la joie. Fête, sociabilité et politique dans les capitales congolaises. In Goerg O (ed.), *Fêtes urbaines en Afrique*. Paris: Karthala, 1999.

72. Yoka L. *Kinshasa, signes de vie*. Paris: L'Harmattan, 1999.

73. Comhaire-Sylvain S. *Femmes de Kinshasa, hier et aujourd'hui*. Paris: Mouton, 1968.

74. Anonymous. Congo: la prostitution se camoufle. *Zaire*, 13 April 1970, 10–11.

75. Anonymous. L'histoire naturelle des filles de joie. *Zaire* (1969), **42**: 10–15.

7 Injections and the transmission of viruses

1. Drucker E et al. The injection century: massive sterile injections and the emergence of human pathogens. *Lancet* (2001), **358**: 1989–92.

2. Morgan D et al. HIV-1 infection in rural Africa: is there a difference in median time to AIDS and survival compared with that in industrialized countries? *AIDS* (2002), **16**: 597–603.

3. Pepin J et al. Parenteral transmission during excision and treatment of tuberculosis and trypanosomiasis may be responsible for the HIV-2 epidemic in Guinea-Bissau. *AIDS* (2006), **20**: 1303–11.

4. Carreira A. *Mandingas da Guiné Portuguesa*. Lisbon: Centre de Estudos da Guiné Portuguesa, 1947.

5. Mast EE et al. Risk factors for perinatal transmission of Hepatitis C virus (HCV) and the natural history of HCV infection acquired in infancy. *J Infect Dis* (2005), **192**: 1880–9.
6. Vandelli C. Lack of evidence of sexual transmission of Hepatitis C among monogamous couples: results of a 10-year prospective follow-up study. *Am J Gastroenterol* (2004), **99**: 855–9.
7. Des Jarlais D et al. HIV-1 infection among intravenous drug users in Manhattan, New York City. *JAMA* (1989), **261**: 1008–12.
8. Robertson JR et al. Epidemic of AIDS related virus (HTLV-III/LAV) infection among intravenous drug users. *Br Med J* (1986), **292**: 527–9.
9. Angarano G et al. Rapid spread of HTLV-III among drug addicts in Italy. *Lancet* (1985), **2**: 1302.
10. Rodrigo JM et al. HTLV-III antibodies in drug addicts in Spain. *Lancet* (1985), **2**: 156–7.
11. Robert CF et al. Behavioural changes in intravenous drug users in Geneva: rise and fall of HIV infection, 1980–1989. *AIDS* (1990), **4**: 657–60.
12. Nicolosi A et al. Incidence and prevalence trends of HIV infection in intravenous drug users attending treatment centers in Milan and Northern Italy. *JAIDS* (1992), **5**: 365–73.
13. Choopanya K et al. Risk factors and HIV seropositivity among injecting drug users in Bangkok. *AIDS* (1991), **5**: 1509–13.
14. Strathdee SA et al. Needle exchange is not enough: lessons from the Vancouver injecting drug use study. *AIDS* (1997), **11**: F59–F65.
15. Emmanuel F et al. Factors associated with an explosive HIV epidemic among injecting drug users in Sargodha, Pakistan. *JAIDS* (2009), **51**: 85–90.
16. Kaplan EH et al. A model-based estimate of HIV infection via needle sharing. *JAIDS* (1992), **5**: 1116–18.
17. Hudgens MG et al. Subtype-specific transmission probabilities for HIV-1 among injecting drug users in Bangkok. *Am J Epidemiol* (2002), **155**: 159–68.
18. Mathers BM et al. Global epidemiology of injecting drug use and HIV among people who inject drugs: a systematic review. *Lancet* (2008), **372**: 1733–45.
19. Patrascu IV et al. HIV-1 infection in Romanian children. *Lancet* (1990), **1**: 672.
20. Hersh B et al. AIDS in Romania. *Lancet* (1991), **338**: 645–9.
21. Hersh B et al. The epidemiology of HIV and AIDS in Romania. *AIDS* (1991), **5**: S87–S92.
22. Hersh B et al. Risk factors for HIV infection among abandoned Romanian children. *AIDS* (1993), **7**: 1617–24.

23. Kozinetz CA et al. The burden of pediatric HIV/AIDS in Constanta, Romania: a cross-sectional study. *BMC Infect Dis* (2001), **1**: 7.

24. Apetrei C et al. HIV-1 diversity in Romania. *AIDS* (1998), **12**: 1079–85.

25. Guimaraes ML et al. Close phylogenetic relationship between Angolan and Romanian HIV-1 subtype F1 isolates. *Retrovirology* (2009), **6**: 39.

26. Yerly S et al. Nosocomial outbreak of multiple bloodborne viral infections. *J Infect Dis* (2001), **184**: 369–72.

27. Visco-Comandini U et al. Monophyletic HIV type 1 CRF02_AG in a nosocomial outbreak in Benghazi, Libya. *AIDS Res Hum Retrovir* (2002), **18**: 727–32.

28. Hirsch M. Justice in Libya? Let scientific evidence prevail. *J Infect Dis* (2007), **195**: 467–8.

29. de Oliveira T et al. HIV-1 and HCV sequences from Libyan outbreak. *Nature* (2006), **44**: 836–7.

30. Bobkov A et al. Molecular epidemiology of HIV-1 in the former Soviet Union: analysis of *env* V3 sequences and their correlation with epidemiologic data. *AIDS* (1994), **8**: 619–24.

31. Frank C et al. The role of parenteral antischistosomal therapy in the spread of hepatitis C virus in Egypt. *Lancet* (2000), **355**: 887–91.

32. Strickland GT. Liver disease in Egypt: Hepatitis C superseded schistosomiasis as a result of iatrogenic and biological factors. *Hepatology* (2006), **43**: 915–22.

33. Pybus OG et al. The epidemiology and iatrogenic transmission of hepatitis C virus in Egypt: a Bayesian coalescent approach. *Molecular Biology & Evolution* (2003), **20**: 381–7.

34. Madhava V et al. Epidemiology of chronic hepatitis C virus infection in sub-Saharan Africa. *Lancet Infect Dis* (2002), **2**: 293–302.

35. Nerrienet E et al. Hepatitis C virus infection in Cameroon: a cohort-effect. *J Med Virol* (2005), **76**: 208–14.

36. Delaporte E et al. Hepatitis C in remote populations of southern Cameroon. *Ann Trop Med Parasitol* (1994), **88**: 97–8.

37. Louis F et al. Grandes variations de la prévalence de l'infection par le virus C des hépatites en Afrique centrale. *Med Trop (Mars)* (1994), **54**: 277–8.

38. Kowo M et al. Prevalence of hepatitis C virus and other blood-borne viruses in Pygmies and neighbouring Bantus in southern Cameroon. *Trans R Soc Trop Med Hyg* (1995), **89**: 484–6.

39. Nkengasong J et al. A pilot study of the prevalence of hepatitis C virus antibodies and hepatitis C virus RNA in southern Cameroon. *Am J Trop Med Hyg* (1995), **52**: 98–100.

40. Njouom R et al. High rate of hepatitis C virus infection and predominance of genotype 4 among elderly inhabitants of a remote village of the rain forest of South Cameroon. *J Med Virol* (2003), **71**: 219–25.

41. Laurent C et al. HIV and hepatitis C virus coinfection, Cameroon. *Emerg Infect Dis* (2007), **13**: 514–16.

42. Njouom R et al. The hepatitis C virus epidemic in Cameroon: genetic evidence for rapid transmission between 1920 and 1960. *Infect Gen Evol* (2007), **7**: 361–7.

43. Ndong-Atome G et al. High prevalence of hepatitis C virus infection and predominance of genotype 4 in rural Gabon. *J Med Virol* (2008), **80**: 1581–7.

44. Louis F et al. High prevalence of anti-hepatitis C virus antibodies in a Cameroon rural forest area. *Trans R Soc Trop Med Hyg* (1994), **88**: 53–4.

45. Delaporte E et al. High level of hepatitis C endemicity in Gabon, Equatorial Africa. *Trans R Soc Trop Med Hyg* (1993), **87**: 636–7.

46. Pepin J et al. Noble goals, unforeseen consequences: the control of tropical diseases in colonial Central Africa and the iatrogenic transmission of blood-borne viruses. *Trop Med Inter Health* (2008), **13**: 744–53.

47. Yazdanpanah Y et al. Risk factors for hepatitis C virus transmission to health care workers after occupational exposure: a European case-control study. *Clin Infect Dis* (2005), **41**: 1423–30.

48. Jagger J et al. Occupational transmission of Hepatitis C virus. *JAMA* (2002), **288**: 1469–70.

49. Apetrei C et al. Potential for HIV transmission through unsafe injections. *AIDS* (2006), **20**: 1074–6.

50. Blanchard M. *Précis d'épidémiologie. Médecine préventive et hygiène coloniales*. Paris: Vigot, 1938.

51. Levaditi C et al. *Les ultravirus des maladies humaines*. Paris: Maloine, 1948.

52. Reynes V. *Précis d'épidémiologie et prophylaxie des grandes endémies tropicales*. Marseilles: Éditions M. Leconte, 1950.

53. Vaucel M. *Médecine Tropicale*. Paris: Flammarion, 1952.

54. Bigger JW. Jaundice in syphilitics under treatment. *Lancet* (1943), **1**: 457–8.

55. Salaman MH et al. Prevention of jaundice resulting from antisyphilitic treatment. *Lancet* (1944), **2**: 7–8.

56. Sheehan HL. Epidemiology of infective hepatitis. *Lancet* (1944), **2**: 8–11.

57. Laird SM. Syringe-transmitted hepatitis. *Glasgow Med J* (1947), **28**: 199–219.

58. Hughes RR. Post-penicillin jaundice. *Br Med J* (1946), **1**: 685–8.

59. Seeff L et al. A serologic follow-up of the 1942 epidemic of post-vaccination hepatitis in the United States army. *N Eng J Med* (1987), **316**: 965–70.

60. Zuckerman AJ. Syringe-transmitted hepatitis. *Br Med J* (1978), **2**: 696.
61. Ledentu. *Cours technique des infirmiers de l'Assistance Médicale Indigène.* Paris: Agence Économique de l'Afrique Équatoriale Française, 1931.

8 The legacies of colonial medicine I: French Equatorial Africa and Cameroun

1. Lapeyssonie L. *La médecine coloniale. Mythes et réalités.* Paris: Seghers, 1988.
2. Eyidi MB. *Le vainqueur de la maladie du sommeil. Le Docteur Eugène Jamot (1879–1937).* Paris, 1950.
3. Lapeyssonie L. *Moi, Jamot, le vainqueur de la maladie du sommeil.* Brussels: Éditions Louis Musin, 1987.
4. Ducloux M. Eugène Jamot: un fils du Limousin. *Bull Soc Pathol Exot* (1988), **81**: 419–26.
5. Milleiri JM. Jamot, cet inconnu. *Bull Soc Pathol Exot* (2004), **97**: 213–22.
6. Jamot E. Essai de prophylaxie médicale de la maladie du sommeil dans l'Oubangui-Chari. *Bull Soc Pathol Exot* (1920), **13**: 343–76.
7. Naval Intelligence Division. Geographical Handbook Series. *The Belgian Congo.* Oxford, 1944.
8. Kérandel J. Un cas de trypanosomiase chez un médecin (auto-observation). *Bull Soc Pathol Exot* (1910), **3**: 644–62.
9. David J. Observation de trypanose humaine. *Ann Soc Bel Med Trop* (1922), **2**: 227–30.
10. Pepin J et al. Noble goals, unforeseen consequences: the control of tropical diseases in colonial Central Africa and the iatrogenic transmission of blood-borne viruses. *Trop Med Inter Health* (2008), **13**: 744–53.
11. Cameroun Français. Service de Santé & Services de santé publique. Rapport annuel. Yaoundé, 1936, 1939 to 1951, 1955 to 1959.
12. Moyen-Congo [Colonie du; Territoire du]. Rapport annuel. Brazzavillle, 1930, 1931, 1933, 1934, 1945, 1947 to 1954, 1955 to 1958.
13. Oubangui-Chari [Colonie de l'; Territoire de l']. Service de Santé & Direction de la santé publique. Rapport annuel. Bangui, 1932, 1933, 1945, 1946, 1948, 1950 to 1957, 1959.
14. Gabon [Colonie du; Territoire du] (1931–57) Service de Santé. Rapport annuel. Libreville, 1931 to 1933, 1945, 1947 to 1950, 1952 to 1957.
15. Afrique Équatoriale Française. Rapport médical sur le fonctionnement durant l'année 1935 des services sanitaires et médicaux civils de l'Afrique Équatoriale Française. Brazzaville, 1936.
16. Afrique Équatoriale Française. Inspection Générale des Services Sanitaires et Médicaux. Rapport annuel. Brazzaville, 1936–44.

17. Afrique Équatoriale Française. Direction Générale de la Santé Publique. Rapport annuel. Brazzaville, 1945–56.

18. Afrique Équatoriale Française. Service Général d'Hygiène Mobile et de Prophylaxie de l'Afrique Équatoriale Française. Rapport annuel. Brazzaville, 1947–58.

19. Gouvernement français. *Rapport annuel adressé par le gouvernement français au conseil de la Société des Nations conformément à l'article 22 du pacte sur l'administration sous mandat du territoire du Cameroun pour l'année*. Paris, 1921 to 1938.

20. Gouvernement français. *Rapport annuel du gouvernement français aux Nations-Unies sur l'administration du Cameroun placé sous la tutelle de la France*. Paris, 1947 to 1957.

21. Rousseau;Hermant;Ledentu;Lefèvre;Marque;Grosfillez;Peltier;Vogel;Le Rouzic;Riou (1927–38) Les maladies transmissibles observées dans les colonies françaises et territoires sous mandat. Annales de Médecine et de Pharmacie Coloniales. Available at: http://web2.bium.univ-paris5.fr/livanc/?cote=131132&do=livre.

22. Ministère de la France d'Outre-Mer. Direction du Service de Santé. Statistique médicale de l'année. Paris, 1946–9.

23. Ministère de la France d'Outre-Mer. Situation médicale des territoires français d'outre-mer. Paris, 1950–6.

24. Letonturier et al. La prophylaxie de la maladie du sommeil au Cameroun dans les secteurs du Haut-Nyong et de Doumé. *Ann Instit Past* (1924), **38**: 1053–110.

25. Jamot E. La maladie du sommeil au Cameroun en janvier 1929. *Bull Soc Pathol Exot* (1929), **22**: 473–96.

26. Muraz G. État actuel des traitements chimiothérapiques de la maladie du sommeil. In *Les grandes endémies tropicales*. Paris: Vigot Frères, 1936.

27. Vamos S. Traitement de trypanosomés dans un secteur du Moyen-Chari (AEF): étude de 3705 observations. *Bull Soc Pathol Exot* (1936), **29**: 1015–22.

28. Millous. Le traitement de la maladie du sommeil au Cameroun. *Ann Med Pharm Col* (1936), **34**: 966–95.

29. Jamot E. La lutte contre la maladie du sommeil au Cameroun. *Ann Instit Past* (1932), **48**: 481–539.

30. Vaucel M. État de la maladie du sommeil au Cameroun en 1939. *Ann Instit Past* (1941), **67**: 189–215.

31. Demarchi J. Rapport sur la chimioprophylaxie de la trypanosomiase à *T. gambiense*. In International Scientific Committee for Trypanosomiasis Research, Seventh Meeting. Brussels, 1958.

32. Waddy BB. Chemoprophylaxis of human trypanosomiasis. In Mulligan HW and Potts WH (eds.), *The African trypanosomiases*. London: George Allen and Unwin, 1970.

33. Richet P. Quelques considérations sur la chimio-prophylaxie de la trypanosomiase humaine en AEF. In International Scientific Committee for Trypanosomiasis Research, Fifth Meeting. Pretoria, 1954.

34. Haut Commissariat de la République en Afrique Équatoriale Française. Direction Générale de la Santé Publique, Rapport confidentiel 707/DGSP. 22 April 1953. Brazzaville.

35. Cartron. Le pian et sa répartition dans les colonies françaises. Considérations étiologiques, cliniques, sérologiques, thérapeutiques et prophylactiques. *Ann Med Pharm Col* (1937), **35**: 5–73.

36. Vaucel MA. Le pian dans les territoires français. *Bull World Health Organ* (1953), **8**: 183–204.

37. Joyeux C. *Précis de médecine tropicale*. Paris: Masson, 1944.

38. Montel M. *Mémento thérapeutique du praticien colonial*. Paris: Masson, 1945.

39. Vaucel M. *Médecine Tropicale*. Paris: Flammarion, 1952.

40. De Baudre. *Le danger vénérien*. Yaoundé: Imprimerie du Gouvernement, 1928.

41. Richet P. Une question d'actualité: la maladie de Hansen en AEF. *Ann Soc Bel Med Trop* (1954), **34**: 589–602.

42. Gaud J. Les bilharzioses en Afrique occidentale et en Afrique centrale. *Bull World Health Organ* (1955), **13**: 209–58.

43. Brunel M. La tuberculose pulmonaire au Cameroun en 1958, endémie tuberculeuse, formes cliniques, traitement prophylaxie. *Bull Soc Pathol Exot* (1958), **51**: 920–35.

44. Echenberg M. For their own good: the Pasteur Institute and the quest for an anti-yellow fever vaccine in French Colonial Africa. In Bado JP (ed.), *Conquêtes médicales. Histoire de la médecine moderne et des maladies en Afrique*. Paris: Karthala, 2005.

45. Hackett CJ. Extent and nature of the yaws problem in Africa. *Bull World Health Organ* (1953), **8**: 129–82.

46. Direccion general de marruecos y colonias. Seccion de estadistica de la delegacion del trabajo del gobierno general de los territorios espanoles del golfo de Guinea. Resumenes de los anos: 1944 to 1953.

47. Alonso C. Diferentes aspectos de la tripanosomiasis africana (su importancia en Africa y Guinea ecuatorial espanola). *Med Trop (Madr)* (1966), **42**: 157–83.

48. Vicente G et al. Importancia de las grandes enfermedades transmisibles en la sanidad publica de Guinea ecuatorial y su relacion con las grandes campanas de masas. *Med Trop (Madr)* (1968), **44**: 282–97.

49. Yazdanpanah Y et al. Risk factors for hepatitis C virus transmission to health care workers after occupational exposure: a European case-control study. *Clin Infect Dis* (2005), **41**: 1423–30.

50. Moudgil K et al. Global overview of the prevalence of hepatitis B virus markers (HBsAg and anti-HBs) in leprosy patients. *Trop Gastroenterol* (1988), **9**: 184–90.

51. Verdier M et al. Antibodies to human T lymphotropic virus type 1 in patients with leprosy in tropical areas. *J Infect Dis* (1990), **161**: 1309–10.

52. Denis F et al. Prevalence of antibodies to hepatitis C virus among patients with leprosy in several African countries and the Yemen. *J Med Virol* (1994), **43**: 1–4.

53. Lechat M et al. Decreased survival of HTLV-I carriers in leprosy patients from the Democratic Republic of the Congo: a historical prospective study. *JAIDS* (1997), **15**: 387–90.

54. Moraes Braga A et al. Leprosy and confinement due to leprosy show high association with hepatitis C in Southern Brazil. *Acta Trop* (2006), **97**: 88–93.

55. Louis F et al. Grandes variations de la prévalence de l'infection par le virus C des hépatites en Afrique centrale. *Med Trop (Mars)* (1994), **54**: 277–8.

56. Kowo M et al. Prevalence of hepatitis C virus and other blood-borne viruses in Pygmies and neighbouring Bantus in southern Cameroon. *Trans R Soc Trop Med Hyg* (1995), **89**: 484–6.

57. Delaporte E et al. Seroepidemiological survey of HTLV-I infection among randomized populations of western central African countries. *JAIDS* (1989), **2**: 410–13.

58. Louis J et al. Epidemiological features of retroviral infection by HTLV-1 in central Africa. *Bull Soc Pathol Exot* (1993), **86**: 163–8.

59. Hay S et al. Annual *Plasmodium falciparum* entomological inoculation rates across Africa: literature survey, internet access and review. *Trans R Soc Trop Med Hyg* (2000), **94**: 113–27.

60. Hay S et al. Urbanization, malaria transmission and disease burden in Africa. *Nature Rev* (2005), **3**: 81–90.

61. Hay S et al. A world malaria map: *Plasmodium falciparum* endemicity in 2007. *PLoS Med* (2009), **6**: e1000048.

62. Pepin J et al. HCV transmission during medical interventions and traditional practices in colonial Cameroon: potential implications for the emergence of HIV-1. *Clin Infect Dis* (2010), **51**: 768–76.

63. Pepin J et al. Iatrogenic transmission of human retrovirus HTLV-1 and of Hepatitis C virus through parenteral treatment and chemoprophylaxis of sleeping sickness in colonial Equatorial Africa. *Clin Infect Dis* (2010), **51**: 777–84.

9 The legacies of colonial medicine II: the Belgian Congo

1. Schwetz J. *L'évolution de la médecine au Congo Belge.* Brussels: Office de Publicité, 1946.
2. Fédération pour la défense des intérêts belges à l'étranger. *L'assistance médicale dans l'État Indépendant du Congo.* Brussels: Bulens Frères, 1907.
3. Rodhain J. La maladie du sommeil dans l'Ouellé. *Bull Soc Pathol Exot* (1916), **9**: 38–72.
4. Schwetz J. Rapport sur les travaux de la mission médicale antitrypanosomique du Kwango-Kasaï 1920–1923. *Ann Soc Bel Med Trop* (1924), **4**: 1–138.
5. Janssens PG. Eugène Jamot et Émile Lejeune, pages d'histoire. *Ann Soc Bel Med Trop* (1995), **75**: 1–12.
6. Congo Belge. Rapport annuel de la direction générale des services médicaux du Congo Belge. Léopoldville, 1958.
7. Congo Belge. Rapport sur l'Hygiène. Années 1940, 1941–4, 1945, 1946, 1947, 1948, 1949. Brussels.
8. Congo Belge. Rapport sur l'Hygiène. Brussels, 1924 to 1930.
9. David J. *Vade-mecum à l'usage des infirmiers et des assistants médicaux indigènes.* Brussels: Vromant & Co., 1931.
10. Chesterman C. *Manuel du dispensaire tropical.* London: Lutterworth Press, 1947.
11. Ministère des Colonies. *Rapport de la Commission de la Lèpre.* Brussels, 1939.
12. Dupuy L. L'endémie pianique au cours de l'année 1934 dans les territoires soumis à l'action du Fonds Reine Elisabeth pour l'assistance médicale aux indigènes du Congo Belge. *Ann Soc Bel Med Trop* (1936), **16**: 189–97.
13. Kivits M et al. Le traitement du pian par voie buccale au STB et au Stovarsol. *Ann Soc Bel Med Trop* (1951), **31**: 37–49.
14. Gillet J et al. Les bilharzioses humaines au Congo Belge et au Ruanda-Urundi. *Bull World Health Organ* (1954), **10**: 315–419.
15. Dubois A. *La lèpre au Congo Belge en 1938.* Brussels: Académie Royale de Belgique, 1940.
16. Kivits M. *La lutte contre la lèpre au Congo belge en 1955.* Brussels: Académie Royale des Sciences Coloniales, 1956.
17. Duren A. *Un essai d'étude d'ensemble du paludisme au Congo Belge.* Brussels: Institut Royal Colonial Belge, 1937.
18. Duren A. Essai d'étude sur l'importance du paludisme dans la mortalité au Congo Belge. *Ann Soc Bel Med Trop* (1951), **31**: 129–47.
19. Gillet J. *Le paludisme au Congo Belge et au Ruanda Burundi.* Brussels: Institut Royal Colonial Belge, 1953.

20. Gillet J. *Atlas général du Congo et du Ruanda-Urundi. Carte nosologique et notice de la carte nosologique du Congo belge et du Ruanda-Urundi.* Brussels: Institut Royal Colonial Belge, 1954.
21. Congo Belge. Rapport des services médicaux. Brussels, 1958.
22. Duren A. La santé des Européens au Congo. *Arch Med Soc Hyg* (1940), **5**: 385–97.
23. Mense. *Rapport de l'état sanitaire de Léopoldville de novembre 1885 à mars 1887.* Brussels: Publications de l'État Indépendant du Congo, 1888.
24. Pierquin L. *Historique du Laboratoire Médical de l'Institut de Médecine Tropicale Princesse Astrid à Léopoldville.* Léopoldville: Graphicongo, 1958.
25. Whyms. *Les services médicaux et sanitaires de Léopoldville.* Brussels: Office de Publicité, 1952.
26. Van Hoof L. Immunité et guérison spontanée de singes cercopithèques infectés par *Trypanosoma gambiense. Bull Soc Pathol Exot* (1934), **27**: 167–9.
27. Van Hoof L et al. Guérisons spontanées, état réfractaire et immunité des singes pour certains trypanosomes pathogènes. *Bull Soc Pathol Exot* (1937), **30**: 727–37.
28. Peel E et al. Sur des filaridés de chimpanzés *Pan paniscus* et *Pan satyrus* au Congo Belge. *Ann Soc Bel Med Trop* (1946), **26**: 117–56.
29. Van Hoof L et al. Contribution à l'épidémiologie de la maladie du sommeil au Congo Belge. *Ann Soc Bel Med Trop* (1938), **18**: 143–201.
30. Arnaud. Vaccin antigonococcique actif contre l'écoulement. *Ann Soc Bel Med Trop* (1934), **14**: 5–6.
31. Brutsaert P. La méningite cérébrospinale au Katanga (Congo Belge). Résultats de la vaccination prophylactique et de la sérothérapie anti-méningococciques obtenus à l'Union Minière du Haut-Katanga. *Ann Soc Bel Med Trop* (1931), **11**: 11–39.
32. Anonymous. Le laboratoire de Léopoldville. *Congo Illustré* (1941): 5–9.
33. Dedet JP. *Les Instituts Pasteur d'outre-mer. Cent vingt ans de microbiologie française dans le monde.* Paris: L'Harmattan, 2002.
34. Bosmans E and Janssens PG. Laboratoires médicaux et d'hygiène. In Janssens PG (ed.), *Médecine et hygiène en Afrique centrale de 1885 à nos jours.* Brussels: Fondation Roi Beaudoin, 1992.
35. Congo Belge. Province Orientale. Service Médical. Rapport annuel. Stanleyville, 1952 to 1957.
36. Rodhain J. Nécrologie. Lucien Van Hoof. *Ann Soc Bel Med Trop* (1948), **28**: 381–4.
37. Thomas AC. Hommage au Docteur L. Van Hoof. *Ann Soc Bel Med Trop* (1954), **34**: 559–67.

38. Duren A. Lucien Van Hoof. *Bulletin des séances de l'Institut Royal Colonial Belge* (1949), **20**: 147–54.

39. Kivits M. Lucien Van Hoof. Biographie belge d'outre-mer. Brussels: Académie Royale des Sciences d'Outre-Mer, 1968.

40. Rodhain J et al. Contribution à l'étude des plasmodiums des singes africains. *Ann Soc Bel Med Trop* (1938), **18**: 237–53.

41. Van Hoof L. Observations on trypanosomiasis in the Belgian Congo. *Trans R Soc Trop Med Hyg* (1947), **40**: 728–54.

42. Van Hoof L et al. Chimioprophylaxie de la maladie du sommeil par la pentamidine. *Ann Soc Bel Med Trop* (1946), **26**: 371–84.

43. Van Hoof L et al. Pentamidine in the prevention and treatment of trypanosomiasis. *Trans R Soc Trop Med Hyg* (1944), **37**: 271–80.

44. Van Hoof L et al. A field experiment on the prophylactic value of pentamidine in sleeping sickness. *Trans R Soc Trop Med Hyg* (1946), **39**: 327–9.

45. Van Hoof L et al. Sur la chimiothérapie de l'onchocercose (note préliminaire). *Ann Soc Bel Med Trop* (1947), **27**: 173–7.

46. Mouchet R. Le problème de la tuberculose humaine en Afrique tropicale et spécialement au Congo Belge. *Ann Soc Bel Med Trop* (1937), **17**: 509–54.

47. Congo Belge. Service d'Hygiène du District Urbain de Léopoldville. Rapport annuel. Léopoldville, 1949, 1950, 1951, 1956, 1958.

48. Michiels A. *L'œuvre de la Croix-Rouge au Congo belge.* Université Libre de Bruxelles, 2000.

49. Anonymous. Du sang en conserve. *Zaire*, 31 January 1972, 12–17.

50. Dubois A. *La Croix-Rouge du Congo.* Brussels: Académie Royale des Sciences d'Outre-Mer, 1969.

51. Croix Rouge du Congo. Rapport annuel. Brussels, 1929 to 1959.

52. Beheyt P. Contribution à l'étude des hépatites en Afrique. L'hépatite épidémique et l'hépatite par inoculation. *Ann Soc Bel Med Trop* (1953), **33**: 297–340.

53. Institut d'Hygiène Marcel Wanson. Rapport annuel. Léopoldville, 1956.

54. Congo Belge. Rapport des Services Médicaux de la Province de Léopoldville. Léopoldville, 1957.

55. Congo Belge. Service d'Hygiène du District Urbain de Léopoldville. Rapport annuel. Léopoldville, 1958.

10 The other human immunodeficiency viruses

1. De Leys R et al. Isolation and partial characterization of an unusual human immunodeficiency retrovirus from two persons of west-central African origin. *J Virol* (1990), **64**: 1207–16.

2. Loussert-Ajaka I et al. Variability of HIV-1 group O strains isolated from Cameroonian patients living in France. *J Virol* (1995), **69**: 5640–9.

3. Nkengasong J et al. Antigenic evidence of the presence of the aberrant HIV-1ant70 virus in Cameroon and Gabon. *AIDS* (1993), 7: 1536–8.

4. Peeters M et al. Geographical distribution of HIV-1 group O viruses in Africa. *AIDS* (1997), **11**: 493–8.

5. Mauclère P et al. Serological and virological characterization of HIV-1 group O infection in Cameroon. *AIDS* (1997), **11**: 445–53.

6. Ayouba A et al. HIV-1 group O infection in Cameroon, 1986–1998. *Emerg Infect Dis* (2001), 7: 466–7.

7. Brennan C et al. The prevalence of diverse HIV-1 strains was stable in Cameroonian blood donors from 1996 to 2004. *JAIDS* (2008), **49**: 432–9.

8. Barin F et al. Prevalence of HIV-2 and HIV-1 group O infections among new HIV diagnoses in France: 2003–2006. *AIDS* (2007), **21**: 2351–3.

9. Arien KK et al. The replicative fitness of primary HIV-1 group M, HIV-1 group O, and HIV-2 isolates. *J Virol* (2005), **79**: 8979–90.

10. Vergne L et al. Biological and genetic characteristics of HIV infections in Cameroon reveals dual group M and O infections and a correlation between SI-inducing phenotype of the predominant CRF02_AG variant and disease stage. *Virology* (2003), **310**: 254–66.

11. Lemey P et al. The molecular population genetics of HIV-1 group O. *Genetics* (2004), **167**: 1059–68.

12. Roques P et al. Phylogenetic analysis of 49 newly derived HIV-1 group O strains: high viral diversity but no group M-like subtype structure. *Virology* (2002), **302**: 259–73.

13. Yamaguchi J et al. Near full-length genomes of 15 HIV-1 group O isolates. *AIDS Res Hum Retrovir* (2003), **19**: 979–88.

14. Simon F et al. Identification of a new HIV-1 distinct from group M and group O. *Nat Med* (1998), **4**: 1032–7.

15. Yamaguchi J et al. Identification of HIV-1 group N infections in a husband and wife in Cameroon: viral genome sequences provide evidence for horizontal transmission. *AIDS Res Hum Retrovir* (2006), **22**: 83–92.

16. Corbet A et al. *env* sequences of SIV from chimpanzees in Cameroon are strongly related to those of HIV group N from the same geographic area. *J Virol* (2000), **74**: 529–34.

17. Vallari A et al. Four new HIV-1 group N isolates from Cameroon: prevalence continues to be low. *AIDS Res Hum Retrovir* (2010), **26**: 109–15.

18. Takehisa J et al. Origin and biology of SIV in wild-living western gorillas. *J Virol* (2009), **83**: 1635–48.

19. Neel C et al. Molecular epidemiology of simian immunodeficiency virus infection in wild-living gorillas. *J Virol* (2010), **84**: 1464–76.
20. Plantier JC et al. A new human immunodeficiency virus derived from gorillas. *Nature Med* (2009), **15**: 871–2.
21. Clavel F et al. Isolation of a new human retrovirus from West African patients with AIDS. *Science* (1986), **233**: 343–6.
22. Clavel F et al. HIV-2 infection associated with AIDS in West Africa. *N Eng J Med* (1987), **316**: 1180–5.
23. Hirsch V et al. An African primate lentivirus (SIV$_{sm}$) closely related to HIV-2. *Nature* (1989), **339**: 389–91.
24. Marx PA et al. Isolation of a simian immunodeficiency virus related to HIV-2 from a west African pet sooty mangabey. *J Virol* (1991), **65**: 4480–5.
25. Gao F et al. Human infection by genetically diverse SIV$_{sm}$–related HIV-2 in West Africa. *Nature* (1992), **358**: 495–9.
26. Rey-Cuillé MA et al. SIV replicates to high levels in sooty mangabeys without inducing disease. *J Virol* (1998), **72**: 3872–86.
27. Santiago ML et al. Simian immunodeficiency virus infection in free-ranging sooty mangabeys (*Cercocebus atys atys*) from the Tai forest, Côte d'Ivoire: implications for the origin of epidemic HIV-2. *J Virol* (2005), **79**: 12515–27.
28. Chen Z et al. Genetic characterization of new West African SIV$_{sm}$: geographic clustering of household-derived SIV strains with HIV-2 subtypes and genetically diverse viruses from a single feral sooty mangabey troop. *J Virol* (1996), **70**: 3617–27.
29. Chen Z et al. HIV-2 seroprevalence and characterization of a distinct HIV-2 subtype from the natural range of SIV-infected sooty mangabey. *J Virol* (1997), **71**: 3953–60.
30. Poulsen AG et al. Prevalence of and mortality from HIV-2 in Bissau, West Africa. *Lancet* (1989), **1**: 827–31.
31. Poulsen AG et al. 9-year HIV-2 associated mortality in an urban community in Bissau, west Africa. *Lancet* (1997), **349**: 911–14.
32. Ricard D et al. The effects of HIV-2 in a rural area of Guinea-Bissau. *AIDS* (1994), **8**: 977–82.
33. Gottlieb GS et al. Lower levels of HIV-1 RNA in semen in HIV-2 compared with HIV-1 infection: implications for differences in transmission. *AIDS* (2006), **20**: 895–900.
34. Ghys P et al. The association between cervicovaginal HIV shedding, sexually transmitted diseases and immunosuppression in female sex workers in Abidjan, Côte d'Ivoire. *AIDS* (1997), **11**: F85–F93.
35. Van der Loeff M et al. Towards a better understanding of the epidemiology of HIV-2. *AIDS* (1999), **13**: S69–S84.

36. Poulsen AG et al. Risk factors of HIV-2 seropositivity among older people in Guinea-Bissau. A search for the early history of HIV-2 infection. *Scand J Infect Dis* (2000), **32**: 169–75.

37. Norrgren H et al. HIV-1, HIV-2, HTLV-I/II and *Treponema pallidum* infections: incidence, prevalence and HIV-2 associated mortality in an occupational cohort in Guinea-Bissau. *JAIDS* (1995), **9**: 422–8.

38. Wilkins A et al. The epidemiology of HIV infection in a rural area of Guinea-Bissau. *AIDS* (1993), **7**: 1119–22.

39. Larsen O et al. Declining HIV-2 prevalence and incidence among men in a community study from Guinea-Bissau. *AIDS* (1998), **12**: 1707–14.

40. Holmgren B et al. Dual infections with HIV-1, HIV-2 and HTLV-I are more common in older women than in men in Guinea-Bissau. *AIDS* (2003), **17**: 241–53.

41. Da Silva ZJ et al. Changes in prevalence and incidence of HIV-1, HIV-2 and dual infections in urban areas of Bissau, Guinea-Bissau: is HIV-2 disappearing? *AIDS* (2008), **22**: 1195–202.

42. Spiegel P et al. Prevalence of HIV infection in conflict affected and displaced people in seven sub-Saharan countries: a systematic review. *Lancet* (1997), **369**: 2187–95.

43. Gomes P et al. Transmission of HIV-2. *Lancet Infect Dis* (2003), **3**: 683–4.

44. Supervie V et al. Assessing the impact of mass rape on the incidence of HIV in conflict-affected countries. *AIDS* (2010), **24**: 2481–7.

45. Piedade J. Longstanding presence of HIV-2 in Guinea-Bissau (west Africa). *Acta Trop* (2000), **76**: 119–24.

46. Kawamura M et al. HIV-2 in West Africa in 1966. *Lancet* (1989), **1**: 385.

47. US Census Bureau. *HIV/AIDS surveillance data base*. Washington, 2006.

48. Bryceson A et al. HIV-2 associated AIDS in the 1970s. *Lancet* (1988), **2**: 221.

49. Saimot AG et al. HIV-2/LAV-2 in Portuguese man with AIDS (Paris, 1978) who had served in Angola in 1968–74. *Lancet* (1987), **1**: 688.

50. Ancelle R et al. Long incubation period for HIV-2 infection. *Lancet* (1987), **1**: 688–9.

51. Mota-Miranda A et al. HIV-2 infection with a long asymptomatic report. *J Infect* (1995), **31**: 163–4.

52. Lemey P et al. Tracing the origin and history of the HIV-2 epidemic. *Proc Natl Acad Sci U S A* (2003), **100**: 6588–92.

53. Wertheim JO et al. Dating the age of the SIV lineages that gave rise to HIV-1 and HIV-2. *PLoS Comput Biol* (2009), **5**: e1000377.

54. Mansson F et al. Trends of HIV-1 and HIV-2 prevalence among pregnant women in Guinea-Bissau, West Africa: possible effect of the civil war 1998–1999. *Sex Transm Infect* (2007), **83**: 463–7.

55. Pepin J et al. Parenteral transmission during excision and treatment of tuberculosis and trypanosomiasis may be responsible for the HIV-2 epidemic in Guinea-Bissau. *AIDS* (2006), **20**: 1303–11.

56. Ferreira FS. História da doença do sono na Guiné Portuguesa: IV-período de 1927 a 1932. *Boletim cultural da Guiné Portuguesa* (1961), **16**: 139–57.

57. Ferreira FS. História da doença do sono na Guiné Portuguesa: V- período de 1933 a 1946. *Boletim cultural da Guiné Portuguesa* (1961), **16**: 313–47.

58. Ferreira FS. História da doença do sono na Guiné Portuguesa: VII- período de 1947 a 1956. *Boletim cultural da Guiné Portuguesa* (1961), **16**: 569–606.

59. Carreira A. *Mandingas da Guiné Portuguesa*. Lisbon: Centre de Estudos da Guiné Portuguesa, 1947.

60. Johnson MC. Becoming a Muslim, becoming a person: female circumcision, religious identity, and personhood in Guinea-Bissau. In Shell-Duncan B and Hernlund Y (eds.), *Female circumcision in Africa. Culture, Controversy and Change*. Boulder: Lynne Rienner Publishers, 2000.

61. Jamot E. La lutte contre la maladie du sommeil au Cameroun. *Ann Instit Pasteur (Paris)* (1938), **48**: 481–539.

62. Pepin J et al. Noble goals, unforeseen consequences: the control of tropical diseases in colonial Central Africa and the iatrogenic transmission of blood-borne viruses. *Trop Med Inter Health* (2008), **13**: 744–53.

63. Pinto AR. Relatório sobre a actividade da missão permanente de estudo e combate da doença do sono e outros endemas na Guiné Portuguesa: referente ao ano de 1955. *An Inst Med Trop (Lisb)* (1956), **13**: 275–332.

64. Pinto AR. Relatório anual da missão permanente de estudo e combate da doença do sono e outros endemas na Guiné Portuguesa (1958). *An Inst Med Trop (Lisb)* (1960), **17**: 817–905.

65. Pinto AR and da Costa FC. La lutte contre la lèpre en Guinée Portuguaise. *Boletim cultural da Guiné Portuguesa* (1959), **14**: 603–32.

11   From the Congo to the Caribbean

1. Bezy F. Principes pour l'organisation du développement économique au Congo. *Zaire* (1959), **13**: 3–55.

2. Romaniuk A. *Démographie congolaise au milieu du XXe siècle*. Presses Universitaires de Louvain, 2006.

3. Gondola C. *The history of Congo*. Westport: Greenwood Press, 2002.

4. Romaniuk A. *La fécondité des populations congolaises*. Paris: Mouton, 1967.

5. Schwers GA. Quand y aura-t-il des médecins noirs en Afrique centrale? *Bulletin du Centre d'Études des Problèmes Sociaux Indigènes* (1952), **19**: 91–111.
6. MacGaffey G et al. *US Army area handbook for the Republic of Congo (Leopoldville)*. Washington: The American University, 1962.
7. Ndaywel è Nziem I. *Histoire générale du Congo. De l'héritage ancien à la République Démocratique*. Paris: Duculot, 1996.
8. Bouvier P. *L'accession du Congo belge à l'indépendance. Essai d'analyse sociologique*. Université Libre de Bruxelles, 1965.
9. Ministère des Affaires Africaines. *La situation économique du Congo belge et du Ruanda-Urundi en 1959*. Brussels, 1960.
10. Gordon K. *The United Nations in the Congo. A quest for peace.* Washington: Carnegie Endowment for International Peace, 1962.
11. Ryelandt B. Inflation et structure des prix en période de décolonisation. *Cah Econ Soc* (1965), **3**: 3–48.
12. Willame JC. *Patrice Lumumba. La crise congolaise revisitée*. Paris: Karthala, 1990.
13. De Witte L. *The assassination of Lumumba*. London: Verso, 2001.
14. Caprasse P et al. Les conditions de vie des familles d'enseignants à Léopoldville. *Cah Econ Soc* (1965), **3**: 411–54.
15. Houyoux C et al. Les conditions de vie dans soixante familles à Kinshasa. *Cah Econ Soc* (1970), **8**: 99–132.
16. Huybrechts A et al. *Du Congo au Zaire, 1960–1980. Essai de bilan*. Brussels: CRISP, 1980.
17. House A. *The UN in the Congo. The political and civilian efforts.* Washington: University Press of America, 1978.
18. Gendebien PH. *L'intervention des Nations Unies au Congo, 1960–1964*. Paris: Mouton, 1967.
19. Centre de Recherche et d'information socio-politique. *Congo 1963*. Brussels: CRISP, 1964.
20. Shilts R. *And the band played on. Politics, people and the AIDS epidemic*. New York: Penguin Books, 1987.
21. Fullerton G. *L'UNESCO au Congo*. Paris: UNESCO, 1964.
22. Kuyu C. *Les Haitiens au Congo*. Paris: L'Harmattan, 2006.
23. Kuyu C, personal communication.
24. République démocratique du Congo. *Étude socio-démographique de Kinshasa 1967*. Kinshasa, 1969.
25. Rotberg R. *Haiti. The politics of squalor*. Boston: Houghton Mifflin, 1971.
26. Verhaegen B. *Femmes zairoises de Kisangani. Combats pour la survie*. Louvain-la-Neuve: Centre d'Histoire de l'Afrique, 1990.

27. Denis J. Léopoldville. Étude de géographie urbaine et sociale. *Zaire* (1956), **10**: 563–611.

28. Sonnet J et al. Early AIDS cases originating from Zaire and Burundi (1962–1976). *Scand J Infect Dis* (1987), **19**: 511–17.

29. Kolonga Molei. *Kinshasa, ce village d'hier*. Kinshasa, 1979.

30. Findlay T. *The Blue Helmets' first war. Use of force by the UN in the Congo, 1960–64*. Clementsport: Canadian Peacekeeping Press, 1999.

31. Van Grunderbeeck R et al. *Quarante-six hommes en colère. Violations par l'ONU au Katanga*. Brussels: Guyot, 1962.

32. Spooner KA. *Canada, the Congo crisis, and the UN peacekeeping, 1960–64*. Vancouver: UBC Press, 2009.

33. Centers for Disease Control. Opportunistic infections and Kaposi's sarcoma among Haitians in the United States. *MMWR* (1982), **31**: 353–61.

34. Vieira J et al. Opportunistic infections in previously healthy Haitian immigrants. *N Eng J Med* (1983), **308**: 125–9.

35. Moskowitz LB et al. Unusual cause of death in Haitians residing in Miami: high prevalence of opportunistic infections. *JAMA* (1983), **250**: 1187–91.

36. Malebranche R et al. Acquired immunodeficiencies syndrome with severe gastrointestinal manifestations in Haiti. *Lancet* (1983), **2**: 873–8.

37. Pitchenik A et al. Opportunistic infections and Kaposi's sarcoma among Haitians: evidence of a new acquired immunodeficiency state. *Ann Int Med* (1983), **98**: 277–84.

38. Laverdière M et al. AIDS in Haitian immigrants and in a Caucasian woman closely associated with Haitians. *Can Med Assoc J* (1983), **129**: 1209–12.

39. Farmer P. *AIDS and accusation. Haiti and the geography of blame*. Berkeley: University of California Press, 2006.

40. Francisque E. *La structure économique et sociale d'Haiti*. Port-au-Prince: Imprimerie Henri Deschamps, 1986.

41. Barros J. *Haiti. De 1804 à nos jours (2 volumes)*. Paris: L'Harmattan, 1984.

42. Jaffe H. AIDS in the United States: the first 1000 cases. *J Infect Dis* (1983), **148**: 339–45.

43. Boncy M et al. Acquired immunodeficiency in Haitians. *N Eng J Med* (1983), **308**: 1419–20.

44. Greco R. Haiti and the stigma of AIDS. *Lancet* (1983), **2**: 515–16.

45. Gold H. *Best nightmare on Earth. A life in Haiti*. New York: Prentice Hall Press, 1991.

46. Péan LJR. *Haiti, économie politique de la corruption. IV: L'ensauvagement macoute et ses conséquences 1957–1990*. Paris: Maisonneuve et Larose, 2007.

47. Comhaire-Sylvain S. *Les montagnards de la région de Kenscoff. Une société Kongo au-delà des mers.* Bandundu: CEEBA, 1984.
48. Stanford JD. *Spartacus international gay guide 1982.* Amsterdam: Spartacus, 1982.
49. Stanford JD. *Spartacus 85. Guide for gay men.* Amsterdam: Spartacus, 1985.
50. Fettner AG et al. *The truth about AIDS. Evolution of an epidemic.* New York: Holt, Rinehart and Winston, 1985.
51. Saint-Gérard Y. *L'état de mal.* Toulouse: Eché, 1984.
52. Saint-Gérard Y. *Haiti. Mort d'une dictature.* Toulouse: Privat, 1986.
53. Altema R et al. Only homosexual Haitians, not all Haitians. *Ann Int Med* (1983), **99**: 877–8.
54. Pape J et al. Characteristics of AIDS in Haiti. *N Eng J Med* (1983), **309**: 945–50.
55. Barry M et al. Haiti and the AIDS connection. *J Chron Dis* (1984), **37**: 593–5.
56. Pape J et al. AIDS in Haiti: 1982–1992. *Clin Infect Dis* (1993), **17**: S341–S345.
57. Mitacek E et al. Cancer in Haiti 1979–84: distribution of various forms of cancer according to geographical area and sex. *Int J Cancer* (1986), **38**: 9–16.
58. Liautaud B et al. Le sarcome de Kaposi en Haiti: foyer méconnu ou récemment apparu. *Ann Dermatol Venereol* (1983), **110**: 213–19.
59. Thijs A. L'angiosarcomatose de Kaposi au Congo belge et au Rwanda-Urundi. *Ann Soc Bel Med Trop* (1957), **37**: 295–311.
60. Pélissier A. La maladie de Kaposi en Afrique Noire. A propos de 18 cas. *Bull Soc Pathol Exot* (1953), **46**: 832–9.
61. Gigase PL. Quelques aspects du sarcome de Kaposi en Afrique. *Ann Soc Bel Med Trop* (1965), **45**: 195–210.
62. Hymes K et al. Kaposi's sarcoma in homosexual men – a report of eight cases. *Lancet* (1981), **2**: 598–600.
63. Urmacher C et al. Outbreak of Kaposi's sarcoma with cytomegalovirus infection in young homosexual men. *Am J Med* (1982), **74**: 569–75.
64. Selik RM et al. Acquired immune deficiency syndrome (AIDS) trends in the United States, 1978–1982. *Am J Med* (1984), **76**: 493–500.
65. Bacchetti P et al. Incubation period of AIDS in San Francisco. *Nature* (1989), **338**: 251–3.
66. Beral V et al. Kaposi's sarcoma among persons with AIDS: a sexually transmitted infection? *Lancet* (1990), **335**: 123–8.
67. Noel G. Another case of AIDS in the pre-AIDS era. *Rev Infect Dis* (1988), **10**: 668–9.

68. Johnson W et al. AIDS in Haiti. In Levy J (ed.), *AIDS. Pathogenesis and treatment*. New York: Dekker, 1989.
69. Korber B et al. Timing the ancestor of the HIV-1 pandemic strains. *Science* (2000), **288**: 1789–96.
70. Gilbert M. The emergence of HIV/AIDS in the Americas and beyond. *Proc Natl Acad Sci U S A* (2007), **104**: 18566–70.
71. Robbins K et al. US HIV-1 epidemic: date of origin, population history, and characterization of early strains. *J Virol* (2003), **77**: 6359–66.
72. Pape J et al. The epidemiology of AIDS in Haiti refutes the claims of Gilbert et al. *Proc Natl Acad Sci U S A* (2008), **105**: E13.
73. Worobey M et al. Reply to Pape et al: the phylogeography of HIV-1 group M subtype B. *Proc Natl Acad Sci U S A* (2008), **105**: E16.
74. Boulos R et al. HIV-1 in Haitian women, 1982–88. *JAIDS* (1990), **3**: 721–8.

12 The blood trade

1. Cuthbertson B et al. Safety of albumin preparations manufactured from plasma not tested for HIV antibody. *Lancet* (1987), **2**: 41.
2. Cuthbertson B et al. The viral safety of intravenous immunoglobulin. *J Infect* (1987), **15**: 125–33.
3. Dreskin CA et al. Plasmapheresis-associated hepatitis A outbreak. *MMWR* (1974), **23**: 275–6.
4. Muss N et al. Epidemic outbreak of non-A non-B hepatitis in a plasmapheresis center. I: Epidemiological observations. *Infection* (1985), **113**: 57–60.
5. Laskus T et al. Follow-up of non-A non-B hepatitis oubreak in plasmapheresis unit. *Lancet* (1989), **1**: 391.
6. Avila C et al. The epidemiology of HIV transmission among paid plasma donors, Mexico City, Mexico. *AIDS* (1989), **3**: 631–3.
7. del Rio C et al. AIDS in Mexico: lessons learned and implications for developing countries. *AIDS* (2002), **16**: 1445–57.
8. Volkow P et al. The role of commercial plasmapheresis banks on the AIDS epidemic in Mexico. *Rev Invest Clin* (1998), **50**: 221–6.
9. Volkow P et al. Transfusion-associated HIV infection in Mexico related to paid blood donors; HIV epidemic. *Int J STD AIDS* (2004), **15**: 337–42.
10. Volkow P et al. Plasma trade and the HIV epidemic. *Lancet* (1997), **349**: 327–8.
11. Banerjee K et al. Outbreak of HIV seropositivity among commercial plasma donors in Pune, India. *Lancet* (1989), **2**: 166.

12. Wu Z et al. Prevalence of HIV infection among former commercial plasma donors in rural eastern China. *Health Policy Plan* (2001), **16**: 41–6.

13. Mastro T et al. The legacy of unhygienic plasma collection in China. *AIDS* (2006), **20**: 1451–2.

14. He N et al. The HIV epidemic in China: history, response, and challenge. *Cell Res* (2005), **15**: 825–32.

15. Ji G et al. Correlates of HIV infection among former blood/plasma donors in rural China. *AIDS* (2006), **20**: 585–91.

16. Ferguson J. *Papa Doc, Baby Doc. Haiti and the Duvaliers*. Oxford: Basil Blackwell, 1987.

17. Severo R. Impoverished Haitians sell plasma for use in the US. *New York Times*, 28 January 1972.

18. Abbott E. *Haiti. The Duvaliers and their legacy*. London: Robert Hale, 1988.

19. Sapène R. *Procès à Baby Doc*. Paris: Philippe Daudy, 1973.

20. Anonymous. Dynastic republicanism in Haiti. *Polit Q* (1973), **44**: 77–84.

21. Heinl RD et al. *Written in blood. The story of the Haitian people 1492– 1995*. Lanham: University Press of America, 1996.

22. Hagen PJ. *Blood. Gift of merchandise*. New York: Alan R Liss, 1982.

23. Starr D. *Blood. An epic history of medicine and commerce*. New York: HarperCollins, 2002.

24. Fortuné G. *Haiti, une nation au service d'une minorité*. Brussels: Éditions Vie Ouvrière, 1977.

25. Anonymous. Haiti blood plasma curb poses problems. *The Afro-American*, 18 January 1973.

26. Gold H. *Best nightmare on Earth. A life in Haiti*. New York: Prentice Hall Press, 1991.

27. Deschamps MM et al. HIV infection in Haiti: natural history and disease progression. *AIDS* (2000), **14**: 2515–21.

28. Centers for Disease Control. Opportunistic infections and Kaposi's sarcoma among Haitians in the United States. *MMWR* (1982), **31**: 353–61.

29. Vieira J et al. Opportunistic infections in previously healthy Haitian immigrants. *N Eng J Med* (1983), **308**: 125–9.

30. Moskowitz LB et al. Unusual cause of death in Haitians residing in Miami: high prevalence of opportunistic infections. *JAMA* (1983), **250**: 1187–91.

31. Malebranche R et al. Acquired immunodeficiencies syndrome with severe gastrointestinal manifestations in Haiti. *Lancet* (1983), **2**: 873–8.

32. Pitchenik A. Opportunistic infections and Kaposi's sarcoma among Haitians: evidence of a new acquired immunodeficiency state. *Ann Int Med* (1983), **98**: 277–84.
33. Stanford JD. *Spartacus international gay guide 1982*. Amsterdam: Spartacus, 1982.
34. Pape J et al. Characteristics of AIDS in Haiti. *N Eng J Med* (1983), **309**: 945–50.
35. Fischl M et al. An acquired immunodeficiency syndrome among Haitians: an update. *Ann N Y Acad Sci* (1984), **437**: 325–33.
36. Guerin JM et al. AIDS: specific aspects of the disease in Haiti. *Ann N Y Acad Sci* (1984), **437**: 254–63.
37. Pape J et al. The acquired immunodeficiency syndrome in Haiti. *Ann Int Med* (1985), **103**: 674–8.
38. The Collaborative Study Group of AIDS in Haitian-Americans: risk factors for AIDS among Haitians residing in the United States. *JAMA* (1987), **257**: 635–9.
39. Boulos R et al. HIV-1 in Haitian women, 1982–88. *JAIDS* (1990), **3**: 721–8.
40. Pape J et al. Prevalence of HIV infection and high-risk activities in Haiti. *JAIDS* (1990), **3**: 995–1001.
41. Farmer P. *Infections and inequalities. The modern plagues*. Berkeley: University of California Press, 1999.
42. Desvarieux M et al. HIV and AIDS in Haiti: recent developments. *AIDS Care* (1991), **3**: 271–9.
43. Levine PH. HIV infection in hemophilia. *J Clin Apher* (1993), **8**: 120–5.
44. Levine OH. The acquired immunodeficiency syndrome in persons with hemophilia. *Ann Int Med* (1985), **103**: 723–6.
45. Kroner BL et al. HIV-1 infection incidence among persons with hemophilia in the United States and Western Europe, 1978–1990. *JAIDS* (1994), **7**: 279–86.
46. Cuthbert RJG et al. Five year prospective study of HIV infection in the Edinburgh haemophiliac cohort. *Br Med J* (1990), **301**: 956–61.
47. Fatkenheuer G et al. *Marchands de sang*. Lausanne: Pierre-Marcel Favre, 1986.
48. World Health Organization. International plasma trafficking. *Wkly Epidemiol Rec* (2000), **75**: 289–96.
49. Kumar S. Austria investigates allegations of tainted-blood exports. *Lancet* (2000), **356**: 920.
50. Picard A. Blood trail: Canada still lacks controls on plasma trade, inquiry told. Toronto: Globe and Mail, 14 December 1995.

51. Krever H. Commission of inquiry of the blood system in Canada. Final report. www.hc-sc.gc.ca/ahc-asc/activit/com/krever-eng.php.

13   The globalisation

1. Kawamura M. HIV-2 in West Africa in 1966. *Lancet* (1989), **1**: 385.
2. Dube DK et al. Serological and nucleic acid analyses for HIV and HTLV infection on archival human plasma samples from Zaire. *Virology* (1994), **202**: 379–89.
3. Wendler I et al. Seroepidemiology of HIV in Africa. *Br Med J* (1986), **293**: 782–5.
4. US Census Bureau. *HIV/AIDS surveillance data base.* Washington, 2006.
5. Winkler E et al. Seroepidemiology of human retrovirus in Gabon. *AIDS* (1989), **3**: 106–7.
6. Merlin M et al. Surveillance épidémiologique du syndrome d'immunodépression acquise dans six états d'Afrique centrale. *Med Trop (Mars)* (1988), **48**: 381–9.
7. Clumeck N et al. Seroepidemiological studies of HLTV-III antibody prevalence among selected groups of heterosexual Africans. *JAMA* (1985), **254**: 2599–602.
8. Van de Perre P et al. Female prostitutes: a risk group for infection with HTLV-III. *Lancet* (1985), **2**: 524–7.
9. Vandersypen M. Femmes libres de Kigali. *Cah Etud Afr* (1977), **17**: 95–120.
10. Meheus A et al. Prevalence of gonorrhoea in prostitutes in a Central African town. *Br J Vener Dis* (1974), **50**: 50–2.
11. Larson A. Social context of HIV transmission in Africa: historical and cultural bases of East and Central African relations. *Rev Infect Dis* (1989), **11**: 716–31.
12. Vidal N et al. HIV type 1 diversity and antiretroviral drug resistance mutations in Burundi. *AIDS Res Hum Retrovir* (2007), **23**: 175–80.
13. Servais J et al. HIV type 1 pol gene diversity and archived nevirapine resistance mutation in pregnant women in Rwanda. *AIDS Res Hum Retrovir* (2004), **20**: 279–83.
14. Anonymous. HIV type 1 variation in World Health Organization sponsored vaccine evaluation sites: genetic screening, sequence analysis, and preliminary biological characterization of selected viral strains. *AIDS Res Hum Retrovir* (1994), **10**: 1327–43.
15. Nzila N et al. The prevalence of infection with HIV over a 10-year period in rural Zaire. *N Eng J Med* (1988), **318**: 276–9.

16. Pepin J et al. The impact of HIV infection on the epidemiology and treatment of *Trypanosoma brucei gambiense* sleeping sickness in Nioki, Zaire. *Am J Trop Med Hyg* (1992), **47**: 133–40.

17. Green S et al. Stable seroprevalence of HIV-1 infection in pregnancy in rural Zaire. *AIDS* (1994), **8**: 397–8.

18. Mokili JL et al. Genetic heterogeneity of HIV-1 subtypes in Kimpese, rural Democratic Republic of Congo. *AIDS Res Hum Retrovir* (1999), **15**: 655–64.

19. Vidal N et al. Distribution of HIV-1 variants in the Democratic Republic of Congo suggests increase of subtype C in Kinshasa between 1997 and 2002. *JAIDS* (2005), **40**: 456–62.

20. Gray RR et al. Spatial phylodynamics of HIV-1 epidemic emergence in East Africa. *AIDS* (2009): F9–F17.

21. Dalai SC et al. Evolution and molecular epidemiology of subtype C HIV-1 in Zimbabwe. *AIDS* (2009), **23**: 2523–32.

22. Glynn J et al. The development of the HIV epidemic in Karonga district, Malawi. *AIDS* (2001), **15**: 2025–9.

23. McCormak G et al. Early evolution of the HIV type 1 subtype C epidemic in rural Malawi. *J Virol* (2002), **76**: 12890–9.

24. Robertson C. Women in the urban economy. In Hay MJ and Stichter S (eds.), *African women south of the Sahara*. London: Longman, 1984.

25. Zehender G. Population dynamics of HIV-1 subtype B in a cohort of men-having-sex-with-men in Rome, Italy. *JAIDS* (2010), **55**: 156–60.

26. Brunet JB et al. Epidemiological aspects of AIDS in France. *Ann N Y Acad Sci* (1984), **437**: 334–9.

27. Hué S et al. Genetic analysis reveals the complex structure of HIV-1 transmission within defined risk groups. *Proc Natl Acad Sci U S A* (2005), **102**: 4425–9.

28. Picard A. *The gift of death. Confronting Canada's tainted blood tragedy.* Toronto: HarperCollins, 1998.

29. Lukashov VV et al. Evidence for HIV-1 strain of US intravenous drug users as founders of AIDS epidemic among intravenous drug users in northern Europe. *AIDS Res Hum Retrovir* (1996), **12**: 1179–83.

30. Thomson M. Increasing HIV-1 genetic diversity in Europe. *Clin Infect Dis* (2007), **196**: 1120–4.

31. Paraskevis D et al. Increasing prevalence of HIV-1 subtype A in Greece: estimating epidemic history and origin. *Clin Infect Dis* (2007), **196**: 1167–76.

32. Dietrich U et al. HIV-1 strains from India are highly divergent from prototypic African and US/European strains, but are linked to a South African isolate. *AIDS* (1993), **7**: 23–7.

33. Lakhashe S et al. HIV infection in India: epidemiology, molecular epidemiology and pathogenesis. *J Biosc* (2008), **33**: 515–25.

34. Grez M et al. Genetic analysis of HIV-1 and HIV-2 mixed infections in India reveals a recent spread of HIV-1 and HIV-2 from a single ancestor for each of these viruses. *J Virol* (1994), **68**: 2161–8.

35. Bredell H et al. Genetic characterization of HIV-1 from migrant workers in three South African gold mines. *AIDS Res Hum Retrovir* (1998), **14**: 677–84.

36. Jain MK et al. Epidemiology of HIV and AIDS in India. *AIDS* (1994), **8** (suppl 2): S61–S75.

37. Beyrer C et al. Overland heroin trafficking routes and HIV-1 spread in south and south-east Asia. *AIDS* (2000), **14**: 75–83.

38. Weninger BG et al. The epidemiology of HIV infection and AIDS in Thailand. *AIDS* (1991), **5**(suppl 2): S71–S85.

39. Hemelaar J et al. Global and regional distribution of HIV-1 genetic subtypes and recombinants in 2004. *AIDS* (2006), **20**: W13–W23.

40. Liao H et al. Phylodynamic analysis of the dissemination of HIV-1 CRF01_AE in Vietnam. *Virology* (2009), **391**: 51–6.

41. Li Y et al. Explosive HIV-1 subtype B epidemics in Asia driven by geographic and risk group founder events. *Virology* (2010), **402**: 223–7.

42. Deng X et al. The epidemic origin and molecular properties of B': a founder strain of the HIV-1 transmission in Asia. *AIDS* (2008), **22**: 1851–64.

43. Ligon-Borden BL. Dr Jonathan Mann: champion of human rights in the fight against AIDS. *Sem Pediatr Infect Dis* (2003), **14**: 314–22.

44. Fee E et al. Jonathan Mann, HIV/AIDS, and human rights. *J Public Health Policy* (2008), **29**: 54–71.

45. Camus A. *La peste*. Paris: Gallimard, 1947.

46. Cohen J. The rise and fall of Projet Sida. *Science* (1997), **278**: 1565–8.

47. Ryder RW. Tribute to Jonathan Mann. *AIDS* (1998), **12**: ii–v.

48. Mann J et al. *AIDS in the world. A global report*. Harvard University Press, 1992.

49. Mann J et al. *AIDS in the world II*. Oxford University Press, 1996.

50. Tarantola D et al. Jonathan Mann: founder of the health and human rights movement. *Am J Public Health* (2006), **96**: 1942–3.

14   Assembling the puzzle

1. Neel C et al. Molecular epidemiology of simian immunodeficiency virus infection in wild-living gorillas. *J Virol* (2010), **84**: 1464–76.

2. Wolfe N et al. Exposure to nonhuman primates in rural Cameroon. *Emerg Infect Dis* (2004), **10**: 2094–9.

3. Sautter G. Notes sur la construction du chemin de fer Congo–Océan (1921–1934). *Cah Etud Afr* (1967), **7**: 219–99.
4. Mathers BM et al. Global epidemiology of injecting drug use and HIV among people who inject drugs: a systematic review. *Lancet* (2008), **372**: 1733–45.
5. Muller-Trutwin M et al. Increase of HIV-1 subtype A in Central African Republic. *JAIDS* (1999), **21**: 164–71.
6. Vidal N et al. High genetic diversity of HIV-1 strains in Chad, West Central Africa. *JAIDS* (2003), **33**: 239–46.
7. Butler I et al. HIV genetic diversity: biological and public health consequences. *Curr HIV Res* (2007), **5**: 23–45.
8. Peeters M et al. Genetic diversity of HIV in Africa: impact on diagnosis, treatment, vaccine development and trials. *AIDS* (2003), **17**: 2547–60.
9. Vidal N et al. Unprecedented degree of HIV-1 group M genetic diversity in the Democratic Republic of Congo suggests that the HIV-1 pandemic originated in Central Africa. *J Virol* (2000), **74**: 10498–507.
10. Kalish M et al. Recombinant viruses and early global HIV-1 epidemic. *Emerg Infect Dis* (2004), **10**: 1227–34.
11. Zhu T et al. An African HIV-1 sequence from 1959 and implications for the origin of the epidemic. *Nature* (1998), **391**: 594–7.
12. Worobey M et al. Direct evidence of extensive diversity of HIV-1 in Kinshasa by 1960. *Nature* (2008), **55**: 661–4.
13. Sonnet J et al. Early AIDS cases originating from Zaire and Burundi (1962–1976). *Scand J Infect Dis* (1987), **19**: 511–17.
14. Desmyter J et al. Anti LAV-HTLV-III in Kinshasa mothers in 1970 and 1980. Paris: International Conference on AIDS, June 1985.
15. Merlin M et al. Surveillance épidémiologique du syndrome d'immunodépression acquise dans six états d'Afrique centrale. *Med Trop (Mars)* (1988), **48**: 381–9.
16. Infor-Congo. *Congo Belge et Rwanda-Urundi. Guide du voyageur.* Brussels: Office de l'Information et des Relations Publiques pour le Congo Belge et le Rwanda-Urundi, 1958.
17. Beheyt P. Contribution à l'étude des hépatites en Afrique. L'hépatite épidémique et l'hépatite par inoculation. *Ann Soc Bel Med Trop* (1953), **33**: 297–340.
18. La Fontaine JS. *City politics. A study of Léopoldville, 1962–63.* Cambridge University Press, 1970.
19. Raymaekers P. *L'organisation des zones de squatting. Élément de résorption du chômage structurel dans les milieux urbains des pays en voie de développement. Application au milieu urbain de Léopoldville.* Paris: Éditions Universitaires, 1964.

20. Comhaire-Sylvain S. *Femmes de Kinshasa, hier et aujourd'hui*. Paris: Mouton, 1968.
21. Illiffe J. *The African AIDS epidemic. A history*. Athens: Ohio University Press, 2006.
22. US Census Bureau. *HIV/AIDS surveillance data base*. Washington, 2006.
23. Boulos R et al. HIV-1 in Haitian women, 1982–88. *JAIDS* (1990), **3**: 721–8.
24. Jacquez J et al. Role of the primary infection in epidemics of HIV infection in gay cohorts. *JAIDS* (1994), **7**: 1169–84.
25. Byers R et al. Estimating AIDS infection rates in the San Francisco cohort. *AIDS* (1988), **2**: 207–10.
26. Foley B et al. Apparent founder effect during the early years of the San Francisco HIV-1 epidemic (1978–79). *AIDS Res Hum Retrovir* (2000), **15**: 1463–9.
27. Moore JD et al. HTLV-III seropositivity in 1971–72 parenteral drug abusers – a case of false positives or evidence of viral exposure. *N Eng J Med* (1986), **314**: 1387–8.
28. Des Jarlais DC. Risk reduction for AIDS among intravenous drug users. *Ann Int Med* (1985), **103**: 755–9.
29. Garrett L. *The coming plague. Newly emerging diseases in a world out of balance*. New York: Penguin Books, 1994.
30. Bacchetti P et al. Incubation period of AIDS in San Francisco. *Nature* (1989), **338**: 251–3.
31. Busch MP et al. Risk of HIV transmission by blood transfusions before the implementation of HIV-1 antibody screening. *Transfusion* (1991), **31**: 4–11.
32. Kroner BL et al. HIV-1 infection incidence among persons with hemophilia in the United States and Western Europe, 1978–1990. *JAIDS* (1994), **7**: 279–86.
33. Goedert JJ et al. A prospective study of HIV-1 infection and the development of AIDS in subjects with hemophilia. *N Eng J Med* (1989), **321**: 1141–8.
34. Evatt BL et al. Coincidental appearance of LAV/HTLV-III antibodies in hemophiliacs and the onset of the AIDS epidemic. *N Eng J Med* (1985), **312**: 483–6.
35. Lee CA. The best of times, the worst of times: a story of haemophilia. *Clin Med* (2009), **5**: 453–8.
36. Shilts R. *And the band played on. Politics, people and the AIDS epidemic*. New York: Penguin Books, 1987.
37. Holtgrave DR et al. Updated annual transmission rates in the United States, 1977–2006. *JAIDS* (2009), **50**: 236–8.

APPENDIX
Classification of retroviruses

For readers unfamiliar with virology, this section reviews a few concepts, which are summarised in the table. HIV-1 and HIV-2 are the two human 'retroviruses' that cause AIDS. To replicate, retroviruses transcribe RNA into DNA, which is then integrated into the DNA genome of the human host cells. This process is the reverse of what normally happens (DNA transcripted into RNA), hence their name. Retroviruses are further subdivided into 'lentiviruses' (HIV-1 and HIV-2), 'oncoviruses' (HTLV-I, the first retrovirus isolated from humans, which does not cause AIDS but sometimes cancer or paraplegia) and 'spumaviruses' (not pathogenic).

Of course, the pandemic is caused by HIV-1. HIV-2 differed enough, genetically, from HIV-1 to be considered a distinct virus. It remained confined to West Africa, is less transmissible and less pathogenic than HIV-1 and slowly disappeared while HIV-1 spread throughout the world. HIV-1 infection is 100 times more common than HIV-2; when authors use the term HIV, in practice it generally means HIV-1.

Simian immunodeficiency viruses (SIVs) are a diversified group of retroviruses that infect apes and monkeys. They are a crucial part of the story: both HIV-1 and HIV-2 are simian viruses that managed to spread into human populations. Their name is something of a misnomer, because most apes and monkeys tolerate SIV infections rather well, without developing any immune deficiency, unless the virus is experimentally transmitted to a non-human primate species which is not the normal host of a given type of SIV.

Virus	Groups	Subtypes	Distribution	Disease
HIV-1	group M	subtype A	East Africa, central Africa, Eastern Europe, Pakistan	AIDS
		subtype B	North America, Western Europe, Australia, Thailand, China. Rare in central Africa	AIDS
		subtype C	Southern Africa, central Africa, India, China. Represents 50% of all HIV-1 infections worldwide	AIDS
		subtype D	East Africa, central Africa	AIDS
		CRF01_AE	Thailand, other parts of Asia, central Africa	AIDS
		CRF02_AG	West Africa, parts of central Africa	AIDS
		all other subtypes and recombinants	central Africa, various other regions	AIDS
	group O		Cameroon and adjacent countries	AIDS
	group N		Cameroon	AIDS
	group P		Cameroon	AIDS
HIV-2	group A		Guinea-Bissau, The Gambia, Senegal	AIDS
	group B		Ivory Coast	AIDS
	groups C to H		Sierra Leone, Liberia each found in only one human	unclear
HTLV-I			worldwide	1–5% cancer
				< 5% paraplegia
HTLV-II			Americas, Africa	paraplegia?
simian foamy virus			worldwide among humans exposed to apes or monkeys	none

Index

Abidjan, 85
Abomg-Mbang, 127
Abumonbazi, 9
Accra, 84, 85
Adoumas district, 92
African trypanosomiasis
  clinical characteristics of, 120
  control of, 120, 122–3, 124, 128–31,
    145, 146–7, 156–7, 177
  epidemiology of, 121, 127–8, 138,
    141–2, 146–7, 177
  treatment of, 4, 121–2, 125–8, 139,
    145, 151
  see also arsenical drugs, pentamidine,
    suramin
Afrikaners, 12
Afrique Équatoriale Française, 87–8
  economy of, 228
  hepatitis C in, 112, 140
  history of, xiii, 34, 64–6, 69, 74–5
  Kaposi's sarcoma in, 193
  medical services in, 36–7, 116,
    118–38
  population of, 68, 73
  prostitution in, 93, 97–9
  see also Central African Republic,
    Chad, Congo-Brazzaville, Gabon
Afrique Occidentale Française, 63,
  64, 124
Akonolinga, 127
albumin, 197–8, 206, 232
Al-Fateh Pediatric Hospital, 108
Algeria, 120, 219
Angola, 9, 13–14, 73, 100, 108, 173,
  175, 180
  see also Cabinda
Annabon island, 138
antimonial drugs, 137
antiserum, 55, 152–3, 154, 219

Antonetti, Raphael, 36
Antwerp, 145, 181
Antwerp, Institute of Tropical
  Medicine, 7, 54–5, 143, 152,
  155, 157
Arkansas, 207–8
Armour Pharmaceutical, 202
arsenical drugs, 4, 114–15, 121, 123,
  125, 131, 133, 142, 144–5, 148,
  163–5
  see also atoxyl, melarsoprol,
  orsanine, tryparsamide, trypoxyl
Atlanta, 1, 52
atoxyl, 125, 128
Auclert, Jean, 37, 38
Augouard, Prosper, 63–4, 98
Austria, 207
autopsies, 24, 33, 36–9, 48, 53, 152
Ayos, 122

Babunda, 87
Bacongo district, 98
Bafia, 123
Baholoholo, 88
Bakongo, 59, 71–3, 100, 101
Bakota, 45
Bakula, 77–8
Baluba, 77–8, 87, 95
Bandalungwa district, 101
Bandim, 176
Bangkok, 106
Bangui, 63, 64–5, 70, 73, 210, 212
Bantu, 44, 59, 140, 221
Bapende, 87
Bapoto, 77–8
Bari, 106
Barumbu district, 96, 100, 160, 166
Barumbu, Carte de, 96
Bas-Congo province, 148, 150, 227, 228

Basonge, 77–8
Basuku, 77–8
Batetela, 77–8
Bayaka, 77–8
Bayombe, 45
Beheyt, Paul, 164
Belgian Congo *see* Congo, Democratic
    Republic of
Belgian Red Cross, 158
Belgium
    and the colonisation of the Congo,
        67–8, 73–5
    and the decolonisation of the Congo,
        180–8
    experiments in, 55
    HIV in, 10, 168, 189
    and plasma trade, 207
    and World War II, 159
    see also Antwerp, Belgian Congo,
        Brussels
Belize, 206
Benghazi, 108–10
Benin, 84, 96, 213
beriberi, 36
Berlin treaty, 62, 65
Bioko island, 138
Bismarck, Otto von, 65
bismuth salts, 131, 133, 148, 163
blood banks, 159–60, 204
Blukwa, 153–4
Boma, 70, 76, 91, 144, 158
Bongolo, Henri, 94–5
bonobo, 18, 30–1, 45, 50, 54, 142, 221
Boston, 215
Botswana, 9
Brazil, 60, 140, 206, 215
Brazza, Pierre (Pietro) Savorgnan de,
    61–5, 88
Brazzaville
    economic activity in, 34, 63, 74,
        80–1, 228
    history of, 62, 63–4, 69–70, 74
    HIV in, 61–5, 210–11, 212, 227–9
    medical services in, 32, 36–9, 64, 120,
        153, 217
    population of, 69–70, 73–4, 75,
        80, 82
    prostitution in, 93, 97–9
bridewealth, 75, 87, 90, 91, 92, 95, 97
brothels, 92, 99, 100–1, 102, 190

Brussels, 68, 121, 182–3
Bucharest, 108
Bujumbura, 77, 211, 231
Bukavu, 76, 148, 154
Bunia, 154
Burkina Faso, 173, 213
Burma, 94
Burundi, 7, 10, 67, 211, 231
Butembo, 154
Bwamanda, 16, 212

Cabinda, 20, 47, 60, 69, 99
Cachexie du Mayombe, 37–9
Cairo, 111
California, 1, 233
Caloncoba, 136, 139, 148
Cambronne, Luckner, 200–3
Cameroon
    chimpanzees in, 20, 25, 27–9,
        46, 47
    hepatitis C in, 111–14, 140–2,
        224, 225
    history of, xiv, 44, 65–6, 82, 228
    HIV in, 14–15, 168–70, 210–11, 212,
        213, 226–7, 228, 231
    medical services in, 116, 118–38, 177,
        210–11, 225
    population of, 47, 68
    prostitution in, 87, 91–2
    slaves from, 60
    see also Douala, Yaoundé
Camp Lindi, 50–1
Campo, 210
Camus, Albert, 216, 218
Canada, 10, 190, 194, 206–8
    see also Montreal, Vancouver
Canadian Red Cross, 208
Cape Verde, 171, 173
Capelle, Emmanuel, 76, 94
Caribbean, 13, 60
Carrefour, 203
Carrel, Alexis, 56
case-finding, 119, 138, 146, 150,
    158, 177
Castro, Fidel, 14
Catholic Church, 63–4, 69, 88–9, 98,
    145, 180, 202
Ceausescu, Nicolae, 107
Centers for Disease Control, 1, 52,
    191, 216

Central African Republic
  chimpanzees in, 20, 29
  economy of, 228
  hepatitis C in, 111–12, 141–2
  history of, xiii, 34–5, 44, 64, 65, 224
  HIV in, 14–15, 29, 141–2, 227, 228
  medical services in, 120, 122, 129,
    136, 141–2
  population of, 47, 68
  prostitution in, 93
  see also Bangui
Centre de Dépistage de la Tuberculose,
  158
Centre de Médecine Sociale, 160
Centre de Prophylaxie, 102
Cercocebus atys atys, 171
  see also sooty mangabey
Cercopithecus, 152
Chad
  hepatitis C in, 112
  history of, xiii, 34–6, 63, 64
  HIV in, 15, 169, 175, 227
  medical services in, 34, 120, 132, 137
Chamorro, Pedro Joaquin, 206
chancroid, 85
CHAT vaccine *see* oral poliomyelitis
  vaccine
chaulmoogra, 134–6, 139, 148, 154
Chemin de Fer Congo-Océan, 34–8, 93,
  98, 224, 228
China, 200, 203, 207, 215
chlamydia, 91, 163, 165
chloroquine, 137
circulating recombinant forms, 11–16,
  40, 108–10, 213, 215, 227, 231
circumcision, 211, 222
Cité Soleil, 196, 204
coagulation factor concentrates, 106,
  197–8, 205–6, 208, 214, 233
  see also haemophiliacs
Collège de France, 55, 57
Colombia, 206
Comhaire-Sylvain, Suzanne, 94, 101, 192
Compania Centroamericana de
  Plasmaferesis, 206
condoms, 85, 219
Congo, Democratic Republic of
  chimpanzees in, 18–20, 30–1, 45,
    50–3
  Haitians in, 187–9

  history of, 61–2, 67–82, 180–90
  HIV in, 6–7, 10–11, 14–16, 40–1,
    166–7, 211–12, 216–17, 228–31
  hunting in, 44–5
  medical services in, 143–66
  prostitution in, 87–91, 93–7, 99–102,
    158–66, 212
  sexually transmitted diseases in, 91,
    158–66
  slaves from, 62
  tuberculosis in, 157–8
  see also Kinshasa
Congo Français, 62–4
  see also Afrique Équatoriale Française
Congo Free State *see* Congo,
  Democratic Republic of
Congo River, 18–20, 30, 59–62,
  80–1, 228
Congo-Brazzaville
  chimpanzees in, 20, 47
  economy of, 228
  history of, xiii, 34, 44, 64,
    181, 224
  HIV in, 16, 209, 210
  medical services in, 34, 136, 225
  population of, 47, 68, 82
  see also Brazzaville, Pointe-Noire
Congo-Kinshasa *see* Congo,
  Democratic Republic of
Congo-Léopoldville *see* Congo,
  Democratic Republic of
Connaught Laboratories, 207–8
Constanta, 108
Continental Pharma Cryosan, 206–8
Coquilhatville, 76, 153–4
Costa Rica, 206
Costermansville *see* Bukavu
Cotonou, 84, 96
Croix-Rouge du Congo, 158–65
Cross River, 18–20
cross-species transmission, 2, 18–20, 41,
  47–58, 169–70, 172, 175, 210
cryoprecipitates, 205, 232
  see also haemophiliacs
Cuba, 13–14, 180, 193
Curtis, Tom, 50
Cutter Laboratories, 202

Dade Reagents, 202
Dakar, 65, 124, 181

Danish surgeon, 9, 187
Dar es Salaam, 212
decolonisation, 180–3
dengue fever, 194
Denmark, 190
Dispensaire Antivénérien de
    Léopoldville, 160–6, 229
Dja River, 228
Dominican Republic, 60,
    192, 206
Douala, 66, 70, 82, 91, 210, 212
Douala tribe, 65
Doumé, 127
Dow Chemical, 202
DRC60, 10–11, 41
Du Bois Institute, 60
Dubois, Albert, 159
Duvalier, François, 188, 201–2
Duvalier, Jean-Claude, 192, 202
Duvalierville, 201
dysentery, 36, 65, 152, 153, 155

Ebola fever, 7–8, 20, 43, 153
Ebolowa, 141
Éboué, Félix, 74
École du Pharo, 34, 39, 118
Ecuador, 60
Edinburgh, 106
Egypt, 110–11, 145, 155, 190
El Salvador, 206
Elisabethville *see* Lubumbashi
emetine, 137
Equateur province, 7, 16, 45, 211
Equatorial Guinea
    chimpanzees in, 20
    history of, 66
    HIV in, 14–15, 210
    malaria in, 140
    medical services in, 138–9
    population of, 47, 68
Estonia, 107
Ethiopia, 14, 145, 190
excision, 104, 176, 177, 178

Fernando Poo island, 138
Ferris, Lieutenant-Colonel, 36
FIMA ferries, 80
firearms, 44–6, 222
    see also hunting
flamingos, 100–1

Florida, 190
    see also Miami
Food and Drug Administration, 207–8
Force Publique, 94, 144, 145, 155
founder effect, 12, 13, 17, 196, 211
France
    and Afrique Équatoriale Française,
        62–4
    and Cameroun, xiv, 44, 66, 92
    colonial medicine in, 118–19
    and Congo-Brazzaville, 36, 62, 74
    HIV in, 168, 169, 170, 175
    and plasma trade, 207
Franceville, 23, 210
Free French Forces, 74
free women *see* prostitution

Gabon
    chimpanzees in, 20, 23, 45, 56
    economy of, 61, 228
    hepatitis C in, 111–12, 225
    history of, xiii, 61, 63, 64
    HIV in, 168, 175, 209–10, 213, 226,
        227, 231
    medical services in, 116, 129–31,
        133, 225
    population of, 47, 68, 91, 92
    prostitution in, 61, 92–3
    slaves from, 60
    see also Libreville, Port-Gentil
Gabon River, 61
The Gambia, 3, 172–3
Garrett, Laurie, 1
gas gangrene, 129–31
gay men *see* homosexuals
gender imbalance, 71–3, 75, 76–8,
    79–80, 95, 211, 213
genetic diversity of HIV, 13–16, 169,
    172, 227
Geneva, 106
Gentil, Emile, xiii, 64
Georgia, 233
Germany, 62, 65–6, 199, 202
Ghana, 8, 173, 175, 181, 190, 213
    see also Accra
Gide, André, 36
Gold, Herbert, 192
Gombe reserve, 18, 22, 26, 29, 48
gonorrhoea, 91, 152, 162, 163, 165
gorillas, 27, 29, 45, 46–7, 169–70

Gorinstein, Joseph, 201
Guatemala, 60, 206
Guiné Portuguesa *see* Guinea-Bissau
Guinea, 20, 55, 56–7, 173, 190
Guinea Espanola *see* Equatorial Guinea
Guinea-Bissau, 104, 170–4
Guyana, 60, 74

haemophiliacs, 194, 200–3, 208, 214,
    233–4
Haiti, 60, 188–9, 190–6, 200–5, 231–3
    see also Port-au-Prince
Hammarskjold, Dag, 185
Harvard School of Public Health, 218
Health Management Associates, 207–8
healthcare workers, occupational
    exposure of, 49, 112–13, 122, 223
Hemo-Caribbean, 200–3, 204–5,
    206, 232
hepatitis, 51, 114, 216
hepatitis A, 116, 197, 199
hepatitis B
    epidemiology of, 104, 105, 111,
        197–9
    iatrogenic transmission of, 115–16,
        140, 164, 166, 207–8, 230
    and the slave trade, 60
hepatitis C
    epidemiology of, 104–5
    iatrogenic transmission of, 105,
        110–16, 125, 128, 139, 140–2,
        164, 198, 208, 224, 225
    and intravenous drug use, 106
    among plasma donors, 199, 200
    and the slave trade, 60
Herpes B virus, 43
histopathology, 33, 154, 193, 194
HIV-1 group M, 11, 14, 24, 28–9, 40–1,
    50, 168–70, 226, 228
HIV-1 group N, 29, 168–70, 226
HIV-1 group O, 9, 28–9, 168–70
HIV-1 group P, 170
HIV-1 subtypes, 39–40, 41, 108, 168,
    169, 195–6, 211–13, 231
HIV-2, 9, 11, 24, 50, 61, 104, 168,
    170–4, 209, 213, 226
Homo sapiens, 12, 52
homosexual tourism, 191–3
homosexuals, 1, 8, 12, 191–4, 210, 214,
    233, 234

Hooper, Edward, 2, 50–3
Hôpital des Blancs in Léopoldville, 91
Hôpital des Congolais in Léopoldville,
    164
Hôpital des Noirs in Boma, 144
Hôpital des Noirs in Léopoldville, 152
Hôpital Mama Yemo, 6, 32, 217
hormones, 55–7
human herpesvirus 8 *see* Kaposi's
    sarcoma
human T-cell lymphotropic virus type 1,
    60, 118, 140, 141, 157
hunting, 20, 43–6, 49, 223
    see also firearms
hydnocarpus oil, 148

iatrogenic
    Ebola fever, 8
    epidemic of hepatitis C in Egypt,
        110–11
    epidemics of hepatitis B, 115–16
    epidemics of hepatitis C in Cameroon,
        111–14
    epidemics of HIV, 107–10
    gas gangrene, 131
    transmission of viruses, 103–5
Illiffe, John, 2
immunoglobulins, 197–8, 206, 232
incidence, 7, 209
India, 173, 175, 190, 199, 207, 214
Indochina, 62, 135
Indonesia, 107, 190
infertility, 78, 91, 98
Institut Pasteur, 52, 53, 55, 171
Institut Pasteur de Bangui, 227
Institut Pasteur de Brazzaville, 37, 69,
    120, 153
International Union for Conservation
    of Nature, 18–20
internationalistas, 13
intravenous drug users, 8, 12, 103–7,
    214–15, 225, 233, 234
Italy, 106, 208
Ivory Coast, 8, 20, 85, 172–3, 174–5,
    231

Jadotville, 76
Jamot, Eugène, 120–7, 146, 177
Janssens, Émile, 184
Japan, 208, 218

Kampala, 181, 212
Kapita, Bila, 32
Kaposi's sarcoma, 154, 193–4
Karolinska Institute, 52
Kasaï province, 87, 95, 146, 148
Kasaï River, 30
Kasavubu, Joseph, 183–5
Katanga province, 67, 75, 148, 153,
    185–6, 212, 231
Kenscoff, 192
Kenya, 9, 14, 85, 96
    see also Nairobi
Kigali, 6, 211, 230
Kikongo, 101
Kikwit, 146
King Baudouin, 182, 184
King Leopold II, 62, 67
Kinshasa
    economic activity in, 30
    Haitians in, 188
    history of, 69–82, 181–9, 189–90
    HIV in, 6–7, 9–11, 16, 32, 40–1,
        166–7, 189, 209–10, 211, 212,
        216–17, 227, 230
    malaria in, 140
    medical services in, 144, 150–3,
        158–66
    population of, 79–80, 211
    prostitution in, 86, 91, 93–7, 99–102,
        189, 212
Kisangani
    history of, 61–2, 76, 93, 182–3,
        186, 189
    HIV in, 212, 231
    medical services in, 144
    population of, 76
    public health laboratory of, 50–3,
        153–4, 154–5
Kisenso district, 79
Kisumu, 96
Kivu province, 148, 151
Koprowski, Hilary, 50, 51
Krever Commission, 207–8
Kribi region, 225
Kuyu, Camille, 188
Kwango region, 79, 87, 145, 156

La Fontaine, Jean, 100
La Semaine de l'AEF, 99
Lake Albert, 154

Lake Tanganyika, 88
Lake Tchad, 59
Lambaréné, 210
Lambotte, Claude, 159
Lasnet, Alexandre, 36
League of Nations, 44, 66–7, 155
Leclerc, Philippe de Hautecloque dit, 74
Legrand, Jeanne, 159
Lemba district, 7
Léopoldville *see* Kinshasa
Leplae, Edmond, 44
leprosy *see also Caloncoba*,
        chaulmoogra, methylene blue,
        sulphones
    clinical characteristics of, 134
    epidemiology of, 150, 165, 177
    treatment of, 134–6, 139–40, 148,
        154, 177, 224
Lesotho, 9, 207, 213
Lever palm oil company, 70
Liberia, 8, 172–3, 175, 190
Libreville, 61, 63, 69–70, 73, 210
Libya, 74, 99, 108–10
Lingala, 76, 90, 101
Lisbon, 171
liver cancer, 154
Liverpool, 121
Loango, 60, 63
London, 121, 217
Londres, Albert, 36
Los Alamos National Laboratory, 40
Los Angeles, 1
Louisiana, 208
Lovanium university, 181
Lubero, 154
Lubumbashi, 76–7, 94, 95, 153–4,
        181, 212
Luluabourg, 76, 154
Lumumba, Patrice, 76, 183–6
Lusaka, 212
lymphatic filariasis, 60

Madame Rose, 99
Mahale park, 26
Mahler, Halfdan, 217–18
Mai-Ndombe region, 3
Makala district, 79, 100
malaria
    in chimpanzees, 53–5
    epidemiology of, 136–7

malaria (cont.)
  treatment of, 136–7, 140–1, 150–1, 224
  see also chloroquine, quinacrine, quinine
Malawi, 9, 212, 231
Malaysia, 190
Malebo Pool, 62
Malembo, 60
Mali, 8, 57, 173, 175, 190, 213
Managua, 206
Mann, Jonathan, 215–20
Marburg haemorrhagic fever, 43
Marseilles, 34, 37, 118, 120, 121, 124
Martinique, 60
Matadi, 64, 76, 182, 184
Matadi–Léopoldville railway, 34, 36, 63, 69
Matete district, 100, 101
Max Planck Institute, 52
Mayo Kebbi district, 137
Mayombe, 20, 34–6, 37–9, 47, 148, 150
Mbuji-Mayi, 16, 212
Medical Research Council Laboratories, 3
melarsoprol, 4, 128, 176
ménagères, 88–9
mercury salts, 131, 133
methylene blue, 135–6, 139, 148
Mexico, 60, 199, 203
Mfoa, 63
Miami, 190, 195, 201, 202–3, 204
migrants
  in Abidjan, 213
  in Brazzaville, 80–2, 98
  in Douala, 82
  in Europe, 214
  from Haiti, 190
  HIV among, 176
  in Léopoldville, 70–1, 74, 75, 80–2, 102, 160–2, 165–6, 227, 228–9
  in North America, 13
Milan, 106
military medicine, 118–20
Mimongo district, 92
Mobutu, Joseph Désiré (Mobutu Sese Seko), 6, 82, 184–7
molecular clocks, 39–42, 109, 111, 175, 195
monkeypox, 43
monkeys, 31, 43, 46, 51
Montpellier, 120

Montreal, 190, 194, 206
Morbidity and Mortality Weekly Report, 1, 234
Morocco, 66
Moscow, 186
Mouvement National des Congolais, 183
Mouvement Populaire de la Révolution, 217
Mozambique, 9, 173, 175, 213
mulattoes, 89, 98, 159
Musée de l'Homme, 34

Nachtigal, Gustav, 65–6
Nairobi, 85, 102, 211, 212
Nakajima, Hiroshi, 218
National Institute for Biological Standards and Control, 52
Ndjili airport, 79
Ndola, 96
ndumbas see prostitution
New Mexico, 216
New York, 1, 106, 190, 191, 204, 214, 233
New York Times, 201–3
New York University School of Medicine, 52
Ngiri-Ngiri district, 100
Ngoko River, 228
Nicaragua, 206
Niger, 8, 175
Niger delta, 65
Nigeria
  chimpanzees in, 19
  history of, 66, 155, 190
  HIV in, 8, 9, 14, 15, 168, 173, 175, 214, 231
  slaves from, 60
Nile delta, 110–11, 150
Nilodin, 150
Nioki, 3, 32, 212
Nkoltang, 131
Nola, 141–2
northern Rhodesia *see* Zambia
Norway, 190
Norwegian sailor, 9, 170, 196
Ntem region, 225
nucleotide sequencing, 11, 13, 22–3, 39, 168–70
Nyungwe reserve, 26

Ogooué River, 61
onchocerciasis, 156
oral poliomyelitis vaccine, 50–3
Oran, 218
Organisation des Nations-Unies au Congo, 185–8, 190
orsanine, 125, 128
Osterrieth, Paul, 51
Otraco transportation utility, 70
Ouagadougou, 124
Oubangui-Chari *see* Central African Republic

Pakistan, 106, 190
palaeopathology, 33–4
Pales, Léon, 33–9
Pan paniscus see bonobo
Pan troglodytes ellioti, 18–22, 26, 27, 41
Pan troglodytes schweinfurthii, 18–22, 24–30, 45, 48, 50, 52, 54
Pan troglodytes troglodytes, 15
habitat of, 58, 76, 138, 148, 157, 224, 227, 228
HTLV-1 and, 60
SIV$_{cpz}$ in, 2, 18–22, 24–30, 46–8, 169, 221
Pan troglodytes verus, 18–22, 26, 41, 54, 55, 58
parenteral, 103–5
Paris, 55
Paulis, 154
Pearce, Louise, 151
penicillin, 115, 131, 133–4, 152–3, 163, 165, 177
pentamidine, 1, 128–31, 141, 156–7, 176
Pettit, Auguste, 55
phylogenetic trees, 22–3, 40, 52, 169, 195
physiological misery, 36
pimps, 90, 102
Piot, Peter, 7
plague, 152, 154, 216–20
The plague, 216
plasma, 116, 197
plasma pimps, 200
plasma trade, 198–203, 205–8, 214, 232
plasmapheresis, 198–205, 232
Pliny the Elder, 6

pneumococcus, 36, 37, 152–3
Pneumocystis jiroveci (carinii), 1, 9, 128
pneumonia, 36–7, 153
Pointe-Noire, 34, 70, 73, 93, 212, 228
Poland, 51, 199
poliomyelitis, 22, 50–3, 55, 153, 154
Port-au-Prince, 191–2, 196, 200–5, 206, 214, 231–2
see also Carrefour, Cité Soleil
Port-Gentil, xiii, 70, 73, 210
Portugal, 60, 62, 100, 138, 170–9, 189
Poto-Poto district, 98
prevalence, 6–7, 209
Princess Astrid Institute of Tropical Medicine, 152
prisoners, 197, 207–8
Projet Sida, 6, 16, 152, 216–17
prostitution
in the Belgian Congo, 71, 76, 78, 87–91, 93–7, 158–66, 229
in Benin, 84–5, 96
in Cameroon, 9, 87, 91–2, 96
in Congo-Brazzaville, 36, 38, 88, 92–3, 97–9
in the DRC, 99–102, 186, 189, 212, 230
in Gabon, 87, 92–3
gender imbalance and, 70, 76
in Ghana, 84–5
in Guinea-Bissau, 173–4
in Haiti, 191–3, 212, 231–2
HIV prevalence among women who practise, 6, 9, 84–5, 212, 213, 217
and infertility, 78
in Ivory Coast, 213
in Kenya, 9, 85, 96
in Oubangui-Chari, 93
in Rwanda, 212
and sexually transmitted diseases, 90–1
in Thailand, 215, 219
types of, 84–7
in Zambia, 96
Puerto Rico, 203, 206
Pune, 199
Punjab, 106
pygmies, 44, 46, 59, 140, 209, 221

quinacrine, 137
quinine, 63, 136–7, 141, 150–1, 178

Raymaekers, Paul, 100–1
Renkin, Jules, 67
Rhodesia *see* Zimbabwe
Rieux, Dr, 216, 219–20
Rio Muni, 138
Roche Molecular Systems, 52
Rockefeller Institute, 125
Rodhain, Jérôme, 54–5, 155, 157
Rolling Stone, 50
Romania, 107–8
Romaniuk, Anatole, 100
Royal Canadian Mounted Police, 207
Ruanda *see* Rwanda
Russia, 55, 58, 107
Ruzizi valley, 50
Rwanda
    chimpanzees in, 20, 26
    history of, 67
    HIV in, 6–7, 211, 230
Ryckmans, Pierre, 75

Sabin, Albert, 50
Sacramento, 138
Sahara desert, 74
Saigon, 135
San Francisco, 191, 214
Sanaga River, 18, 20
Sanaga-Maritime region, 225
Sangha, 210
Sangha River, 228
Sargodha, 106
schistosomiasis, 60, 110–11, 137,
    148–50, 154
    see also antimonial drugs, Nilodin,
    tartar emetic
Schwarz, Alf, 100
Schwetz, Jacques, 143, 147
Scotland, 106, 206
Selembao district, 79
Senegal, 8, 14, 19, 57, 172–3, 175, 213
    see also Dakar
sex workers *see* prostitution
sexual tourism, 191–3
sexually transmitted diseases
    in the Belgian Congo, 91, 95–6,
        158–66
    in Cameroon, 91–2
    in Congo-Brazzaville, 36, 92, 93
    in Gabon, 90–1, 92–3
    HIV among patients with, 9, 85, 211

and infertility, 78
in Oubangui-Chari, 93
among prostitutes, 90–3
    see also chancroid, chlamydia,
    gonorrhoea, syphilis
Shilts, Randy, 1
Sierra Leone, 8, 53, 120, 172–3,
    175, 190
Simao Mendes national hospital, 176
simian foamy virus, 43, 46
simian vacuolating virus, 50
SIV_{cpz}, 23–31, 41, 46–50, 52, 169–70,
    221–5, 227–8
SIV_{smm}, 50, 171–2, 178
slave trade, 35, 59–61, 62, 120, 222
sleeping sickness *see* African
    trypanosomiasis
Société de Construction des
    Batignolles, 35
Société Générale de Belgique, 67
Somoza, Anastasio, 206
Sonnet, Jean, 189
sooty mangabey, 104, 171–2, 175
South Africa, 2, 9, 12, 207, 213,
    214–15, 231
South-West Africa, 66
Soviet Union, 110, 185, 215
Spain, 107, 199
    see also Equatorial Guinea
Spartacus Gay Guide, 192, 203
Stanleyville *see* Kisangani
streptomycin, 4, 104, 138, 163,
    176–7
strongyloidiasis, 53
Sudan, 20, 190
sulphones, 136, 150, 177
suramin, 128, 137, 156
Swaziland, 9, 213
Sweden, 10, 190, 202
syphilis
    control of, 102, 124, 156, 160–3,
        166
    epidemiology of, 92–3, 131–3, 138,
        148, 165, 177, 204
    history of, 54, 114–15, 121
    treatment of, 90–1, 114–15, 131,
        133, 144–5, 148, 160–3, 166,
        229–30
    see also arsenical drugs, bismuth salts,
    mercury salts, penicillin

Taï Forest, 172
Taiwan, 206
Tanganyika, 66
Tanzania, 9, 14, 18, 20, 21, 26, 52
tartar emetic, 110–11, 125, 128, 148
Tchad *see* Chad
testicular transplants, 55–8
Thailand, 40, 107, 206, 215, 219
Thysville, 184
Togo, 8, 66, 175
Tontons Macoutes, 201
transfusions, 159–60, 204, 217, 234
tryparsamide, 123, 125, 128, 139, 151
trypoxyl, 128
Tshombe, Moise, 82
tuberculosis
   clinical characteristics of, 32–3,
      37–8, 154
   epidemiology of, 138, 157–8, 160, 194
   history of, 235
   treatment of, 4, 104, 176
   see also streptomycin

Ubangui River, 18–20, 227
Uele region, 145
Uganda, 9, 14, 20, 26, 52, 193
   see also Kampala
Union Minière du Haut-Katanga, 67
United Nations, 66, 92, 101, 185,
   187–8, 217–18
United Nations Education, Science and
   Culture Organization, 188
Université Catholique de Louvain,
   44, 181
University of Kinshasa, 10
Upper Nyong region, 124
urbanisation, 65, 66, 70–80, 158
Urundi *see* Burundi
Usumbura *see* Bujumbura

vaccines, 52, 104, 108, 138, 152, 153–4,
   163, 197–8
Valencia, 106, 199
Van Bilsen, Jef, 181
Van Hoof, Lucien, 154–7

Van Wing, Joseph, 71, 94
Vancouver, 106
Venezuela, 60
Verhaegen, Benoit, 189
Vermeersch, Arthur, 88
viraemia, 12, 47–8, 85, 107, 173, 179
Voix du Congolais, 96–7
von Puttkamer, Jesko, 66
Voronoff, Serge, 55–8

Winterbottom, Thomas, 120
Wistar Institute, 50–2
World Health Organization, 187–8,
   207, 217–18
World War I, 56, 66, 67, 120, 155
World War II, 73–5, 99, 115–16, 145,
   152–3, 155, 159, 189–90

Yambuku, 7–8, 209
Yaoundé
   hepatitis C in, 112, 140
   history of, 82, 228
   HIV in, 168, 210–11, 212
   population of, 70, 75
   prostitution in, 96
yaws
   clinical characteristics of, 131
   control of, 156, 224
   epidemiology of, 131–3, 138, 140,
      141, 148, 165–6, 177
   treatment of, 131–4, 144–5, 148,
      162–3, 177
yellow fever, 60, 115–16, 138,
   152–4, 175
Yonda, 209
   see also arsenical drugs, bismuth salts,
     mercury salts, penicillin

Zaire *see* Congo, Democratic
   Republic of
Zambia, 9, 14, 96, 186, 212, 231
Zanzibar, 61
Zimbabwe, 9, 212, 231
ZR59, 10–11, 40, 41
Zulus, 12